Gerhard Winkler

Image Analysis, Random Fields and Dynamic Monte Carlo Methods

A Mathematical Introduction

With 59 Figures

Springer

Gerhard Winkler

Mathematical Institute, Ludwig-Maximilians Universität,
Theresienstraße 39, D-80333 München, Germany

Mathematics Subject Classification (1991):
68U10, 68U20, 65C05, 93Exx, 65K10, 65Y05, 60J20, 62M40

ISBN-13: 978-3-642-97524-0 e-ISBN-13: 978-3-642-97522-6
DOI: 10.1007/978-3-642-97522-6

Library of Congress Cataloging-in-Publication Data.
Winkler, Gerhard, 1946-
Image analysis, random fields and dynamic Monte Carlo methods: a mathematical introduction
Gerhard Winkler. p. cm. (Applications of mathematics; 27)
Includes bibliographical references and index.
ISBN-13: 978-3-642-97524-0
1. Image analysis–Statistical methods. 2. Markov random fields. 3. Monte Carlo method.
I. Title. II. Series. TA1637.W56 1995 621.36'7'015192–dc20 94-24251 CIP

Softcover reprint of the hardcover 1st edition 1995

Typesetting: Data conversion by Springer-Verlag
SPIN: 10078306 41/3140 - 5 4 3 2 1 0 – Printed on acid-free paper

Stochastic Mechanics
Random Media
Signal Processing and Image Synthesis
Mathematical Economics
Stochastic Optimization
Stochastic Control

Applications of Mathematics

Stochastic Modelling and Applied Probability

27

Applications of Mathematics

1 Fleming/Rishel, **Deterministic and Stochastic Optimal Control** (1975)
2 Marchuk, **Methods of Numerical Mathematics,** Second Edition (1982)
3 Balakrishnan, **Applied Functional Analysis,** Second Edition (1981)
4 Borovkov, **Stochastic Processes in Queueing Theory** (1976)
5 Liptser/Shiryayev, **Statistics of Random Processes I: General Theory** (1977)
6 Liptser/Shiryayev, **Statistics of Random Processes II: Applications** (1978)
7 Vorob'ev, **Game Theory: Lectures for Economists and Systems Scientists** (1977)
8 Shiryayev, **Optimal Stopping Rules** (1978)
9 Ibragimov/Rozanov, **Gaussian Random Processes** (1978)
10 Wonham, **Linear Multivariable Control: A Geometric Approach,** Third Edition (1985)
11 Hida, **Brownian Motion** (1980)
12 Hestenes, **Conjugate Direction Methods in Optimization** (1980)
13 Kallianpur, **Stochastic Filtering Theory** (1980)
14 Krylov, **Controlled Diffusion Processes** (1980)
15 Prabhu, **Stochastic Storage Processes: Queues, Insurance Risk, and Dams** (1980)
16 Ibragimov/Has'minskii, **Statistical Estimation: Asymptotic Theory** (1981)
17 Cesari, **Optimization: Theory and Applications** (1982)
18 Elliott, **Stochastic Calculus and Applications** (1982)
19 Marchuk/Shaidourov, **Difference Methods and Their Extrapolations** (1983)
20 Hijab, **Stabilization of Control Systems** (1986)
21 Protter, **Stochastic Integration and Differential Equations** (1990)
22 Benveniste/Métivier/Priouret, **Adaptive Algorithms and Stochastic Approximations** (1990)
23 Kloeden/Platen, **Numerical Solution of Stochastic Differential Equations** (1992)
24 Kushner/Dupuis, **Numerical Methods for Stochastic Control Problems in Continuous Time** (1992)
25 Fleming/Soner, **Controlled Markov Processes and Viscosity Solutions** (1993)
26 Baccelli/Brémaud, **Elements of Queueing Theory** (1994)
27 Winkler, **Image Analysis, Random Fields and Dynamic Monte Carlo Methods** (1995)

To my parents, Daniel and Micki

Preface

This text is concerned with a probabilistic approach to image analysis as initiated by U. GRENANDER, D. and S. GEMAN, B.R. HUNT and many others, and developed and popularized by D. and S. GEMAN in a paper from 1984. It formally adopts the Bayesian paradigm and therefore is referred to as 'Bayesian Image Analysis'.

There has been considerable and still growing interest in prior models and, in particular, in discrete Markov random field methods. Whereas image analysis is replete with ad hoc techniques, Bayesian image analysis provides a general framework encompassing various problems from imaging. Among those are such 'classical' applications like restoration, edge detection, texture discrimination, motion analysis and tomographic reconstruction. The subject is rapidly developing and in the near future is likely to deal with high-level applications like object recognition. Fascinating experiments by Y. CHOW, U. GRENANDER and D.M. KEENAN (1987), (1990) strongly support this belief.

Optimal estimators for solutions to such problems cannot in general be computed analytically, since the space of possible configurations is discrete and very large. Therefore, dynamic Monte Carlo methods currently receive much attention and stochastic relaxation algorithms, like simulated annealing and various dynamic samplers, have to be studied. This makes up a major section of this text. A cautionary remark is in order here: There is scepticism about annealing in the optimization community. We shall not advocate annealing as it stands as a universal remedy, but discuss its weak points and merits. Relaxation algorithms will serve as a flexible tool for inference and a useful substitute for exact or more reliable algorithms where such are not available.

Incorporating information gained by statistical inference on the data or 'training' the models is a further important aspect. Conventional methods must be modified to become computationally feasible or new methods must be invented. This is a field of current research inspired for instance by the work of A. BENVENISTE, M. MÉTIVIER and P. PRIOURET (1990), L. YOUNES (1989) and R. AZENCOTT (1990)–(1992). There is a close connection to learning algorithms for Neural Networks which again underlines the importance of such studies.

The text is intended to serve as an introduction to the mathematical aspects rather than as a survey. The organization and choice of the topics are made from the author's personal (didactic) point of view rather than in a systematic way. Most of the study is restricted to finite spaces. Besides a series of simple examples, some more involved applications are discussed, mainly to restoration, texture segmentation and classification. Nevertheless, the emphasis is on general principles and theory rather than on the details of concrete applications. We roughly follow the classical mathematical scheme: motivation, definition, lemma, theorem, proof, example. The proofs are thorough and almost all are given in full detail. Some of the background from imaging is given, and the examples hopefully give the necessary intuition. But technical details of image processing definitely are not our concern here.

Given basic concepts from linear algebra and real analysis, the text is self-contained. No previous knowledge of image analysis is required. Knowledge of elementary probability theory and statistics is certainly beneficial, but not absolutely necessary. The text should be suitable for students and scientists from various fields including mathematics, physics, statistics and computer science. Readers are encouraged to carry out their own experiments and some of the examples can be run on a simple home computer. The appendix reviews the techniques necessary for the computer simulations. The text can also serve as a source of examples and exercises for more abstract lectures or seminars since the single parts are reasonably selfcontained.

The general model is introduced in Chapter 1. To give a realistic idea of the subject a specific model for restauration of noisy images is developed step by step in Chapter 2. Basic facts about Markov chains and their multi-dimensional analogue – the random fields – are collected in Chapters 3 and 4. A simple version of stochastic relaxation and simulated annealing, a generally applicable optimization algorithm based on the Gibbs sampler, is developed in Chapters 4 through 6. This is sufficient for readers to do their own experiments, perhaps following the guide line in the appendix. Chapter 7 deals with the law of large numbers and generalizations. Metropolis type algorithms are discussed in Chapter 8. It also indicates the connection with combinatorial optimization. So far the theory of dynamic Monte Carlo methods is based on DOBRUSHIN's contraction technique. Chapter 9 introduces to the method of 'second largest eigenvalues' and points to recent literature. Some remarks on parallel implementation can be found in Chapter 10. It is followed by a few examples of segmentation and classification of textures in Chapters 11 and 12. They mainly serve as a motivation for parameter estimation by the pseudo-likelihood method addressed in Chapters 13 and 14. Chapter 15 applies random field methods to simple neural networks. In particular, a popular learning rule is presented in the framework of maximum likelihood estimation. The final Chapter 16 contains a selected collection of other typical applications, hopefully opening prospects to higher level problems.

The text emerged from the notes of a series of lectures and seminars the author gave at the universities of Kaiserslautern, München, Heidelberg, Augsburg and Jena. In the late summer of 1990, D. Geman kindly gave us a copy of his survey article (1990): plainly, there is some overlap in the selection of topics. On the other hand, the introductory character of these notes is quite different.

The book was written while the author was lecturing at the universities named above and Erlangen-Nürnberg. He is indebted to H.G. Kellerer, H. Rost and K.H. Fichtner for giving him the opportunity to hold this series of lectures on image analysis. Finally, he would like to thank G.P. Douglas for proof-reading parts of the manuscript and, last but not least, D. Geman for his helpful comments on Part I.

Gerhard Winkler

Table of Contents

Part III. More on Sampling and Annealing

Introduction

In this first chapter, basic ideas behind the Bayesian approach to image analysis are introduced in an informal way. We freely use some notions from elementary probability theory and other fields with which the reader is perhaps not perfectly familiar. She or he should not worry about that – all concepts will be made thoroughly precise where they are needed.

This text is concerned with *digital image analysis*. It focuses on the extraction of information implicit in recorded digital image data by automatic devices aiming at an interpretation of the data, i.e. an explicit (partial) description of the real world. It may be considered as a special discipline in *image processing*. The latter encompasses fields like image digitization, enhancement and restoration, encoding, segmentation, representation and description (we refer the reader to standard texts like ANDREWS and HUNT (1977), PRATT (1978), HORN (1986), GONZALEZ and WINTZ (1987) or HARALICK and SHAPIRO (1992)).

Image analysis is sometimes referred to as 'inverse optics'. Inverse problems generally are underdetermined. Similarly, various interpretations may be more or less compatible with the data and the art of image analysis is to select those of interest. *Image synthesis*, i.e. the 'direct problem' of mapping a real scene to a digital image will not be dicussed in this text.

Here is a selection of typical problems :

- Image restoration: Recover a 'true' two-dimensional scene from noisy data.
- Boundary detection: Locate boundaries corresponding to sudden changes of physical properties of the true three-dimensional scene such as surface, shape, depth or texture.
- Tomographic reconstruction: Showers of atomic particles pass through the body in various directions (transmission tomography). Reconstruct the distribution of tissue in an internal organ from the 'shadows' cast by the particles onto an array of sensors. Similar problems arise in emission tomography.
- Shape from shading: Reconstruct a three-dimensional scene from the observed two-dimensional image.
- Motion analysis: Estimate the velocity of objects from a sequence of images.
- Analysis of biological shape: Recognize biological shapes or detect anomalies.

We shall comment on such applications in Chapter 2 and in Parts IV and VI. Concise introductions are GEMAN and GIDAS (1991), D. GEMAN (1990). For shape from shading and the related problem of shape from texture see GIDAS and TORREAO (1989). A collection of such (and many other) applications can be found in CHELLAPA and JAIN (1993). Similar problems arise in fields apparently not related to image analysis:

- Reconstruct the locations of archeological sites from measurements of the phosphate concentration over a study region (the phosphate content of soil is the result of decomposition of organic matter).
- Map the risk for a particular disease based on observed incidence rates.

Study of such problems in the Bayesian framework is quite recent, cf. BESAG, YORK and MOLLIÉ (1991).

The techniques mentioned will hopefully be helpful in high-level vision like object recognition and navigation in realistic environments.

Whereas image analysis is replete with ad hoc techniques one may believe that there is a need for theory as well. Analysis should be based on precisely formulated mathematical models which allow one to study the performance of algorithms analytically or even to design optimal methods. The probabilistic approach introduced in this text is a promising attempt to give such a basis. One characterization is to say it is Bayesian. As always in Bayesian inference, there are two types of information: prior knowledge and empirical data. Or, conversely, there are two sources of uncertainty or randomness since empirical data are distorted ideal data and prior knowledge usually is incomplete.

In the next paragraphs, these two concepts will be illustrated in the context of restoration, i.e. 'reconstruction' of a real scene from degraded observations. Given an observed image, one looks for a 'restored image' hopefully being a better represention of the true scene than was provided by the original records. The problem can be stated with a minimum of notation and therefore is chosen as the introductory example.

In general, one does not observe the ideal image but rather a distorted version. There may be a loss of information caused by some deterministic noninvertible transformation like blur or a masking deformation where only a portion of the image is recorded and the rest is hidden to the observer. Observations may also be subject to measurement errors or unpredictable influences arising from physical sources like sensor noise, film grain irregularities and atmospheric light fluctuations. Formally, the mechanism of distortion is a deterministic or random transformation $y = f(x)$ of the true scene x to the observed image y. 'Undoing' the degradations or 'restoring' the image ideally amounts to the inversion of f. This raises severe problems associated with invertibility and stability. Already in the simple linear model $y = Bx$, where the true and observed images are represented by vectors x and y, respectively, and the matrix B represents some linear 'blur operator', B is in general highly noninvertible and solutions x of the equation can be far apart. Other difficulties come in since y is determined by physical sampling and the elements of B are specified independently by system modeling. Thus the system of equations may be inconsistent in practice and have no solution at all. Therefore an error term enters the model, for example in the additive form $y = Bx + e(x)$.

Restoration is the object of many conventional methods. Among those one finds *ad hoc* methods like 'noise cleaning' via smoothing by weighted moving averages or – more generally – application of various linear filters to the image. Surprising results can be obtained by such methods and linear filtering is a highly developed discipline in engineering. On the other hand, linear filters only transform an image (possibly under loss of information), hopefully, to a better representation, but there is no possibility of *analysis*.

Another example is inverse filtering. A primitive example is least-square inverse filtering: For simplicity, suppose that the ideal and the distorted image are represented by rectangular arrays or real functions x and y on the plane giving the distribution of light intensity. Let $y = Bx + \eta$ for some linear operator B and a noise term η. An image $\hat{x}$ is a candidate for a 'restoration' of y if it minimizes the distance between y and Bx in the L^2-norm; i.e. the function $x \mapsto \|y - Bx\|_2^2$ (for an array $z = (z_s)_{s \in S}$, $\|z\|_2^2 = \sum_s z_s^2$). This amounts to the criterion to minimize the noise variance $\|\eta\|_2^2 = \|y - Bx\|_2^2$. A final solution is determined according to additional criteria. The method can be interpreted as minimization of the quadratic function $z \mapsto \|y - z\|_2^2$ under the 'rigid' constraint $z = Bx$ and the choice of some $\hat{x}$ satisfying $\hat{z} = B\hat{x}$ for the solution $\hat{z}$. The constraint $z = Bx$ mathematically expresses the prior information that x is transformed to Bx.

If the noise variance is known one can minimize $x \mapsto \|y - x\|_2^2$ under the constraint $\|y - Bx\|_2^2 = \sigma^2$ where σ^2 denotes noise variance. This is a simple example of constrained smoothing.

Bayesian methods differ from most of these methods in at least two respects: (i) they require full information about the (probabilistic) mechanism which degrades the original scene, (ii) rigid constraints are replaced by weak ones. These are more flexible: instead of classifying the objects in question into allowed and forbidden ones they are weighted by an 'acceptance function' quantifying the degree to which they are desired or not. Proper normalization yields a probability measure on the set of objects - called the 'prior distribution' or prior. The Bayesian paradigm allows one to consistently combine this 'weak constraint measure' with the data. This results in a modification of the prior called *posterior distribution* or posterior. Here the more or less rigid expectations compete with faithfulness to the data. By a suitable decision rule a solution to the inverse problem is selected, i.e. an image hopefully in proper balance between prior expectations and fidelity to the data.

To prevent fruitless discussions on the Bayesian philosophy, let us stress that though the model formally is Bayesian, the prior distribution can be just considered as a flexible substitute for rigid constraints and, from this point of view, it is at least in the present context an analytical rather than a probabilistic concept. Nevertheless, the name 'Bayesian image analysis' is common for this approach. Besides its formal merits the Bayesian framework has several substantial advantages. Methods from this mature field of statistics can be adopted or at least serve as a guideline for the development of more specific methods. In particular, this is helpful for the estimation of optimal solutions. Or, in texture classification, where the prior can only be specified up to a set of parameters, statistical inference can be adopted to adjust the parameters to a special texture.

All of this is a bit general. Though of no practical importance, the following simple example may give you a flavour of what is to come.

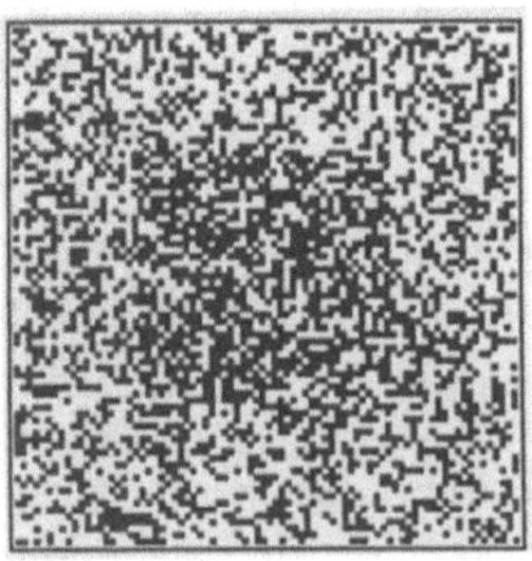

Fig. 0.1. A degraded image

Consider black and white pictures as displayed on a computer screen. They will be represented by arrays $(x_s)_{s\in S}$; S is a finite rectangular grid of 'pixels' s, $x_s = 1$ corresponds to a black spot in pixel s and $x_s = 0$ means that s is white. Somebody (nature ?) displays some image y (Fig. 1).

We are given two pieces of information about the generating algorithm: (i) it started from an image x composed of large connected patches of black and white, (ii) the colours in the' pixels were independently flipped with probability p each. We accept a bet to construct a machine which roughly recovers the original image. There are 2^σ possible combinations of black and white spots, where σ is the number of pixels. In the figures we chose $\sigma = 80 \times 80$ and hence $2^\sigma \sim 10^{192}$; in the more realistic case $\sigma = 256 \times 256$ one has $2^\sigma \sim 10^{19,660}$. We want to restrict our search to a small subset using the information in (i). It is not obvious how to state (i) in precise mathematical terms. We may start selecting only the two extreme images which are either totally white or totally black (Fig. 2). Formally, this amounts to the choice of a feasible subset of the space $\mathbf{X} = \{0,1\}^S$ consisting of two elements. This is a poor formulation of (i) since it does not express the degrees to which for instance Fig. 3(a) and (b) are in accordance with the requirement: both are forbidden. Thus let us introduce the local constraints

- $x_s = x_t$ for all pixels s and t adjacent in the horizontal, vertical or diagonal directions.

In the example, we have $n = 80$ rows and columns, respectively, and hence $2n(n-1) = 12,640$ adjacent pairs s, t in the horizontal or vertical directions, and the same number of diagonally adjacent pairs. The feasible set is the same as before but weighting configurations x by the number $A(x)$ of valid constraints gives a measure of smoothness. Fig. 3(a) differs from the black

Fig. 0.2. Two very smooth images

image only by a single white dot and thus violates only 8 of the 25, 280 local constraints whereas (b) violates one half of the local constraints. By the rigid constraints both are forbidden whereas A differentiates between them. This way the rigid constraints are relaxed to 'weak constraints'. Hopefully, the reader will agree that the latter is a more adequate formulation of piecewise smoothness in (i) than the rigid ones.

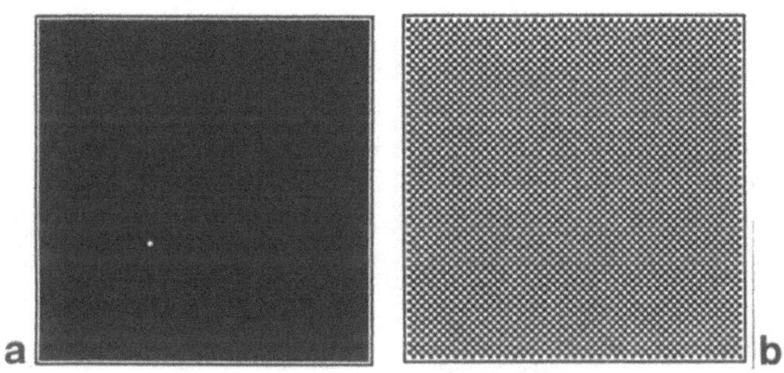

Fig. 0.3. (**a**) Violates few, (**b**) violates many local constraints

More generally, one may define local acceptor functions by

$$A_{st}(x_s, x_t) = \begin{cases} a_{st} & if \quad x_s = x_t \\ r_{st} & if \quad x_s \neq x_t \end{cases}$$

(a for 'attractive' and r for 'repulsive'). The numbers a_{st} and r_{st} control the degree to which the rigid local constraints are fulfilled. For the present, they are not completely specified. But if we agree that $A_{st}(x_s, x_t) > A_{st}(x'_s, x'_t)$

means that (x_s, x_t) is more favourable than (x'_s, x'_t) we must require that $a_{st} > r_{st}$ since smooth images are desired. Forming the product over all horizontal, vertical and diagonal nearest neighbour pairs gives the global acceptor

$$A(x) = \prod A_{st}(x_s, x_t).$$

Since in (i) no direction is preferred, we let $a_{st} = a$ and $r_{st} = r$, $a > r$, in the experiment. Little is lost, if the acceptor is normalized such that $A \geq 0$ and $\sum_x A(x) = 1$. Then A formally is a probability distribution on $\mathbf{X}$ which we call the *prior distribution.*

From (ii) we conclude: Given x the observation y is obtained with probability

$$P(x, y) = \prod_s p^{1_{\{x_s \neq y_s\}}} (1-p)^{1_{\{x_s = y_s\}}}$$

(the function 1_A equals 1 on A and vanishes off A). Given a fixed observation $\hat{y}$, the acceptor A should be modified by the weights $P(x, \hat{y})$ to

$$\hat{A}(x) = A(x)P(x, \hat{y}) = \prod_s \left(\prod_t A_{st}(x_s, x_t) \right) p^{1_{\{x_s \neq \hat{y}_s\}}} (1-p)^{1_{\{x_s = \hat{y}_s\}}}$$

(this rule for modification is borrowed from the Bayesian model). $\hat{A}$ is a new acceptor function and proper normalization gives a probability distribution called the *posterior distribution.* Now two terms compete: A formerly desirable configuration with large $A(x)$ may be weighted down if not compatible with the data, i.e. if $P(x, \hat{y})$ is small, and conversely, an *a priori* less favourable configuration with small $A(x)$ may become acceptable if $P(x, \hat{y})$ is large.

Finally, we need a rule how to decide which image we shall present to our contestant. Let us agree that we take one with highest value of $\hat{A}$. Now

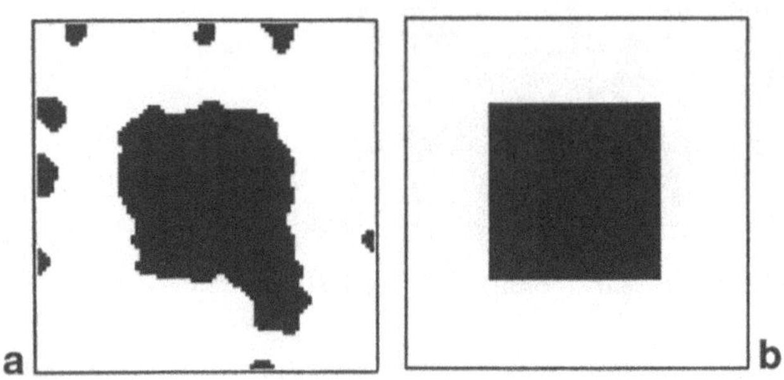

Fig. 0.4. (a) A poor reconstruction of (b)?

we are faced with a new problem: how should we maximize $\hat{A}$? This is in fact another story and thus let us suppose for the present that we have an optimization method and apply it to $\hat{A}$. It generates an image like Fig. 4(a). Now the original image 4(b) is revealed.

At the first glance, this is a bit disappointing, isn't it ? On the other hand, there *is* a large black spot which even resembles the square and thus (i) is met. Moreover, we did *not include any information about shape* into the model and thus we should be suspicious about much better reconstructions with *this* prior. Information about shape can and will be exploited and this will result in almost perfect reconstructions (you may have a look at the figures in Chapter 2).

Just for fun, let us see what happens with a 'wrong' acceptance function A. We tell our reconstruction machine that in the original image there are vertical stripes. To be more precise, we set a_{st} equal to a large number and r_{st} equal to a low number for vertical pixel pairs and, conversely, a_{st} to a low and r_{st} to a large numbers for pairs not in the same coloumn. Then the output is Fig. 5.

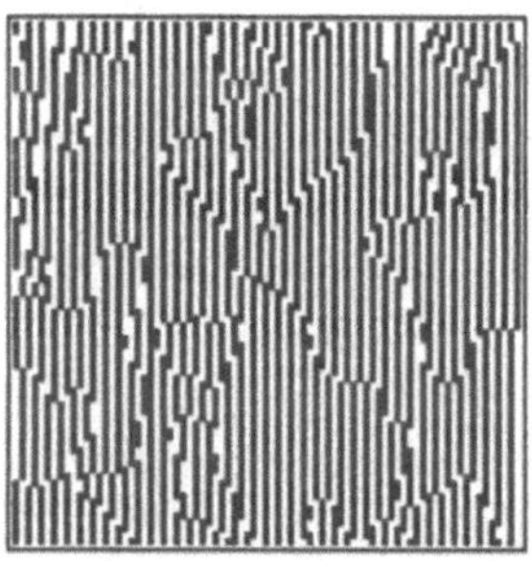

Fig. 0.5. A reconstruction with an impropriate acceptance function

Like the broom of the wizard's apprentice, the machine steadfastly does what it is told to do, or, in other words, it sees what it is prepared to see. This teaches us that we must form a clear idea which kind of information we want to extract from the data and precisely formulate this in the mathematical terms of the acceptor function before we set the restoration machine to work.

Any model is practically useless unless the solution of the reconstruction problem cannot be computed. In the example, the function $x \mapsto \hat{A}(x)$ has to be maximized. Since the space of images is discrete and because of its size this may turn out to be a tough job and, in fact, a great deal of effort is spent on the construction of suitable algorithms in the image analysis community. One may search through the tool box of exact optimization algorithms. Nontrivial considerations show that, for example, the above problem can be transformed into one which can be solved by the well-known Ford-Fulkerson algorithm. But as soon as there are more than two colours or one plays around with the acceptor function it will no longer apply. Similarly, most exact algorithms are tailored for rather restricted applications or they become computationally unfeasible in the imaging context. Hence one is looking for a flexible albeit fast optimization method.

There are several general strategies: one is 'divide and conquer'. The problem is divided into small tractable subproblems which are solved independently. The solutions to the subproblems then have to be patched together consistently. Another design principle for many common heuristics is 'successive augmentation'. In this approach an initially empty structure is successively augmented until it becomes a solution. We shall not pursue these aspects. 'Iterative improvement' is a dynamical approach. Pixels are subsequently selected following some systematic or random strategy and at each step the configuration (i.e. image) is changed at the current pixel. 'Greedy' algorithms, for example, select the colour which improves the objective function $\hat{A}$ the most. They permanently move uphill and thus get stuck in local maxima which are global maxima only in very special cases. Therefore it is customary to repeat the process several times starting from different, for instance randomly chosen configurations, and to save the best result. Since the objective functions in image analysis will have a very large number of local maxima and the set of initial configurations necessarily is rather thin in the very large space of all configurations this trick will help in special cases only. The dynamic Monte Carlo approach – which will be adopted here – replaces the chain of systematic updates by a temporal stochastic process: at each pixel a dye is tossed and thus a new colour picked at random. The probabilities depend on the value of $\hat{A}$ for the respective colours and a control parameter β. Colours giving high values are selected with higher probability than those giving low values. Thus there is a tendency uphill but there is also a chance for descent. In principle, routes through the configuration space designed by such a procedure will find a way out of local maxima. The parameter β controls the actual probabilites of the colours: let $p(\beta_0)$ be the uniform distribution on all colours and let $p(\beta_\infty)$ be the degenerate distribution concentrated on the locally optimal colours. Selection of a colour w.r.t. $p(\beta_\infty)$ amounts to the choice of a colour maximizing the local acceptor function, i.e. to a locally maximal ascent. If updating is started with $p(\beta_0)$ then the process will randomly stagger around in the space of images. While β varies from β_0 to β_∞ the uniform distribution is continuously transformed into $p(\beta_\infty)$: Favourable colours become more and more probable and the updating rule changes from a completely random search to maximal ascent. The trick is to vary β in such a fashion that, on the one hand, ascent is fast enough to run into maxima, and, on the other hand, to keep the procedure random enough to escape from local maxima before it has reached a global one.

Plainly, one cannot expect a universal remedy by such methods. One has to put up with a tradeoff between accuracy, precision, speed and flexibility. We shall study these aspects in some detail.

Our primitive reconstruction machine still is not complete. It does not know how to choose the parameters $a_{st} = a$ and $r_{st} = r$. The requirement $a > r$ corresponds to smoothness but it does not say anything about the *degree* of smoothness. The latter may for example depend on the approximate number of patches and their shape. We could play around with a and r until a satisfactory result is obtained but this may be tiring already in simple cases and turns out to be impracticable for more complicated patterns. A more substantial problem is that we do not know what 'satisfactory' does mean. Therefore we must gain further information by statistical inference. Conventional estimation techniques frequently require a large number of independent samples. Unfortunately, we have only a single observation where the colours of pixels depend on each other. Hence methods to estimate parameters (or, in more fashionable terms 'learning algorithms') based on dependent observations must be developed. Besides modeling and optimization, this is the third focal point of activity in image analysis. In summary, we raised the following clusters of problems:

- Design of prior models.
- Statistical inference to specify free parameters.
- Specification of the posterior, in particular the law of the data given the true image.
- Estimation of the true image based on the posterior distribution (presently by maximization).

Specification of the transition probabilites in the third item is more or less a problem of engineering or physics and will not be discussed in detail here. The other three items roughly lay out a program for this text.

Part I

Bayesian Image Analysis: Introduction

1. The Bayesian Paradigm

In this chapter the general model used in Bayesian image analysis is introduced.

1.1 The Space of Images

A monochrome digital picture can be represented by a finite set of numbers corresponding to the intensity of light. But an image is much more. An array of numbers may be visualized by a transformation to a pattern of grey levels on a computer screen. As soon as one realizes that there is a cat shown on the screen this pattern achieves a new quality. There has been some sort of high-level image processing in our eyes and brain producing the association 'cat'. We shall not philosophize on this but notice that information hidden in the data is extracted. Such informations should be included in the description of the image.

Which kind of information has to be taken into account depends on the special task one is faced with. Most examples in this text deal with problems like restoration of degraded images, edge detection or texture discrimination. Hence besides intensities, attributes like boundary elements or labels marking certain types of texture will be relevant. The former are observable up to degradation while the latter are not and correspond to some interpretation of the data.

In summary, an image will be described by an array

$$x = (x^P, x^L, x^B, \ldots)$$

where the single components correspond to the various attributes of interest. Usually they are multi-dimensional themselves. Let us give some first examples of such attributes and their meaning.

Let S^P denote a finite square lattice - say with 256×256-lattice points - each point representing a pixel on a screen. Let G be the set of grey values, typically $|G| = 256$ (the symbol $|G|$ denotes the number of elements of G) and for $s \in S^P$ let x_s^P denote the grey value in pixel s. The vector $x^P = (x_s^P)_{s \in S^P}$ represents a pattern or configuration of grey values. In this example there are $256^{256^2} \sim 10^{157,826}$ possible patterns and these large numbers cause many of the problems in image processing.

Remark 1.1.1. Grey values may be replaced by any kind of observable quantities. Let us mention a few:

- intensities of any sort of radiant energy;
- the numbers of photons hitting the cells of a CCD-camera (cf. Chapter 2);
- tristimulus: in additive colour matching the contributions of primary colours - say red, green and blue light - to the colour of a pixel, usually normalized by their contribution to a reference colour like 'white' (Pratt (1978), Chapter 3));
- depth, i.e. at each point the distance from the viewer; such depth maps may be produced by stereopsis or processing of optical flow (cf. Marr (1982));
- transforms of the original intensity pattern like discrete Fourier- or Hough-transforms.

In *texture classification* blocks of pixels are labeled as belonging to one of several given textures like 'meadow', 'wood' or 'damadged wood'. A pattern of such labels is represented by an array $x^L = (x_s^L)_{s \in S^L}$ where S^L is a set of pixel blocks and $x_s^L = l \in L$ is the label of block s, for instance 'damadged wood'. The blocks may overlap or not. Frequently, blocks center around pixels on some subgrid of S^P and then S^L usually is identified with this subgrid. The labeling is not an observable but rather an interpretation of the intensity pattern. We must find rules how to pick a reasonable labeling from the set L^{S^L} of possible ones.

Image boundaries or edges are useful primitive features indicating sudden changes of image attributes. They may separate regions of dark or bright pixels, regions of different texture or creases in a depth map. They can be represented by strings of small edge elements, for example microedges between adjacent pixels:

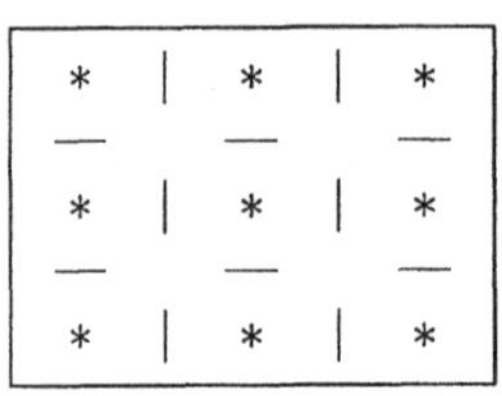

$*$: pixel

— : microedge

Let S^E be the set of microedges in S^P. For $s \in S^E$ set $x_s^E = 1$ if the microedge represents a piece of a boundary (it is 'on') and $x_s^E = 0$ otherwise (it is 'off').

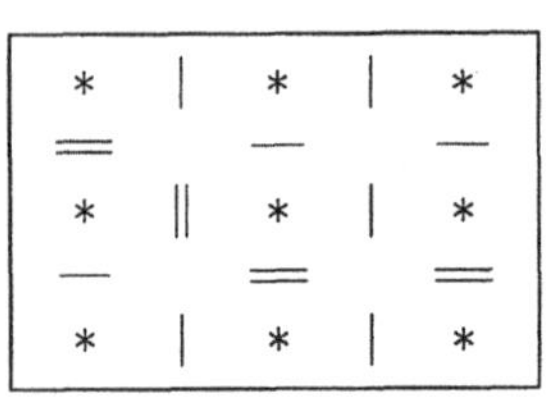

$\|$: microedge is 'on'

$|$: microedge is 'off'

Again, the configuration x^E is not observable. An edge element can be switched on for example if the contrast of grey levels nearby exceeds a certain threshold or if the adjacent textures are different. But local criteria alone are not sufficient to characterize boundaries. Usually they are smooth or connected and this should be taken into account.

These simple examples of image attributes should suffice to motivate the concepts to be introduced now.

1.2 The Space of Observations

Statistical inference will be based on 'observations' or 'data' y. They are assumed to be some deterministic or random function Y of the 'true' image x. To determine this function in concrete applications is a problem of engineering and statistics. Here we introduce some notation and give a few simple examples.

The space of data will be denoted by $\mathbf{Y}$ and the space of images by $\mathbf{X}$. Given $x \in \mathbf{X}$, the law of Y will be denoted by $P(x, \cdot)$.

If $\mathbf{Y}$ is finite we shall write $P(x,y)$ for the probability of observing $Y = y$ if x is the correct image. Thus for each $x \in \mathbf{X}$, $P(x, \cdot)$ is a probability distribution on $\mathbf{Y}$, i.e. $P(x,y) \geq 0$ and $\sum_y P(x,y) = 1$. Such **transition probabilities** (or **Markov kernels**) can be represented by a matrix where $P(x,y)$ is the element in the x-th row and the y-th column.

Frequently, it is more natural to assume observations in a continuous space $\mathbf{Y}$, for example in an Euclidean space R^d and then the distributions $P(x, \cdot)$ will be given by probability densities $f_x(y)$. More precisely, for each measurable subset B of R^d,

$$P(x,B) = \int_B f_x(y)\,dy$$

where f_x is a nonnegative function on $\mathbf{Y}$ such that $\int f_x(y)dy = 1$.

Example 1.2.1. Here are some simple examples of discrete and continuous transition probabilities.

(a) Suppose we are interested in labeling a grey value picture. An image is then represented by an array $x = (x^P, x^L)$ as introduced above. If undegraded grey values are observed then $y = x^P$ and 'degradation' simply means that the information about the second component x^L of x is missing. The transition probability then is degenerate:

$$P(x,y) = \begin{cases} 1 & \text{if } \ y = x^P \\ 0 & \text{otherwise} \end{cases} .$$

For edge detection based on perfectly observed grey values where $x = (x^P, x^E)$, the transition kernel P has the same form.

(b) The grey values may be degraded by noise in many ways. A particularly simple case is additive noise. Given $x = x^P$ one observes a realization of the random variable

$$Y = x + \eta$$

where $\eta = (\eta_s)_{s \in S^P}$ is a family of real-valued random noise variables. If the random variables η_s are independent and identically distributed with a Gaussian law of mean 0 and variance σ^2 then η is called **white Gaussian noise**. The law $P(x, \cdot)$ of Y has density

$$f_x(y) = \frac{1}{\sqrt[d]{2\pi\sigma^2}} \exp\left(\frac{1}{2\sigma^2} \sum_s (y_s - x_s)^2\right)$$

where $d = |S^P|$. Thermal noise, for example, is Gaussian. While quantum noise obeys a (signal dependent) Poisson law, at high intensities a Gaussian approximation is feasible. We shall discuss this in Chapter 2. In a strict sense, the Gaussian assumption is unrealistic since negative grey values appear with positive probability. But for positive grey values sufficiently larger than the variance of noise the positivity restriction on light intensity is violated infrequently.

(c) Let us finally give an example for multiplicative noise. Suppose that the pattern x, $x_s \in \{-1, 1\}$, is transmitted through a channel which independently flips the values with probability p. Then $Y_s = x_s \cdot \eta_s$ with independent Bernoulli variables η_s which take the value -1 with probability p and the value 1 with probability $1 - p$. The transition probability is

$$P(x, y) = p^{|\{s \in S: y_s = -x_s\}|}(1 - p)^{|\{s \in S: y_s = x_s\}|}.$$

This kind of degradation will be referred to as **channel noise** .

More background information and more realistic examples will be given in the next chapter.

1.3 Prior and Posterior Distribution

As indicated in the introduction, prior expectations may first be formulated as rigid constraints on the ideal image. These may be relaxed in various ways. The degree to which an image fulfills the rigid regularity conditions and constraints finally is expressed by a function $\Pi(x)$ on the space $\mathbf{X}$ of images. By convention, $\Pi(x) > \Pi(x')$ means that x' is less favourable than x. For convenience, we assume that Π is nonnegative and normalized, i.e. Π is a probability distribution. Since Π does not depend on the data it can be designed before data are recorded and hence it is called the **prior distribution**.

We shall not require foreknowledge from measure theory and therefore most of the analysis will be carried out for finite spaces $\mathbf{X}$. In some applications it is more reasonable to allow ranges like R_+ or R^d. Most concepts introduced here easily carry over to the continuous case.

The choice of the prior is problem dependent and one of the main problems in Bayesian image analysis. There is not too much to say about it in the present general context. Chapter 2 will be devoted exclusively to the design of a prior in a special situation. Later on, more prior distributions will be discussed. For the present, we simply assume that some prior is fixed.

The second ingredient is the distributions $P(x,\cdot)$ of the data y given x. Assume for the moment that $\mathbf{Y}$ is finite. The prior Π and the transition probabilities P determine the joint distribution of data and images on the product space $\mathbf{X}\times\mathbf{Y}$ by

$$\mathsf{P}(x,y) = \Pi(x)P(x,y),\ x\in\mathbf{X},\ y\in\mathbf{Y}.$$

This number is interpreted as the probability that x is the correct image *and* that y is observed.

The distribution P is the law of a pair (X,Y) of random variables with values in $\mathbf{X}\times\mathbf{Y}$ where X has the law Π and Y has a law Γ given by $\Gamma(Y=y)=\sum_x \mathsf{P}(x,y)$. We shall use symbols like P and Γ for the law of random variables as well as for the underlying probabilities and hence write $\mathsf{P}(x,y)$ or $\mathsf{P}(X=x,Y=y)$ if convenient. There is no danger of confusion since we can define suitable random variables by $X(x,y)=x$ and $Y(x,y)=y$. Recall that the **conditional probability** of an event (i.e. a subset) E in $\mathbf{X}\times\mathbf{Y}$ given an event F is defined by $\mathsf{P}(E|F)=\mathsf{P}(E\cap F)/\mathsf{P}(F)$ (provided the denominator does not vanish). Setting $E=y$ and $F=x$ shows immediately that $\mathsf{P}(y|x)=P(x,y)$.

Assume now that data $\hat{y}$ are observed. Then the conditional probability of $x\in\mathbf{X}$ is given by

$$\mathsf{P}(x|\hat{y}) = \frac{\mathsf{P}(x,\hat{y})}{\mathsf{P}(\{(z,\hat{y}):z\in\mathbf{X}\})} = \frac{\Pi(x)P(x,\hat{y})}{\sum_z \Pi(z)P(z,\hat{y})}.$$

(we have tacitly assumed that the denominators do not vanish). Since $\mathsf{P}(\cdot|\hat{y})$ can be interpreted as an adjustment of Π to the data (*after* the observation) it is called the **posterior distribution** of x given $\hat{y}$.

For continuous data, the discrete distributions $P(x,\cdot)$ are replaced by densities f_x and in this case, the joint distribution is given by

$$\mathsf{P}(\{x\}\times B) = \Pi(x)\int_B f_x(y)\,dy$$

for $x\in\mathbf{X}$ and a measurable subset B of $\mathbf{Y}$ (e.g. a cube).

The prior distribution Π will always have the **Gibbsian form**

$$\Pi(x) = Z^{-1}\exp(-H(x)),\ Z=\sum_{z\in\mathbf{X}}\exp(-H(z)) \tag{1.1}$$

with some real-valued function

$$H:\mathbf{X}\longrightarrow \mathsf{R},\ x\longmapsto H(x).$$

In accordance with statistical physics, H is called the **energy function** of Π. This is not too a severe restriction since every strictly positive probability distribution on $\mathbf{X}$ has such a representation: For

$$H(x) = -\ln \Pi(x)$$

one has

$$\Pi(x) = \exp(-H(x))$$

and

$$Z = \sum_z \exp(-H(z)) = \sum_z \Pi(z) = 1$$

and hence (1.1).

Plainly, the quality of x can be measured by H as well as by Π. Large values of H correspond to small values of Π.

In most cases the posterior distribution given $\hat{y}$ is concentrated on some subspace $\hat{\mathbf{X}}$ of $\mathbf{X}$ and the posterior is again of Gibbsian form, i.e. there is a function $H(\cdot|\hat{y})$ on $\hat{\mathbf{X}}$ such that

$$\mathsf{P}(x|\hat{y}) = Z(\hat{y})^{-1} \exp(-H(x|\hat{y}), \ x \in \hat{\mathbf{X}}.$$

Remark 1.3.1. The energy function is connected to the (log-) likelihood function, an important concept in statistics. The posterior energy function can be written in the form

$$H(x|y) = c(y)\ln(P(x,y)) - \ln(\Pi(x)) = \tilde{c}(y) - \ln(P(x,y)) + H(x).$$

The second term in the last expression is interpreted as 'infidelity'; in fact it becomes large if y has low probability $P(x,y)$. The last summand corresponds to 'roughness': If H is designed to favour 'smooth' configurations then it becomes large for more 'rough' ones.

Example 1.3.1. Recall that the posterior distribution $\mathsf{P}(x|y)$ is obtained from the joint distribution $\mathsf{P}(x,y)$ by a normalization in the x-variable. Hence the energy function of the posterior distribution can be read off from the energy function of the joint distribution.

(a) The simplest but nevertheless very important case is that of undegraded observations of one or more components of x.

Suppose that $\mathbf{X} = \mathbf{Y} \times \mathbf{U}$ with elements $x = (y,u)$. For instance, if $x = (x^P, x^L)$ or $x = (x^P, x^E)$ the data are $y = x^P$ and $u = x^L$ or $u = x^E$, respectively. According to Example 1.2.1 (a) $P((y,u),y) = 1$ and $P((y,u),y') = 0$ if $y \neq y'$. Suppose further that an energy function H is given and the prior distribution has the Gibbsian form (1.1). Given y the posterior distribution is then concentrated on the space of those x with first component y. The posterior distribution becomes

$$\mathsf{P}(y,u|y) = \frac{\exp(-H(y,u))}{\sum_z \exp(H(y,z))}.$$

The conditional distribution $\mathsf{P}(u|y) = \mathsf{P}(y,u|y)$ can be considered as a distribution on $\mathbf{U}$ and written in the Gibbsian form (1.1) with energy function $H(u|y) = H(y,u)$.

(b) Let now the patterns $x = x^P$ of grey values be corrupted by additive Gaussian noise like in Example 1.2.1 (b). Let again the prior be given by an energy function H and assume that the variables X and η are independent. Then the joint distribution P of X and Y is given by

$$\mathsf{P}(\{x\} \times B) = \Pi(x)\frac{1}{(2\pi\sigma^2)^{d/2}}\int_B \exp\left(\frac{-\sum_s (y_s - x_s)^2}{2\sigma^2}\right) dy,$$

where B is a measurable set and $d = |S|$. The joint density of X and Y is

$$f(x,y) = const \cdot \exp\left(-\left(H(x) + \frac{\|y-x\|_2^2}{2\sigma^2}\right)\right);$$

($\|x\|_2$ denotes the Euclidean norm of x i.e. $\|x\|_2^2 = \sum_s x_s^2$). Hence the energy function of the posterior is

$$x \longmapsto H(x) - \frac{\|y-x\|_2^2}{2\sigma^2}.$$

(c) For the binary channel in Example 1.2.1 (c) the posterior energy is proportional to

$$x \longmapsto H(x) - |\{s \in S : y_s = -x_s\}| \ln p - |\{s \in S : y_s = x_s\}| \ln(1-p).$$

Since $1_{\{y_s = x_s\}} = \frac{x_s y_s}{2} + \frac{1}{2}$ this function is up to an additive constant equal to

$$x \longmapsto H(x) - \frac{1}{2}\ln\left(\frac{1-p}{p}\right)\sum_s x_s y_s.$$

For further examples and more details see Section 2.1.2.

1.4 Bayesian Decision Rules

A 'good' image has to be selected from the variety of all images compatible with the observed data. For instance, noise or blur have to be removed from a photograph or textures have to be classified. Given data y the problem of determining a configuration x is typically underdetermined. If, for example, in texture discrimination we are given undegraded grey values $x^P = y$ then there are $N = |S^L|$, configurations (y, x^L) compatible with the data. Hence we must watch out for rules how to decide on x. These rules will be based on precise mathematical models. Their general form will be introduced now.

On the one hand, the image should fit the data, on the other hand, it should fulfill quality criteria which depend on the concrete problem to be accomplished. The Bayesian approach allows one to take into account both requirements simultaneously. There are many ways to pick some $\hat{x}$ from $\mathbf{X}$ which hopefully is a good representation of the true image, i.e. which is in proper balance between prior expectation and fidelity to the data.

One possible rule is to choose an $\hat{x}$ for which the pair $(\hat{x}, \hat{y})$ is most favourable w.r.t. P, i.e. to maximize the function $x \mapsto \mathsf{P}((x, \hat{y}))$. One can as well maximize the posterior distribution. Since maximizers of distributions are called **modes** we define

- A mode $\hat{x}$ of the posterior distribution $\mathsf{P}(\cdot|\hat{y})$ is called a **maximum a posteriori estimate** of x given $\hat{y}$, or, in short-hand notation a MAP estimate.

Note that the images x are estimated as a whole. In particular, contextual requirements incorporated in the prior (like connectedness of boundaries or homogeneity of regions) are inherited by the posterior distribution and thus influence $\hat{x}$. Let us illustrate this by way of example. Suppose we are given a digitized aerial photograph of ice flow in the polar sea. We want to label the pixels as belonging to ice or water. We may wish a naturally looking estimate x^L composed of large patches of water or ice. For a suitable prior the estimate will respect these requirements. On the other hand, it may erase existing small or thin ice patches or smooth fuzzy boundaries. This way, some pixels may be misclassified for the sake of regularity.

If one is not interested in regular structures but only in a small error rate then there will be no contextual requirements and it is reasonable to estimate the labels site by site independently of each other. In such a situation the following estimator is frequently adopted: A maximizer $\hat{x}_s$ of the function $x_s \mapsto \mathsf{P}(x_s|\hat{y})$ is called a **marginal posterior mode** and one defines:

- A configuration $\hat{x}$ is called a **marginal posterior mode estimate** (MPME) if each $\hat{x}_s$ is a marginal posterior mode (given $\hat{y}$).

In applications like tomographic reconstruction the mean value or expectation of the posterior distribution is a convenient estimator:

- The configuration $\hat{x} = \sum x\mathsf{P}(x|\hat{y})$ is called the **minimum mean squares estimator** (MMSE).

The name will be explained in the following remark. Note that this estimator makes sense only if $\mathbf{X}$ is a subset of a Euclidean space. Even then the MMSE in general is not an element of the discrete and finite space $\mathbf{X}$ and hence one has to choose the element next to the theoretical MMSE. In this context it is natural to work on continuous spaces. Fortunately, much of the later theory generalizes to continuous spaces.

For continuous data the discrete transition probabilities are replaced by densities. For example, the MAP estimator maximizes

$$x \longmapsto \Pi(x) f_x(\hat{y})$$

and the MMSE is

$$\mathsf{E}(X|\hat{y}) = \frac{\sum_x x\Pi(x)f_x(\hat{y})}{\sum_z \Pi(z)f_z(\hat{y})}.$$

Remark 1.4.1. In estimation theory, estimators are studied in terms of loss functions. Let

$$\hat{X} : \mathbf{Y} \longrightarrow \mathbf{X},\ y \longmapsto \hat{X}(y)$$

be any estimator, i.e. a map on the sample space for which $\hat{x} = \hat{X}(y)$ hopefully is close to the unknown x. The loss of estimating a true x by $\hat{x}$ or the 'distance' between $\hat{x}$ and x is measured by a **loss function** $L(x, \hat{x}) \geq 0$ with the convention $L(x, x) = 0$. The choice of L is problem specific.

The **Bayes risk** of the function $\hat{X}$ is the mean loss

$$\hat{R} = \sum_{x,y} L(x, \hat{X}(y))\mathsf{P}(x, y) = \sum_{x,y} L(x, \hat{X}(y))\Pi(x)P(x, y).$$

An estimator minimizing this risk is called a **Bayes estimator**. The quality of an algorithm depends on both, the prior model and the estimator or loss function. The estimators introduced previously can be identified as Bayes estimators for certain loss functions. One of the reasons why the above estimators were introduced is that they can be computed (or at least approximated).

Consider the simple loss function

$$L(x, \hat{x}) = \begin{cases} 0 & \text{if} \quad x = \hat{x} \\ 1 & \text{if} \quad x \neq \hat{x} \end{cases}. \tag{1.2}$$

This is in fact a rather rough measure since an estimate which differs from the true configuration x everywhere has the same distance from x as one which fails in one site only. The Bayes risk

$$\hat{R} = \sum_y \sum_x L(x, \hat{X}(y))\mathsf{P}(x, y)$$

is minimal if and only if each term of the first sum is minimal; more precisely, if for each y,

$$\sum_x L(x, \hat{X}(y))\mathsf{P}(x, y) = \sum_x \mathsf{P}(x, y) - \mathsf{P}(\hat{X}(y), y)$$

is minimal. Hence MAP estimators are the Bayes estimators for the 0-1 loss function (1.2).

There are arguments against MAP estimators and it is far from clear in which situations they are intrinsically desirable (cf. MARROQUIN, MITTER and POGGIO (1987)). Firstly, the computational problem is enormous, and in fact, quite a bit of space in this text will be taken by this problem. On the other hand, hardware develops faster than mathematical theories and one should not be too worried about that. Some found MAP estimators too 'global', leading to mislabelings or oversmoothing in restoration (cf. Fig. 2.1). In our opinion such phenomena do not necessarily occur for carefully designed priors Π, and criticism frequently stems from the fact that in the past prior models often were chosen for sake of computational simplicity only.

The next loss function is frequently used in classification (labeling) problems:

$$L(x, \hat{x}) = |S|^{-1} \left|\{s \in S : \hat{x}_s \neq x_s\}\right| \tag{1.3}$$

is the **error rate** of the estimate. The number

$$d(x, \hat{x}) = \left|\{s \in S : x_s \neq \hat{x}_s\}\right|$$

is called the **Hamming distance** between x and $\hat{x}$. A computation similar to the last one shows: the corresponding Bayes estimator is given by an $\hat{X}(y)$ for which in each site $s \in S$ the component $\hat{X}(y)_s$ maximizes the marginal posterior distribution $\mathsf{P}(x_s|y)$ in x_s. Hence MPM estimators are the Bayes estimators for the mean error rate (1.3). There are models especially designed for MPM estimation like the Markov mesh models (cf. BESAG (1986), 2.4 and also RIPLEY (1988) and the papers by HJORT et al.).

The MMS estimators are easily seen to be the Bayes estimators for the loss function

$$L(x, \hat{x}) = \sum_s |x_s - \hat{x}_s|^2.$$

They minimize a mean of squares which explains their name.

The general model now is introduced completely and we are going to discuss a concrete example.

2. Cleaning Dirty Pictures

The aim of the present chapter is the illustration and discussion of the previously introduced concepts. We continue with the discussion of noise reduction or image restoration started in the introduction. This specific example is chosen since it can easily be described and there is no need for further theory.

The very core of the chapter are the Examples 2.3.1 and 2.4.1. They are concerned with Bayesian image restoration and boundary extraction and due to S. and D. GEMAN. A slightly more special version of the first one was independently developed by A. BLAKE and A. ZISSERMAN. Simple introductory considerations and examples of smoothing hopefully will awaken the reader's interest. We also give some more examples how images get dirty.

The chapter is not necessary for the logical development of the book. For a rapid idea what the chapter is about, the reader should look over Section 2.2 and then work through Example 2.3.1.

2.1 Distortion of Images

We briefly comment on sources of geometric distortion and noise in a physical imaging system and then compute posterior distributions for distortions by blur, noise and nonlinear degradation.

2.1.1 Physical Digital Imaging Systems

Here is a rough sketch of an optoelectronical imaging system. There are many simplifications and the reader is referred to PRATT (1978) (e.g. pp. 365), GONZALEZ and WINTZ (1987) and to the more specific monographs BIBERMAN and NUDELMAN (1971) for photoelectronic imaging devices and MEES (1954) for the theory of photographic processes.

The driving force is a continuous light distribution $I(u, v)$ on some subset of the Euclidean plane R^2. If there is kind of memory in the system, time-dependence must also be taken into account. The image is recorded and processed by a physical imaging system giving an output $I_0(u, v)$. This observed image is digitized to produce an array y followed by the restoration system generating the digital estimation x of the 'true image'. The function of digital image restoration is to compensate for degradations of the physical imaging system and the digitizer. This is the step we are actually interested in. The output sample of the restoration system may then be interpolated by an image display system to produce a visible continuous image.

Basically, the physical imaging system is composed of an optical system followed by a photodetector and an associated electrical filter. The optical system, consisting of lenses, mirrors and prisms, provides a deterministic transformation of the input light distribution. The output intensity is not exactly a geometric projection of the input. Potential degradations include geometric distortion, defocusing, scattering or blur by motion of objects during the exposure time. The concept can be extended to encompass the spatial propagation of light through free space or some medium causing atmospheric turbulence effects. The simplest model assumes that all intensity contributions in a point add up, i.e. the output at point (u, v) is

$$BI(u,v) = \iint I(u',v')K((u,v),(u',v'))\,du'dv'$$

where $K((u,v),(u',v'))$ is the response at (u,v) to a unit signal at (u',v').

The output BI of the optical system still is a light distribution. A photodetector converts incident photons to electrons, or, optical intensity to a detector current. One example is a CCD detector (*c*harge-*c*oupled *d*evice) which in modern astronomy replace photographic plates. CCD chips also replace tubes in every modern home video camera. These are semiconductor sensors counting indirectly the number of photons hitting the cells of a grid (e.g. of size 512 × 512). In scientific use they are frequently cooled to low temperatures. CCD detectors are far more photosensitive than film or photographic plates. Tubes are more conventional devices. Note that there is a system inherent discretization causing a kind of noise: in CCD chips the plane is divided into cells and in tubes the image is scanned line by line. This results in Moiré and aliasing effects (see below). Scanning or subsequently reading out the cells of a CCD chip results in a signal current i_P varying in time instead of space. The current passes through an electrical filter and creates a voltage across a resistor. In general, the measured current is not a linear function but a power $i_P = const \cdot BI(u,v)^\gamma$ of intensity. The exponent γ is system specific; frequently, $\gamma \sim 0.4$. For many scientific applications a linear dependence is assumed and hence $\gamma = 1$ is chosen. For film the dependence is logarithmic. The most common noise is **thermal noise** caused by irregular electron fluctuations in resistive elements. Thermal noise is reasonably modelled by a Gaussian distribution and for additive noise the resultant current is

$$i_T = i_P + \eta_T$$

where η_T is a zero mean Gaussian variable with variance $\sigma^2 = N_T/R$, N_T the thermal noise power at the system output and R resistance. In the simple case in which the filter is a capacitor placed in parallel with the detector and load resistor, $N_T = kT/RC$, where k is the Boltzmann factor, T temperature and C the capacity of the filter.

There is also measurement uncertainty η_Q resulting from quantum mechanical effects due to the discrete nature of photons. It is governed by a Poisson law with parameter depending on the observation time period τ, the average number u_S of electrons emitted from the detector as a result of the incident illumination and the average number u_H of electron emissions caused by dark current and background radiation:

$$Prob(\eta_Q = kq/\tau) = \frac{\alpha^k}{k!} e^{-\alpha};$$

here q is the charge of an electron and $\alpha = u_S + u_H$. The resulting fluctuation of the detector current is called **shot noise.** In presence of sufficient internal amplification, for example a photomutiplier tube, the shot noise will dominate subsequent thermal noise. Shot noise is of particular importance in applications like emission computer tomography. For large average electron emission, background radiation is negligible and the Poisson distribution can be approximated by a Gaussian distribution with mean $qu_S\tau$ and variance $q^2 u_S/\tau^2$. Generally, thermal noise dominates and shot noise can be neglected.

Finally, this image is converted to a discrete one by a digitizer. There will be no further discussion of the various distortions by digitization. Let us mention only the three main sources of digitization errors.

(i) For a suitable class of images the **Wittacker-Shannon sampling theorem** implies:

Suppose that the image is band-limited, i.e. its Fourier transform vanishes outside a square $[-r, r]^2$. Then the continuous image can completely be reconstructed from the array of its values on a grid of coarseness at most r^{-1}.

For this version, the Fourier transform $\hat{I}$ of I is induced by

$$\hat{I}(\varphi, \psi) = \iint f(u, v) \exp(-2\pi\imath(\varphi u + \psi v))\, dudv.$$

If the hypothesis of this theorem holds - one says that the **Nyquist criterion** is fulfilled – then no information is lost by discrete sampling. A major potential source of error is undersampling, i.e. taking values on a coarser grid. This leads to so-called aliasing errors. Moreover, intensity distributions frequently are not band-limited. A look at the Fourier representation shows that band-limited images cannot have fine structure or sharp contrast.

(ii) Replacing 'sharp' values in sampling by weighted averages over a neighbourhood causes blur.

(iii) There is quantization noise since continuous intensity values are replaced by a finite number of values. Restoration methods designed to compensate for such quantization errors can be found in PRATT (1978).

These few remarks should suffice to illustrate the intricate nature of the various kinds of distortion.

2.1.2 Posterior Distributions

Let x and y be grey value patterns on a finite rectangular grid S. The previous considerations suggest models for the distortion of images of the general form

$$Y = \Phi(BX) \odot \eta$$

where $\odot$ is any composition of two arguments (like '+' or '·'). We shall consider only the special case in which degradation takes place site by site, i.e.

$$Y_s = \Phi((BX)_s) \odot \eta_s \quad \text{for every} \quad s \in S. \tag{2.1}$$

Let us explain this formula.

(i) B is a linear blur operator. Usually it has the form

$$(Bx)_s = \sum_t x_t K(t, s)$$

with a **point spread function** K. $K(t, s)$ is the response at s to a unit signal at t. In the space invariant case, K only depends on the differences $s - t$ and Bx is a convolution

$$(Bx)_s = \sum_t x_t K(s - t).$$

The definition does not make sense on finite lattices. Frequently, finite (rectangular) images are periodically extended to all of $\mathbb{Z}^2$ (or 'wrapped around a torus'). The main reason is that convolution corresponds to multiplication of the Fourier transforms which is helpful for analysis and computation. In the present context, K is assumed to have finite support small compared to the image size and the formula is modified near the boundary. It holds strictly on the interior, i.e. for those s for which all t with $K(s - t) > 0$ are members of the image domain.

Example 2.1.1. The simplest example is convolution with a 'blurring mask' like

$$B(k, l) = \begin{cases} 1/2 & \text{if} \quad k, l = 0 \\ 1/16 & \text{if} \quad |k|, |l| \le 1, (k, l) \ne (0, 0) \end{cases}$$

where (i, j) denotes a lattice point. The blurred image has components

$$(Bx)_{(i,j)} = \sum_{k,l} B(k, l) x_{(i+k, j+l)} \tag{2.2}$$

off the boundary. If one insists on the common definition of convolution with a minus sign one has to modify the indices in B.

(i) The blurred image is pixel by pixel transformed by a possibly nonlinear system specific function Φ (e.g. a power with exponent γ).

(ii) In addition, there is noise η, and finally, one arrives at the above formula where $\odot$ stands for addition or say multiplication according to the nature of the noise.

For the computation of posterior distributions the conditional distribution of the data given the true image, i.e. the transition probabilities P, are needed. To avoid some (minor) technical difficulties we shall assume that all variables take values in finite discrete spaces (the reader familiar with densities can easily fill in the additional details). Let $\mathbf{X} = \mathbf{X}^P \times \mathbf{Z}$ where $x \in \mathbf{X}^P$ is an intensity configuration and $\mathbf{Z}$ is a space of further image attributes. Let $Y = \varphi(X, \eta)$. Let P and Q denote the joint distribution of (X, Z) and Y and of (X, Z) and η, respectively. The distribution of (X, Z) is the prior Π. The law of η will be denoted by Γ.

Lemma 2.1.1. *Let (X, Z) and η be independent, i.e.*

$$\mathsf{Q}((X,Z) = (x,z), \eta = n) = \Pi(x,z)\Gamma(\eta = n).$$

Then

$$\mathsf{P}(Y = y|(X,Z) = (x,z)) = \Gamma(\varphi(x,\eta) = y).$$

Proof. The relation follows from the simple computations

$$\begin{aligned} & \mathsf{P}(Y = y|(X,Z) = (x,z)) = \mathsf{Q}(\varphi(X,\eta) = y|X = x, Z = z) \\ = \quad & \mathsf{Q}(\varphi(x,\eta) = y, X = x, Z = z)/\Pi(x,z) \\ = \quad & \Gamma(\varphi(x,\eta) = y). \end{aligned}$$

Independence of (X, Z) and η was used for last but one equation. For the others the definitions were plugged in. □

Example 1.3.1 covered posterior distributions for the simple case $y = x + \eta$ with white noise and $y_s = x_s \eta_s$ for channel noise. Let us give further examples.

Example 2.1.2. The variables (X, Z) and η will be assumed to be independent.

(a) For additive noise, $Y_s = \Phi(B(X)_s) + \eta_s$. For additive white noise, the lemma yields for the density f_x of $\mathsf{P}(\cdot|x,z)$ that

$$f_x(y) = (2\pi\sigma^2)^{-d/2} \exp\left(-(2\sigma^2)^{-1} \sum_s (y_s - \Phi(B(x)_s))^2\right)$$

where σ^2 is the common variance of the η_s. In the case of centered but correlated Gaussian noise variables the density is

$$f_x(y) = (2\pi \det C)^{-d/2} \exp\left(-(1/2)(y - \Phi(Bx))C^{-1}(y - \Phi(Bx))^*\right.$$

where C is the covariance matrix with elements

$$C(s,t) = \mathsf{cov}(\eta_s, \eta_t) = \mathsf{E}(\eta_s \eta_t),$$

$\det C$ is the determinant of C and a vector u is written as a row vector with transpose u^*.

Under mild restrictions the law of the data can be computed also in the general case. Suppose that a Gibbsian prior distribution with energy H on $\mathbf{X} = \mathbf{X}^P \times \mathbf{Z}$ is given.

Theorem 2.1.1. (S. and D. GEMAN (1984), D. GEMAN (1990)).
Let

$$Y_s = \Phi((BX)_s) \odot \eta_s$$

with white noise η of constant mean μ and variance σ^2, and independent of (X, Z). Assume that for each $\alpha > 0$ the map $\gamma \mapsto v = \alpha \odot \gamma$ has a smooth inverse $\Xi(\alpha, v)$ strictly increasing in v. Then the posterior distribution of (X, Z) given Y is of Gibbsian form with energy function

$$\begin{aligned} H(x, z|y) &= H(x, z) \\ &\quad + (2\sigma^2)^{-1} \sum_s (\Xi(\Phi((Bx)_s), y_s) - \mu)^2 \\ &\quad - \sum_s \ln \frac{\partial}{\partial y_s} \Xi(\Phi((Bx)_s), y_s). \end{aligned}$$

(The result is stated correctly in the second reference.) The previous expressions are simple special cases.

Proof. By the last lemma it is sufficient to compute the density h_x of the vector-valued random variable $(\Phi((Bx)_s) \odot \eta_s)_{s \in S^P}$. Letting $h_{x,s}$ denote the density of the component with index s, by independence of the noise variables,

$$h_x(y) = \prod_s h_{x,s}(y_s).$$

By assumption, the density transformation formula (Appendix (A.4)) applies and yields

$$h_{x,s}(y_s) = g \circ \Xi(\Phi((Bx)_s), y_s) \left| \frac{\partial}{\partial y_s} \Xi(\Phi((Bx)_s), y_s) \right|$$

where g denotes the density of a $\mu - \sigma^2$ real Gaussian variable. This implies the result. □

(b) Shot noise usually obeys a Poisson law, i.e.

$$\Gamma(\eta_s = k) = \mathrm{e}^{-\alpha} \cdot \frac{\alpha^k}{k!}$$

for each nonnegative integer k and a parameter $\alpha > 0$. Expectation and variance equal α. Usually the intensity α depends on the signal. Nevertheless, let us compute the posterior for the simple model $y_s = x_s + \eta_s$. If all variables η_s, $s \in S^P$, and (X, Z) are independent the lemma yields

$$\mathsf{P}(Y = y|(X,Z) = (x,z)) = \mathrm{e}^{-\alpha d} \cdot \prod_s \frac{\alpha^{y_s - x_s}}{(y_s - x_s)!}$$

$$= \exp\left(-\left(\alpha d + \sum_s ((x_s - y_s)\ln\alpha - \ln(y_s - x_s)!)\right)\right)$$

if $y_s \geq x_s$ and 0 otherwise, where $d = |S^P|$. The joint distribution is obtained multiplying by $\Pi(x,z)$ and the posterior by subsequent normalization in the (x,z)-variable. The posterior is not strictly positive on all of $\mathbf{X}$ and hence not Gibbsian. On the other hand, the space $\prod_s \{\{x_s\} \times \mathbf{Z} : x_s \leq y_s\}$ where it is strictly positive has a product structure and on this space the posterior is Gibbsian. Its energy function is given by

$$H(x,z|y) = H(x,z) + \alpha d + \sum_s ((x_s - y_s)\ln\alpha - \ln(y_s - x_s)!).$$

2.2 Smoothing

In general, noise results in patterns rough at small scale. Since real scenes frequently are composed of comparably smooth pieces many restoration techniques smooth the data in one or another way and thus reduce the noise contribution. Global smoothing has the unpleasant property to blur contrast boundaries in the real scene. How to avoid this by boundary preserving methods is dicussed in the next section. The present section is intended to introduce the problem by way of some simple examples.

Consider intensity configurations $(x_s)_{s\in S^P}$ on a finite lattice S^P. A first measure of smoothness is given by

$$H(x) = \beta \sum_{\langle s,t\rangle} (x_s - x_t)^2, \quad \beta > 0, \tag{2.3}$$

where the summation extends over pairs of adjacent pixels, say in the south-north and east-west direction. In fact, H is minimal for constant configurations and maximal for configurations with maximal grey value differences between neighbours.

In presence of white noise the posterior energy function is

$$H(x|y) = \beta \sum_{\langle s,t\rangle} (x_s - x_t)^2 + \frac{1}{2\sigma^2} \sum_s (x_s - y_s)^2. \tag{2.4}$$

Two terms compete: the first one is low for smooth – ideally constant – configurations, and the second one is low for configurations close to – ideally equal to – the presumably rough data. Because of the first term, MAP estimation, i.e. minimization of $H(\cdot|y)$, will result in 'restorations' with blurred grey value steps and smoothed creases. This effect will be reinforced by high β.

Results of a simple experiment are displayed in Figure 2.1 (it will be continued in the next section). The one-dimensional 'image' in Fig. (a) is corrupted by white noise (Fig. (b)) with standard deviation about 6% of the total height. Fig. (c) shows the result of repeated application of a binomial

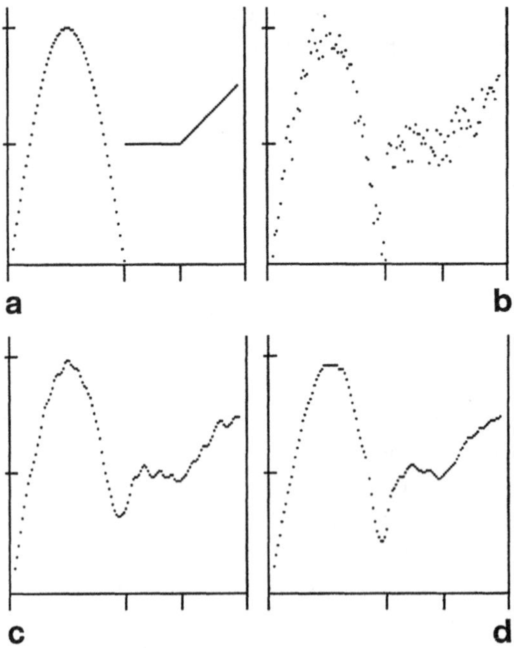

Fig. 2.1. Smoothing: (**a**) Original, (**b**) degraded image, (**c**) binomial filter, (**d**) MAP estimate for (2.3)

filter of length 3, i.e. convolution with the mask $(1/4)(1,2,1)$ (cf. (2.2)). Fig. (d) is an approximate MAP estimate. Both smooth the step in the middle. Note that (d) is much smoother than (c) (e.g. at the top of the mountain).

In binary images there is no blurring of edges and hence they can be used to illustrate the influence of the prior on the organization into patches of similar (here equal) intensity.

S^P is a finite square lattice and $x_s = \pm 1$. Hence the squares in (2.3) can have the two values 0 and 4 only. A suitable choice of β (1/4 of that in (2.3))and addition of a suitable constant (which has no effect on the induced Gibbs field) yields the energy function

$$H(x) = -\beta \sum_{\langle s,t \rangle} x_s x_t$$

which for $\beta > 0$ again favours globally smooth images. In fact, the minima of H are the two constant configurations. In the experiment, summation extends over pairs $\{s,t\}$ of pixels adjacent in the vertical, horizontal or diagonal directions (hence for fixed s there are 8 pixels t in relation $\langle s,t\rangle$; the relation is modified near the boundary of S^P).

The data are created corrupting the 80×80 binary configuration in Fig. 2.2 (a) by channel noise like in Example 1.2.1 (c): the pixels change colour with probability $p = 0.2$ independently of each other. The posterior energy function is

$$H(x|y) = -\beta \sum_{\langle s,t\rangle} x_s x_t - \frac{1}{2} \ln \frac{1-p}{p} \sum_s x_s y_s.$$

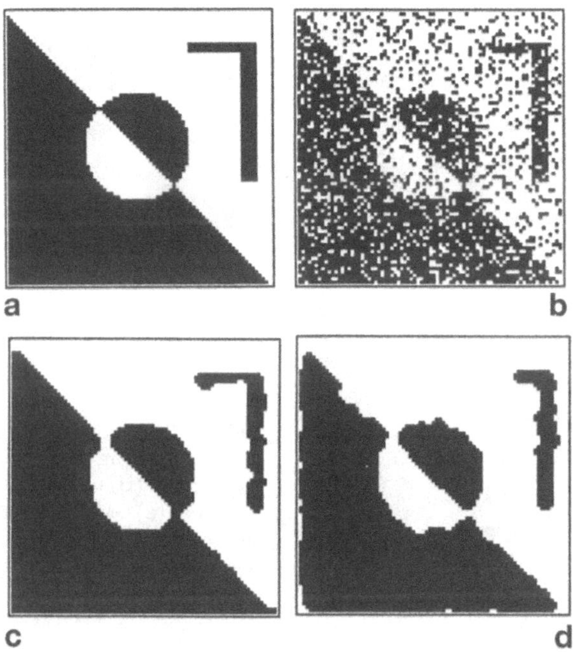

Fig. 2.2. Smoothing of a binary image. (**a**) Original, (**b**) degraded image, (**c**) MAP estimate, (**d**) median filter

The approximate minimum of $H(x|y)$ for $\beta = 1$ in (c) is contrasted with the 'restoration' obtained by the common 'median filter' in Fig. (d). The misclassification rate is not an appropriate quality measure for restoration since it contains no information about the dependence of colours in different pixels. Nevertheless, it is reduced from about 20% in (b) to 1.25% in Fig. (c). The median filter was applied until nothing changed any more, it replaces the colour in each site s by the colour of the majority of sites in a 3×3-block around s. The misclassification rate in (d) is 3.25% (the misclassifications along the border can be avoided if the image is mirrored across the border lines and the median filter is applied to the enlarged image. But one can easily construct images where this trick does not work.)

The next picture (Fig. 2.3(a)) has some fine structure which is lost by MAP estimation for this crude model. For $\beta = 1$ the misclassification rate is about 4% (Fig. (c)). The smaller smoothing parameter $\beta = 0.3$ in (d) gives more fidelity to the data and the misclassification rate of 3.95% is slightly better.

Anyway, Fig. (a) is much nicer than (c) or (d) and playing around with the parameters does not help. Obviously, the prior (2.3) is not appropriate for the restoration of images like 2.3(a). Median filtering resulted in (e) (with 19% error rate).

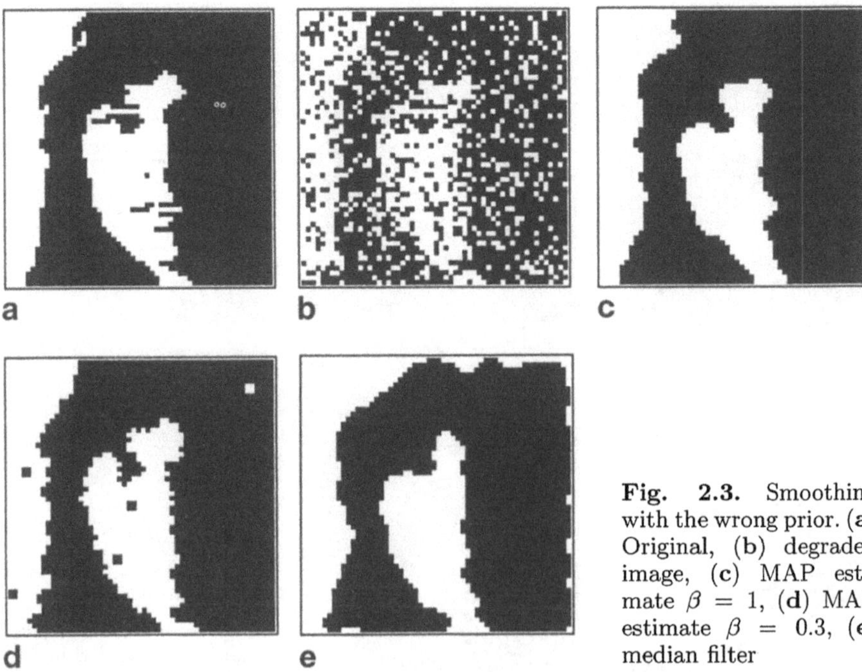

Fig. 2.3. Smoothing with the wrong prior. (**a**) Original, (**b**) degraded image, (**c**) MAP estimate $\beta = 1$, (**d**) MAP estimate $\beta = 0.3$, (**e**) median filter

Remark 2.2.1. Already these primitive examples show that MAP estimation strongly depends on the prior and that the same prior may be appropriate for some scenes but inadequate for others. As SIGERU MASE (1991) puts it,

> we must take into account of underlying spatial structure and relevant knowledges carefully and can not choose a prior because of its mere simplicity and tractability.

In some applications it can at least be checked whether the prior is appropriate or not since there is

> the ability synthetically to degrade images, thus having the 'original' for comparison; or simply having actual digits or road maps for checking algorithms for optical character recognition or automated cartography.

(GEMAN and GEMAN (1991)). In the absence of 'ground truth' (as in archeology, cf. BESAG (1991)), on the other hand, it is not obvious how to demonstrate that a given prior is feasible.

Before we turn to a better method, let us comment on some conventional smoothing techniques.

Example 2.2.1. (a) There are a lot of ad hoc techniques for restoration of dirty images which do not take into account any information about the organization of the ideal image or the nature of degradation. The most simple ones convolve the observed image with 'noise cleaning masks' and this way smooth or blur the noisy image. Due to their simplicity they are frequently used in applied engineering (a classical reference book is PRATT (1978), see also JÄHNE (1991b), in German (1991a)). Perhaps the simplest smoothing technique is running **moving averages**. The image x is convolved with a noise cleaning mask like

$$B_1 = \frac{1}{9}\begin{pmatrix} 1 & 1 & 1 \\ 1 & 1 & 1 \\ 1 & 1 & 1 \end{pmatrix}, \quad B_2 = \frac{1}{16}\begin{pmatrix} 1 & 2 & 1 \\ 2 & 4 & 2 \\ 1 & 2 & 1 \end{pmatrix}$$

(convolution is defined in (2.2)). A variety of such masks (and combinations) can be found in the tool-box of image processing. They should not be applied too optimistically. The first mask, for example, does not only oversmooth, it does not even remove roughness of certain 'wave lengths' (apply it to vertical or horizontal stripes of different width). The 'Binomial mask' B_2 performs much better but there is still oversmoothing. Hence filters have to be carefully designed for specific applications (for example by inspection of Fourier transforms).

Sharp edges are to some extent preserved by the nonlinear **median filter** (cf. Fig. 2.5). The grey values inside an $N \times N$-block around s of odd size are arranged in a vector $(g_1, \ldots, g_{N \cdot N})$ in increasing order. The middle one (with index $(N^2-1)/2+1$) is the new grey value in s (cf. Fig. 2.3). The performance of the median filter is difficult to analyze, cf. TYAN (1981).

(b) Noise enters a model even if it is deterministic at the first glance. Assume that there is blur only and $y = Bx$ for some linear operator B. Theoretically, restoration boils down to solving a system of linear equations. If B is invertible then $x = B^{-1}y$ is the unique solution to the restoration problem. If the system is underdetermined then the solutions form a possibly high dimensional affine space. It is common to restrict the space of solutions imposing further constraints, ideally allowing a single solution only. The method of pseudo inverses provides rules how to do so (cf. PRATT (1978), chapters 8 and 14 for examples, and STRANG (1976) for details). But this is only part of the story. Since y is determined by physical sampling and the elements of B are specified independently by system modeling, the system of equations may be inconsistent in practice and there is no solution at all. Plainly, $y = Bx$

then is the wrong model and one tries $y = Bx + e(x)$ with a hypothetical error term $e(x)$ (which may be called noise).

(c) If there are no prior expectations concerning the true image and little is known about noise, then a Bayesian formulation cannot contribute anything. If, for example, the observed image is $\hat{y} = Bx + \hat{\eta}$ with noise η then one frequently minimizes the function

$$x \mapsto \|\hat{y} - Bx\|_2^2.$$

This is the method of **unconstrained least-squares restoration** or **least-squares inverse filtering.** For identically distributed noise variables of mean 0, the law of large numbers tells us that $\|\hat{\eta}\|_2^2 \sim |S^P|\sigma^2$, where σ^2 is the common variance of the η_s. Hence minimization of the above quadratic form amounts to the minimization of noise variance.

(d) Let us continue with the additive model $y = Bx + \eta$ and assume that the covariance matrix C of η is known. The method of **regression image restoration** minimizes the quadratic form

$$x \mapsto (y - Bx)C^{-1}(y - Bx)^*.$$

Differentiation gives the conditions $B^*C^{-1}Bx = B^*y$. If $B^*C^{-1}B$ is not invertible the minimum is not unique and pseudo inverses can be used.

Since no prior knowledge about the true image was assumed, the Bayesian paradigm is useless. Formally, this is the case where $\Pi(x) = |\mathbf{X}|^{-1}$ and where noise is Gaussian with covariance matrix C. The posterior distribution is proportional to

$$\exp\left(-\ln|\mathbf{X}| - (y - Bx)C^{-1}(y - Bx)^*\right).$$

(e) The method of **constrained smoothing** or **constrained mean-squares filters** exploits prior knowledge and thus can be put into the Bayesian framework. The map

$$x \longmapsto f(x) = xQx^*$$

is minimized under the constraint

$$g(x) = (y - Bx)M(y - Bx)^* = c.$$

Frequently, M is the the inverse C^{-1} of the noise covariance matrix and Q is some smoothing matrix, for example $xQx^* = \sum(x_s - x_t)^2$, summation extending over selected pairs of sites. Here the smoothest image compatible with prescribed fidelity to the data (expressed by the number c) is chosen. The dual problem is to minimize

$$x \longmapsto g(x) = (y - Bx)M(y - Bx)^*$$

under the constraint

$$f(x) = xQx^* = d.$$

For a solution x of these problems it is necessary, that the level sets of f and g are tangential to each other (draw a sketch !) and – since the tangential hyperplanes are perpendicular to the respective gradients – that the gradients $\nabla f(x)$ and $\nabla g(x)$ are colinear:

$$\nabla f(x) = -\lambda \nabla g(x).$$

Solving this equation for each λ and then considering those x which satisfy the constraints provides a necessary condition for the solutions of the above problems (this is the method of Lagrangian multipliers); requiring the gradients to be colinear amounts to the search for a stationary point of

$$x \longmapsto xQx^* + \lambda(((y - Bx)M(y - Bx)^* - c)) \tag{2.5}$$

for the first formulation or

$$x \longmapsto (y - Bx)M(y - Bx)^* + \gamma(xQx^* - d) \tag{2.6}$$

where $\gamma = \lambda^{-1}$ for the second one. For $\gamma = 0$ and $M = C^{-1}$, minimization of (2.6) boiles down to regression restoration. Substitution of $\gamma = 1$, $M = C^{-1}$ and the image covariance Q results in equivalence to the well-known **Wiener estimator**.

If x satisfies the gradient equation for some λ_0 then an x solving the equation for $\lambda_0 + \varepsilon$ satisfies the rigid constraints approximately and thus solutions for various λ-values may be said to fulfill a 'relaxed' constraint. For Gaussian noise with covariance C the solutions of (2.5) correspond to MAP estimates for the prior

$$\Pi(x) \propto \exp(-xQx^*)$$

and

$$P(x, y) = (\pi\lambda^{-1})^{-|S^P|/2} \cdot \exp(\lambda(y - Bx)C^{-1}(y - Bx)^*).$$

Thus there is a close connection between this conventional and the Bayesian method. For a thorough discussion cf. HUNT (1973).

It should be mentioned that the Bayesian approach with additive Gaussian noise and nonlinear Φ in (2.1) and a Gaussian prior was successfully adopted by B.R. HUNT already in 1977.

2.3 Piecewise Smoothing

For images with high contrast a method based on (2.3) will not give anything which deserves the name restoration. The noise will possibly be removed but also all grey value steps will be be blurred. This is caused by the high penalties for large intensity steps. On the other hand, for high signal to noise ratio, large intensity steps are likely to mark sudden changes in the visible surface. For instance, where a surface ends and another begins there usually is a sudden change of intensity called an 'occluding boundary'. To avoid blur, such boundaries must be located and smoothing has to be switched off there. Locating well-organized boundaries combined with smoothing inside the surrounded regions is beyond the abilities of most conventional restoration methods. Here the Bayesian method really can give a new impetus.

In a first step let us replace the sum of squares by a function which smoothes at small scale and preserves high intensity jumps. We consider

$$\sum_{\langle s,t\rangle} \Psi(x_s - x_t)$$

with some function Ψ of the type in Fig. 2.4, for example

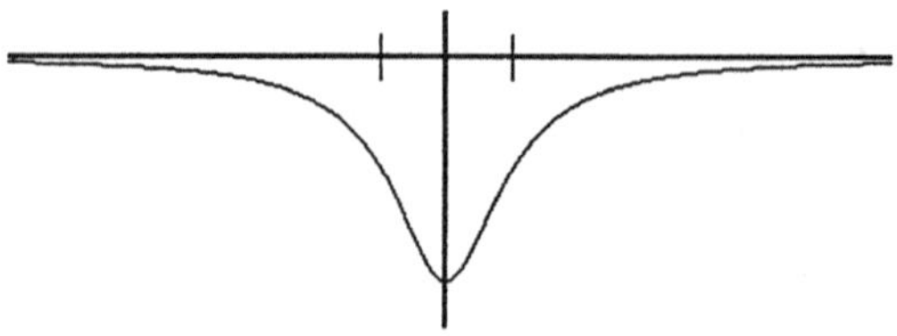

Fig. 2.4. A cup function

$$\Psi(u) = \frac{-1}{1+|u|/\delta} \quad \text{or} \quad \Psi(u) = \frac{-1}{1+(u/\delta)^2}. \tag{2.7}$$

For such functions Ψ, one large step is cheaper than many small ones. The scaling parameter δ controls the height of jumps to be respected and its choice should depend on the variance of the data. If the latter is unknown then δ should be estimated.

If you do not feel happy with this statement cut off the branches of $u \mapsto u^2$ and set

$$\Psi(u) = \frac{|u|^2}{\delta^2} 1_{\{|u|<\delta\}}(u) + 1_{\{|u|\geq\delta\}}(u). \tag{2.8}$$

Set the parameters β, $2\sigma^2$ and δ to 1 and compare the posterior energy functions (2.4) and

$$\tilde{H}(x|y) = \sum_{\langle S,t\rangle} \Psi(x_s - x_t) + \sum_s (x_s - y_s)^2.$$

To be definite, let $S = \{0,1,2,3\} \subset \mathbb{Z}$ with neighbour pairs $\{0,1\}$, $\{1,2\}$ and $\{2,3\}$. To avoid calculations, choose date $y_0 = -1/2 = y_2$, $y_1 = 1/2 = y_3$ and $x_i = 0$ for every i. Then $H(x|y) = 1 = \tilde{H}(x|y)$. This is a low value illustrating the smoothing effect of both functions. On the other hand, set $y_0 = 0 = y_1$ and $y_2 = 3 = y_3$ with a jump between $s = 1$ and $s = 2$. For $x = y$ you get $H(x|y) = 9$ whereas $\tilde{H}(x|y) = 1$! Hence a restoration preserving the intensity step is favourable for $\tilde{H}$ whereas it is penalized by H.

In the following mini-experient two 'edge preserving' methods are applied to the data in Fig. 2.1(b) (= Fig. 2.5(b)). The median filter of length 5 produced Fig. 2.5.(c). It is too short to smooth all the edges caused by noise but at least it respects the jump in the middle. Fig. (d) is a MAP estimate: the squares in H were replaced by the simple 'cup'-function Ψ in (2.8).

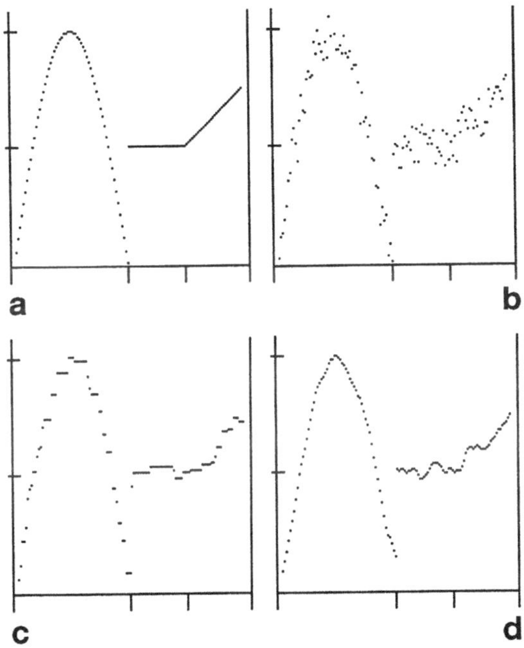

Fig. 2.5. (**a**) Original, (**b**) degraded image, (**c**) median filter, (**d**) MAP with cup function

Piecewise smoothing is closely related to edge detection: accompanied by a simple threshold operation it simultaneously marks locations of sharp contrast. In dimensions higher than one the above method will not work well, since there is no possibility to organize the boundaries. This will be discussed now. The model was proposed in S. GEMAN and D. GEMAN (1984); we follow the survey by D. GEMAN (1990).

Example 2.3.1. Suppose we are given a photograph of a car parked in front of a wall (like those in Figs. 2.10 and 2.11). We observe : (i) In most parts the picture is smooth, i.e. most pixels have a grey value similar to those of their neighbours. (ii) There are thin regions of sharp contrast for example around the wind-screen or the bumper. We shall call them edges. (iii) These edges are organized: they tend to form connected lines and there are only few local edge configurations like double edges, endings or small isolated fragments. How can we allow for these observations in restoring an image degraded by noise, blur and perhaps nonlinear system transformations? Because of (ii) smoothing should be switched off near real (contrast) boundaries. The 'switches' are represented by an edge process which is coupled to the pixel process. This way (iii) can also be taken into account.

Besides the pixel process x an edge or boundary process b is introduced. Let $x = (x_s)_{S^P}$ with a finite lattice S^P represent an intensity pattern and let the symbol $\langle s,t\rangle$ indicate a pair of vertical or horizontal neighbours in S^P. Further let S^B be the set of micro edges defined in Section 1.1. The micro edge between adjacent pixels s and t will also be denoted by $\langle s,t\rangle$ and $S^B = \{\langle s,t\rangle : s,t \in S^P \text{ adjacent}\}$ is the set of edge sites. The edge variables $b_{\langle s,t\rangle}$ will take the values 1 if there is an edge element at $\langle s,t\rangle$ and 0 if there is none. The array $b = (b_{\langle s,t\rangle})_{\langle s,t\rangle\in S^B}$ is a pattern of edge elements. The prior energy function will be composed of two terms:

$$H(x,b) = H_1(x,b) + H_2(b).$$

The first term is responsible for piecewise smoothing and the second one for boundary organization.

For the beginning, let us set

$$H_1(x,b) = \vartheta \sum_{\langle s,t\rangle} \Psi(|x_s - x_t|)(1 - b_{\langle s,t\rangle})$$

with $\vartheta > 0$ and

$$\Psi(0) = -1 \quad \text{and} \quad \Psi(\Delta) = 1 \quad \text{otherwise.}$$

The terms in the sum take values -1, 0 or 1 according to table 2.1:

Table 2.1

edge	contrast no	contrast yes
on	0	0
off	-1	1

If there is high contrast across a micro edge then it is more likely caused by a real edge than by noise (at least if the signal to noise ratio is not too low). Hence the combination 'high contrast' – 'no edge' is unfavourable and its contribution to the energy function is high. Note that Ψ does not play any role if $b_{\langle s,t\rangle} = 1$, i.e. seeding of edges is encouraged where there is contrast.

This disparity functions treats the image like a black-and-white picture and hence is appropriate for small dynamic range – say up to 15 grey values – only. The authors suggest smoothing functions like in Fig. 2.4, for example

$$\Psi(\Delta) = 1 - \frac{2}{1 + (\Delta/\delta)^2} \tag{2.9}$$

for larger dynamic range with a scaling constant $\delta > 0$, $\Psi(\delta) = 0$.

The term $H_2(b) = -\alpha W(b)$, $\alpha > 0$, serves as an organization term for the edges. The function W counts selected local edge configurations weighted with a large factor if desired and with a small one if not. Boundaries should not be set inside smooth surfaces and therefore local configurations of the type

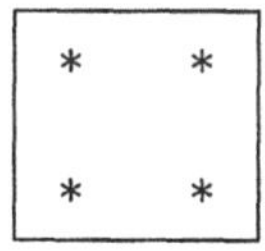

get large weights w_0. Smooth boundaries around smooth patches are welcome and configurations

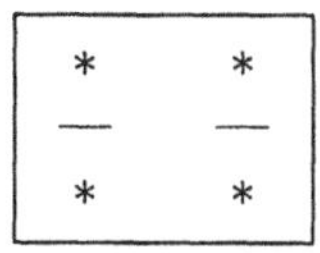

are weighted by $w_1 < w_0$; sharp turns and T-junctions

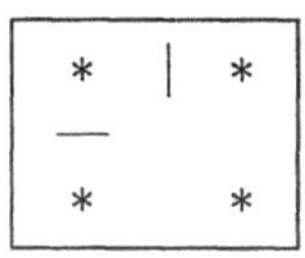 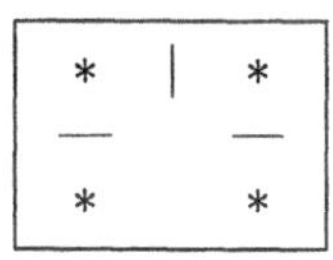

get weights $w_3 \leq w_2 \leq w_1$ and blind endings and crossings

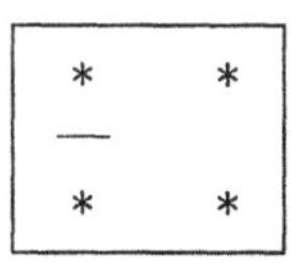 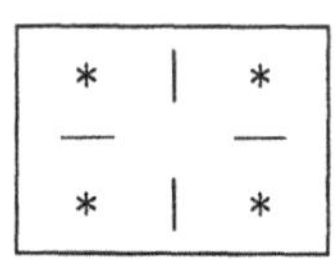

are penalized by weights $w_4 < w_3$. Here organization is reduced to weighting down undesired local configurations. One may add an 'index of connectedness' and further organization terms but this will increase the computational burden. We shall illustrate this aspect once more in the next example.

The prior energy function $H = H_1 + H_2$ is specified now. Given a model for degradation and an observation y of degraded grey values the posterior can be computed (Example 2.1.2) and maximization yields a MAP estimate. Let us finally mention that the MAP estimate depends on the parameters and finding them by trial and error in concrete examples may be cumbersome.

A. Blake and A. Zisserman tackle the problem of restoration from a deterministic point of view (cf. their monograph from 1987). They discuss the analogy of smoothing and fitting an elastic plate to the data such that its elastic energy becomes minimal. To preserve real edges the plate is allowed to break but each break is penalized. By physical reasoning they arrive at an energy function of the form

$$H(x,b) = \lambda^2 \sum_{\langle s,t\rangle} (x_s - x_t)^2 \left(1 - b_{\langle s,t\rangle}\right) + \alpha \sum_{\langle s,t\rangle} b_{\langle s,t\rangle} + \sum_s (x_s - y_s)^2$$

where α is a penalty levied for each break and λ is a measure of elasticity. Obviously, this is a special case of the previous model: the first two terms correspond to $\Psi(\Delta) = \Delta^2 - \alpha$ and the third one to degradation by white noise. Note that there is a term proportional to the total contour length which favours smooth boundaries. For *special energy functions* an exact minimization algorithm called the *g*raduated *n*on-*c*onvexity (GNC) algorithm exists. It does not apply to the more general versions developed above and no blur or nonlinear system function can be incorporated. We shall comment on the GNC algorithm in Chapter 6.

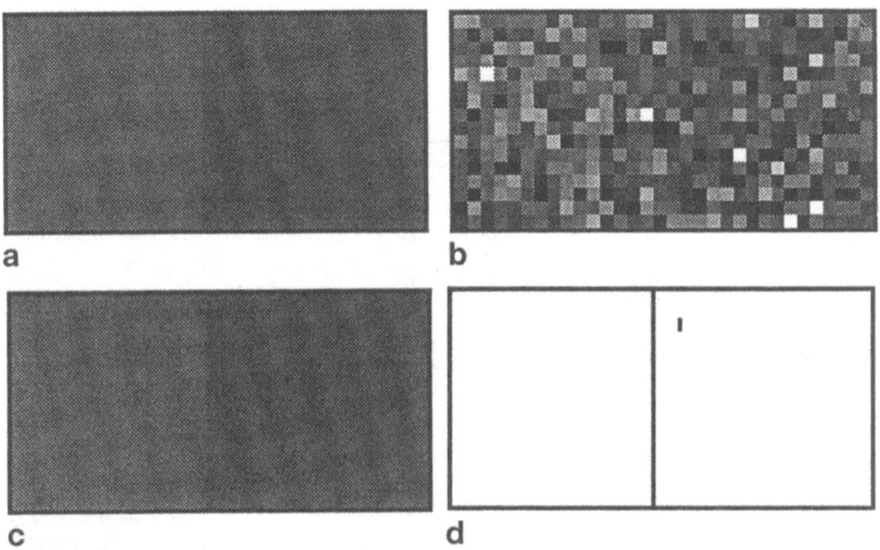

Fig. 2.6. Piecewise smoothing ($\vartheta = 10$, $\delta = 0.75$, $n = 3000$). (**a**) Original, (**b**) degraded image, (**c**) MAP of grey values, (**d**) MAP of edges

Figs. 2.6–2.9 show some results of a series of simple experiments carried out by Y. EDEL in the exercises to my lectures at Heidelberg. Perhaps you may wish to repeat them (after we learn a bit more about algorithms) and therefore reasonable parameters will be listed. For 16 grey values and the disparity function Ψ from (2.9), the following parameters are reasonable: $\vartheta = \alpha$ and $w_0 = 1.3, w_1 = 0.4, w_2 = w_3 = -0.5$ and $w_4 = -1.4$. The other parameters are noted in the captures. The MAP estimates were approximated by simulated annealing (cf. Chapter 5), for completeness we note the number n of sweeps in the caption. All original configurations (displayed respectively in Figs. 2.6(a)–2.9(a)) were degraded by additive white noise of variance $\sigma^2 = 9$ (Figs. (b). For instance the grey values in Fig. 2.6 were perfectly restored after 3000 sweeps of annealing (Fig. 2.6(c)), the edges are nearly perfect, up to a small artefact in the right half (Fig. 2.6(d)). Fig. 2.7 is similar; annealing three times for 5000 sweeps gave two times the perfect reconstructions (c) and

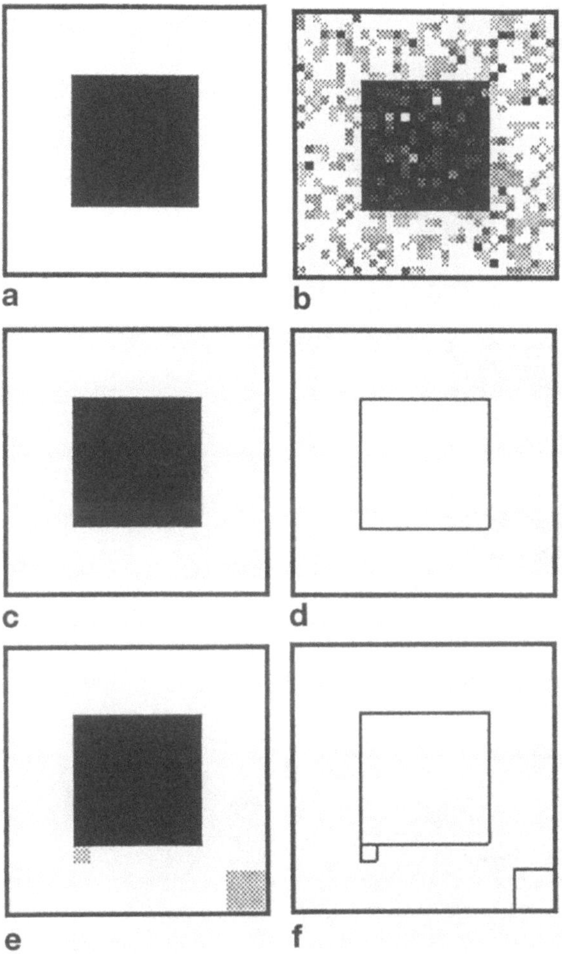

Fig. 2.7. Piecewise smoothing ($\vartheta = 10$, $\delta = 0.1$, $n = 5000$). (**a**) Original, (**b**) degraded image, (**c**), (**d**), (**e**), (**f**) approximate MAP estimates of grey-values and edges

(d) and once (e) and (f) (simulated annealing is a stochastic algorithm and therefore the outcomes may vary). Fig. 2.8 illustrates the dependence on the scaling parameter δ. Finally, Fig. 2.9 shows an undesired effect. The energy function is not isotropic and, for example, treats horizontal and diagonal 'straight' lines in a different way. Since discrete diagonals resemble a staircase they are destroyed by w_3.

This first serious example illustrates a crucial aspect of contextual models. Smoothing, boundary finding and organization are simultaneous and cooperative processes. This distinguishes contextual models as compared to classical ones.

There is a general principle behind the above method. A homogeneous local operation is switched off where there is evidence that it does not make sense. Simultaneously, the set where the operation is switched off is organized

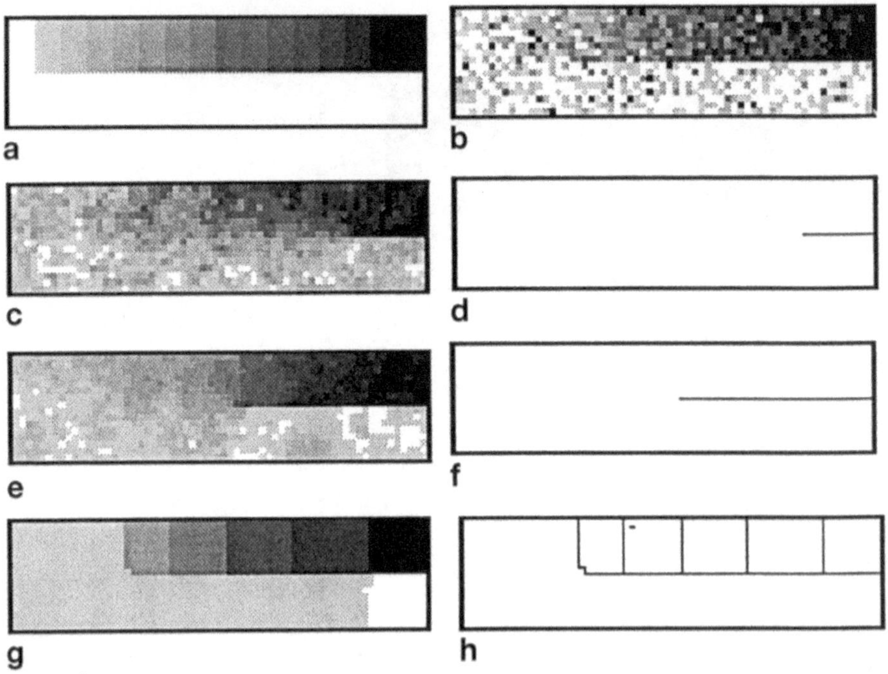

Fig. 2.8. Sensitivity of MAP reconstruction to cup-width ($\vartheta = 8$, $n = 5000$). (**c**), (**d**) $\delta = 5$, (**e**), (**f**) $\delta = 2,5$, (**g**), (**h**) $\delta = 1$

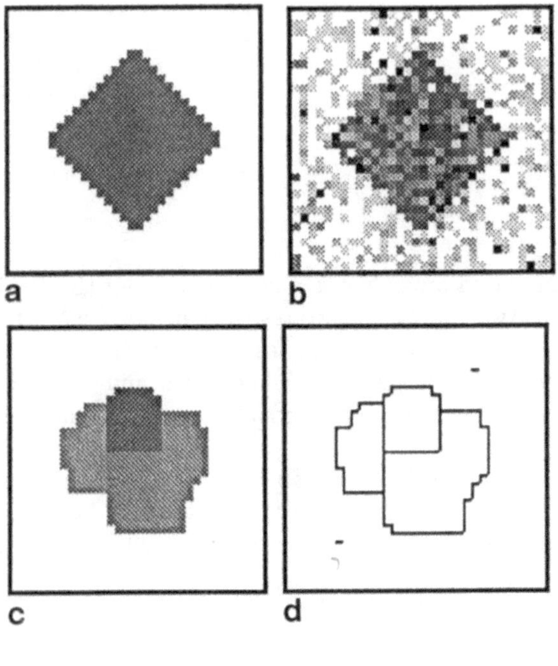

Fig. 2.9. Penalized diagonals. (**a**) Original, (**b**) degraded, (**c**), (**d**) MAPE

according to regularity requirements. We shall meet this principle in various other models for example in texture segmentation (part IV) and estimation of motion (Chapter 16).

2.4 Boundary Extraction

Besides restoration, edge detection or boundary finding is a typical task of image analysis. Edges correspond to sudden changes of an image attribute such as luminance or texture and indicate discontinuities in the actual scene. They are important primitive features; for instance they provide an indication of the extent of objects and hence together with other features may be helpful for higher level processing. We focus now on intensity discontinuities (finding boundaries between regions of different texture will be addressed later). The example is presented here since it is very similar to Example 2.3.1.

Again, there is a variety of filtering techniques for edge detection. Most are based on discrete derivatives, frequently combined with smoothing at small scale to reduce the noise contribution. There are also many ways to do some cosmetics on the extracted raw boundaries, for example erasing loose ends or filling small gaps. More refined methods like fitting step shaped templates locally to the data have been developed but that is beyond the scope of this text (cf. the concise introduction NIEMANN (1990) and also the above mentioned approach by BLAKE and ZISSERMAN (1987)).

While the edge process in Example 2.3.1 mainly serves as an auxiliary tool, it is considered in its own right now. The following example is reported in D. GEMAN (1987) and S. GEMAN, D. GEMAN and CHR. GRAFFIGNE (1987).

Example 2.4.1. The configurations are $(x, b) = (x^P, x^B)$ where S^P is a finite square-lattice of pixels. The possible locations $s \in S^B$ of boundary elements are shown in a sketch:

∘	|	∘	|	∘	|
—	∗	—	∗	—	∗
∘	|	∘	|	∘	|
—	∗	—	∗	—	∗
∘	|	∘	|	∘	|
—	∗	—	∗	—	∗

∘ pixel

— microedge

∗ position of a boundary element

Given perfectly observed grey values x_s and the prior energy function H, the posterior distribution has the form

$$\mathsf{P}(b|x) = Z_x^{-1} \exp(-H(x, b)).$$

H is the sum of two terms:

$$H(x,b) = H_1(x,b) + H_2(b)$$

where H_1 is responsible for seeding boundaries and H_2 for the organization. Seeding is based on contrast and continuation:

$$H_1(x,b) = \vartheta_1 \sum_{\langle s,t \rangle} \Psi(\Delta_{s,t})(1 - b_s b_t) + \vartheta_2 \sum_{s \in S^B} (b_s - \zeta_s(x))^2$$

with positive parameters ϑ_i. In the first term summation extends over pairs of adjacent boundary positions:

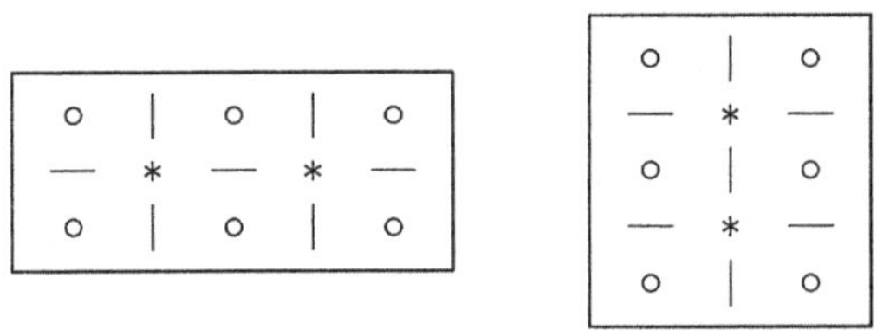

Between two adjacent boundary positions s and t there is a micro edge $\langle s,t \rangle$ separating two pixels. $\Delta_{st}(x)$ is the contrast across this micro edge, i.e. the distance of grey values. Ψ is an increasing function of contrast, for example

$$\Psi(\Delta) = \frac{\Delta^4}{c + \Delta^2}.$$

The second term depends on an index $\zeta(x)$ of connectedness. It is defined as follows: Given thresholds $c_1 < c_2$ a micro edge is called active if either (i) the contrast across the micro edge exceeds c_2 or (ii) the contrast exceeds c_1 and the contrast across one of the neighbouring micro edges exceeds c_1. The index $\zeta_s(x)$ equals 1 if s is inside a string of say four active micro edges and 0 otherwise.

The second term depends on b only and organizes the boundary:

$$H_2(b) = \vartheta_3 \sum_{C \in \mathbf{C}_1} \prod_{s \in C} b_s - \vartheta_4 W(b).$$

The parameters ϑ_3 and ϑ_4 are again positive. The first term penalizes double boundaries counting the local boundary configurations depicted below (and their rotations by 90 degrees):

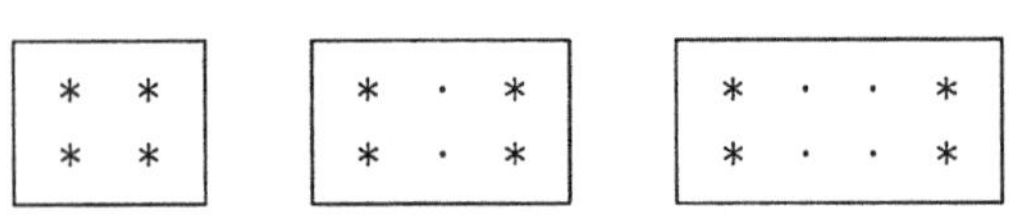

('*' means that there is a boundary element and '·' that there is none). The members C of $\mathbf{C}_1$ are the corresponding sets of boundary sites. Like in Example 2.3.1, the second term penalizes a number of local configurations.

The processes of seeding and organization are entirely cooperative. Low contrast segments may survive if sufficiently well organized and, conversely,

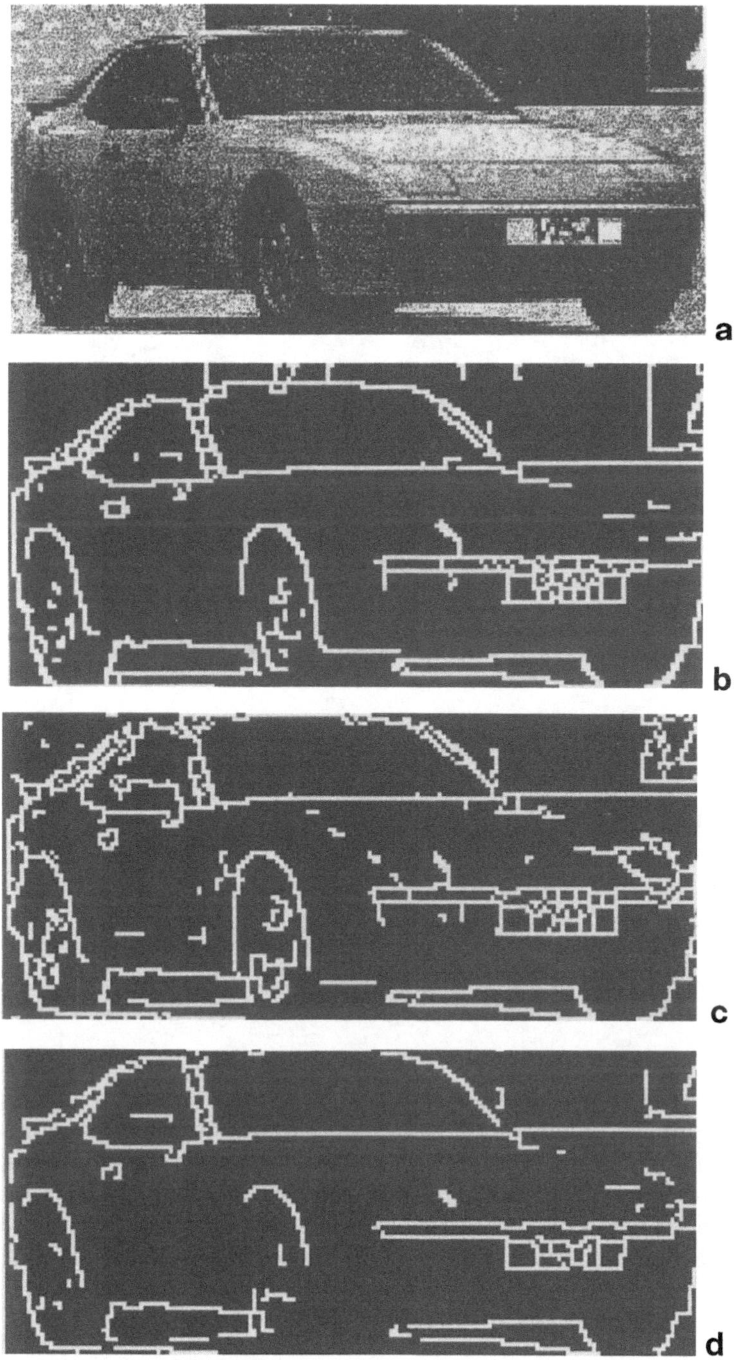

Fig. 2.10. Parameter dependence

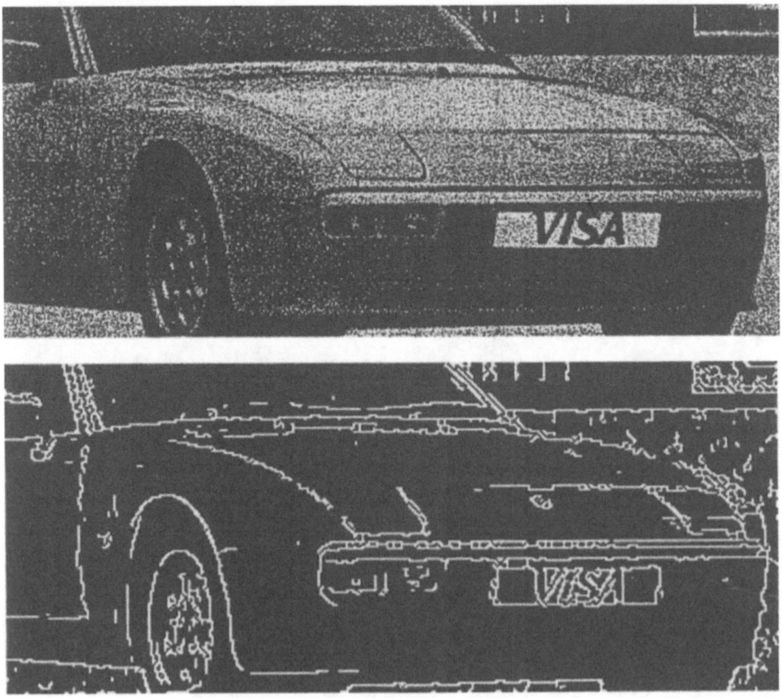

a

b

a

b **Fig. 2.12.** Weak seeding

unstructured boundary segments are removed by the organization terms. Fig. 2.10 shows approximate minima of H for several combinations of the parameters ϑ_1 and ϑ_2 (the term H_2 is switched off). This shows that the results may depend sensitively on the parameters and that a careful choice is crucial for the performance of the algorithms (more on that later). Fig. 2.11 is similar with higher resolution. In Fig. 2.12 the seeding is too weak which results in a small catastrophy. O. Wendlandt, München, wrote the programs and produced the illustrations 2.10–2.12.

3. Random Fields

This chapter will be theoretical and – besides the examples – possibly a bit dry. No doubt, some basic ideas can be imparted without this material. But a deeper understanding, in particular of topics like texture, parameter estimation or parallel algorithms, requires some abstract background and therefore one has to learn random fields. In this chapter, we present some basic notions and elementary results.

3.1 Markov Random Fields

Discrete images were represented by elements of finite product spaces and special probability distributions on the set of such images were discussed. An appropriate abstract setting will now be introduced.

Let S be a finite index set – the set of **sites**; for every site $s \in S$ let $\mathbf{X}_s$ be a finite **space of states** x_s. The product $\mathbf{X} = \prod_{s \in S} \mathbf{X}_s$ is the space of (finite) **configurations** $x = (x_s)_{s \in S}$. We consider **probability measures** or **distributions** Π on $\mathbf{X}$, i.e. vectors $\Pi = (\Pi(x))_{x \in \mathbf{X}}$ such that $\Pi(x) \geq 0$ and $\sum_{x \in \mathbf{X}} \Pi(x) = 1$. Subsets $E \subset \mathbf{X}$ are called **events**; the probability of an event E is given by $\Pi(E) = \sum_{x \in E} \Pi(x)$. A strictly positive probability measure Π on $\mathbf{X}$, i.e. $\Pi(x) > 0$ for every $x \in \mathbf{X}$, is called a **stochastic** or **random field**.

For $A \subset S$ let $\mathbf{X}_A = \prod_{s \in A} \mathbf{X}_s$ denote the space of configurations $x_A = (x_s)_{s \in A}$ on A; the map

$$X_A : \mathbf{X} \longrightarrow \mathbf{X}_A \, , \; x = (x_s)_{s \in S} \longmapsto (x_s)_{s \in A}$$

is the projection of $\mathbf{X}$ onto $\mathbf{X}_A$. We shall use the short-hand notation X_s for $X_{\{s\}}$ and $\{X_A = x_A\}$ for $\{x \in \mathbf{X} : X_A(x) = x_A\}$. Commonly one writes $\{X_A = x_A \, , \; X_B = x_B\}$ for intersections $\{X_A = x_A\} \cap \{X_B = x_B\}$. For a random field Π the random vector $X = (X_s)_{s \in S}$ on the probability space $(\mathbf{X}, \Pi)$ is also frequently called a random field.

For events E and F the **conditional probability** of F given E is defined by $\Pi(F|E) = \Pi(F \cap E)/\Pi(E)$. Conditional probabilities of the form

$$\Pi\left(X_A = x_A \left| X_{S \setminus A} = x_{S \setminus A}\right.\right) \, , \; A \subset S \, , \; x_A \in \mathbf{X}_A \, , \; x_{S \setminus A} \in \mathbf{X}_{S \setminus A} \, ,$$

are called **local characteristics**. They are always defined since random fields are assumed to be strictly positive. They express the probability that the configuration is x_A on A and $x_{S\setminus A}$ on the rest of the world. Later on, we shall use the short-hand notation $\Pi\left(x_A \,|x_{S\setminus A}\right)$.

We compute now local characteristics for a simple random field.

Example 3.1.1. Let $\mathbf{X}_s = \{-1,1\}$ for all $s \in S$. Then

$$\Pi(x) = \frac{1}{Z}\exp\left(\sum_{\langle s,t\rangle} x_s x_t\right),$$

where Z is the normalization constant. The index set S is a finite square lattice and $\langle s,t\rangle$ means that t is the site next to s on the right or left or the next upper or lower site (or more generally, S is a finite undirected graph with bonds $\langle s,t\rangle$). Then

$$\Pi\left(X_t = x_t \mid X_r = x_r,\ r \neq t\right) = \frac{\Pi\left(X_s = x_s \quad \text{for all} \quad s\right)}{\Pi\left(X_s = x_s \quad \text{for all} \quad s \neq t\right)}$$

$$= \frac{\exp\left(\sum_{\langle s,t\rangle} x_s x_t\right)\exp\left(\sum_{\langle r,s\rangle, r\neq t, s\neq t} x_r x_s\right)}{\sum_{x_t'\in\mathbf{X}_t}\exp\left(\sum_{\langle s,t\rangle} x_t' x_s\right)\exp\left(\sum_{\langle r,s\rangle, r\neq t, s\neq t} x_r x_s\right)}$$

$$= \frac{\exp\left(x_t \sum_{\langle s,t\rangle} x_s\right)}{\sum_{x_t'\in\mathbf{X}_t}\exp\left(x_t' \sum_{\langle s,t\rangle} x_s\right)}.$$

Hence the conditional probabilities have a particularly simple form; for example,

$$\Pi\left(X_t = -1 \mid X_r = x_r,\ r \neq t\right) = \frac{1}{1+\exp\left(2\sum_{\langle t,r\rangle} x_r\right)}.$$

This shows: The probability for the state x_t in t given the configuration on the rest of S depends on the states on the (four) neighbours of t only. It is not affected by a change of colours in sites which are no neighbours of t .

The local characteristics of the other distributions in the last chapter also depend only on a small number of neighbouring sites. If so, conditional distributions can be computed in reasonable time whereas the computing time would not be feasible for dependence say on all states if the underlaying space is large. Later on, we shall develop algorithms for the approximate computation of MAP estimates. They will depend on the iterative computation of local characteristics and there local dependence will be crucial. We shall discuss local dependence in more detail now.

Those sites which possibly influence the local characteristic at a site s will be called the neighbours of s. The relation 's and t are neighbours' should fulfill some axioms.

Definition 3.1.1. *A collection $\partial = \{\partial(s) : s \in S\}$ of subsets of S is called a* **neighbourhood system**, *if (i) $s \notin \partial(s)$ and (ii) $s \in \partial(t)$ if and only if $t \in \partial(s)$. The sites $s \in \partial(t)$ are called* **neighbours** *of t. A subset C of S is called a* **clique** *if two different elements of C are always neighbours. The set of cliques will be denoted by $\mathbf{C}$. We shall frequently write $\langle s,t\rangle$ if s and t are neighbours of each other.*

Remark 3.1.1. The neighbourhood relation induces an undirected graph with vertices $s \in S$ and a bond between s and t if and only if s and t are neighbours. Conversely, an undirected graph induces a neighbourhood system. The 'complete' sets in the graph correspond to the cliques.

Example 3.1.2. (a) A degenerate neighbourhood system is given by $\partial(s) = \emptyset$ for all $s \in S$. There are no nonempty cliques and the sites act independently of each other.

(b) The other extreme is $\partial(s) = S\backslash\{s\}$ for all $s \in S$. All subsets of S are cliques and all sites influence each other.

(c) Some of the neighbourhood systems used in the last chapter are of the following type: The index set is a finite lattice

$$S = \{(i,j) \in \mathsf{Z} \times \mathsf{Z} : -m \leq i,j \leq m\}$$

and

$$\partial\left((i,j)\right) = \left\{(k,l) : 0 < (k-i)^2 + (l-j)^2 \leq C\right\}.$$

Up to modifications near the boundary, a site $*$ has for $C = 1$ the upper, lower, left and right site as neighbours; in this case the cliques are

$$\boxed{\emptyset\,, \quad *\,, \quad *\!-\!* \quad \text{and} \quad \begin{array}{c} * \\ | \\ * \end{array}}\,.$$

For $C = 2$ and sites (i,j), $i,j \notin \{-m,m\}$, the neighbours $\circ$ of $*$ are:

$$\boxed{\begin{array}{ccc} \circ & \circ & \circ \\ \circ & * & \circ \\ \circ & \circ & \circ \end{array}}\,.$$

The corresponding cliques are:

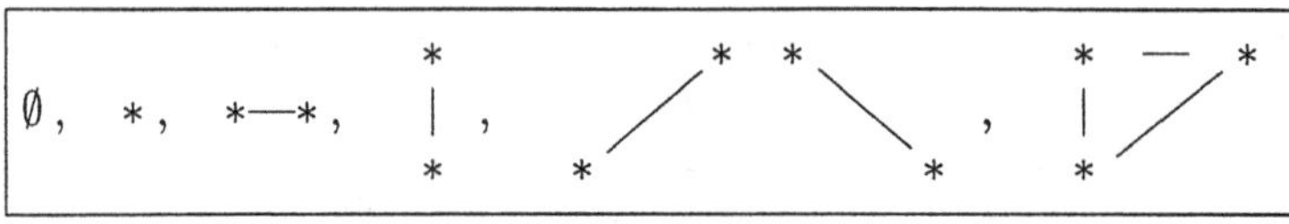 and rotations,

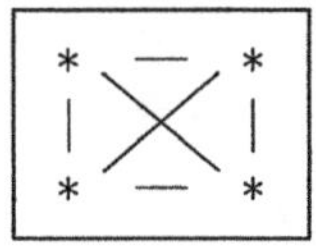 .

For sites near the boundary the cliques are smaller which may cause some trouble in programming the algorithms.

(d) If there is a pixel and an edge process there may be interaction between pixels, between edges and between pixels and edges. If S^P is a lattice of pixels and S^E the set of microedges then the index set for $\left(x^P, x^E\right)$ is $S = S^P \cup S^E$. There may be a neighbourhood system on S^P as in (c) and microedges can be neighbours of pixels and vice versa. For example, pixel $*$ can have neighbouring edges | or — like 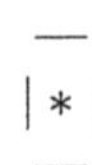 .

Now we can formalize local dependence as indicated in Example 3.1.1.

Definition 3.1.2. *The random field Π is a* **Markov field** *w.r.t. the neighbourhood system ∂ if for all $x \in \mathbf{X}$,*

$$\Pi\left(X_s = x_s \,|X_r = x_r\,,\ r \neq s\right) = \Pi\left(X_s = x_s \,|X_r = x_r\,,\ r \in \partial(s)\right).$$

This definition takes only single site local characteristics into account. The others inherit this property by 3.3.2(b).

Remark 3.1.2. For finite product spaces $\mathbf{X}$ the above conditions are in principle no restriction since *every* random field is a Markov field for the neighbourhood system 3.1.2 where all different sites are neighbours. But we are looking for random fields which are Markov for small neighbourhoods. For instance, the Markov property for the neighbourhood system $\partial(s) = \emptyset$ boiles down to

$$\Pi\left(X_s = x_s \,|X_r = x_r\,,\ r \neq s\right) = \Pi\left(X_s = x_s\right).$$

Since for events $E_1, \ldots, E_k$ with nonempty intersection,

$$\Pi\left(E_1 \cap \ldots \cap E_k\right) = \Pi\left(E_1\right) \cdot \Pi\left(E_2 \,|E_1\right) \cdot \ldots \cdot \Pi\left(E_k \,|E_1 \cap \ldots \cap E_{k-1}\right)$$

this implies that the random variables X_s are independent. Large neighbourhoods correspond to long-range dependence.

3.2 Gibbs Fields and Potentials

Now we turn to the representation of random fields in the Gibbsian form (1.1). It is particularly useful for the calculation of (conditional) probabilities. The idea and hence most of the terminology is borrowed from statistical mechanics where Gibbs fields are used as models for the equilibrium states of large physical systems (cf. Example 3.2.1).

Probability measures of the form

$$\Pi(x) = \frac{\exp(-H(x))}{\sum_{z \in \mathbf{X}} \exp(-H(z))}$$

are always strictly positive and hence random fields. Π is called the **Gibbs field** (or **measure**) induced by the **energy function** H and the numerator is called the **partition function**. *Every* random field Π can be written in this form. In fact, setting $H(x) = -\ln \Pi(x) - \ln Z$, one gets $\exp(-H(x)) = \Pi(x)Z$ and Z necessarily is the partition function of H. Moreover, the energy function for Π is unique up to an additive constant; if H and H' are energy functions for Π then

$$H(x) - H'(x) = \ln Z' - \ln Z$$

for every $x \in \mathbf{X}$. It is common to enforce uniqueness choosing some reference or 'vacuum' configuration $o \in \mathbf{X}$ and requiring $Z = \Pi(o)^{-1}$, or, equivalently, $H(o) = 0$.

Hence we restrict attention to Gibbs fields. It is convenient to decompose the energy into the contributions of the configurations on subsets of S. Let $\emptyset$ denote the empty set.

Definition 3.2.1. *A* **potential** *is a family* $\{U_A : A \subset S\}$ *of functions on* $\mathbf{X}$ *such that*

(i) $U_\emptyset = 0$,
(ii) $U_A(x) = U_A(y)$ *if* $X_A(x) = X_A(y)$.

The **energy** *of the potential* U *is given by*

$$H_U = \sum_{A \subset S} U_A.$$

Given a neighbourhood system ∂ *a potential* U *is called a* **neighbour potential** *w.r.t.* ∂ *if* $U_A = 0$ *whenever* A *is not a clique. If* $U_A = 0$ *for* $|A| > 2$ *then* U *is a* **pair potential**.

Potentials define energy functions and thus random fields.

Definition 3.2.2. *A random field* Π *is a* **Gibbs field** *or* **Gibbs measure for the potential** U, *if it is of the form (3.2) and* H *is the energy* H_U *of a potential* U. *If* U *is a neighbour potential then* Π *is called a* **neighbour Gibbs field**.

We give some examples.

Example 3.2.1. (a) The **Ising model** is particularly simple. But it shows phenomena which are also typical for more complex models. Hence it is frequently the starting point for the study of deep questions about Markov fields. It will be used as an example throughout this text.

S is a finite square lattice and the neighbours of $s \in S$ are the sites with Euclidean distance one (which is the case $C = 1$ in Example 3.1.2(c)). The possible states are -1 and 1 for every site. In the simplest case the energy function is given by

$$H(x) = -\beta \sum_{\langle s,t \rangle} x_s x_t$$

where $\langle s,t \rangle$ indicates that s and t are neighbours. Hence H is the energy function of a neighbour potential (in fact, of a pair potential). The configurations of minimal energy are the constant configurations with states -1 and 1, respectively.

Physicists study a slightly more general model: index set, neighbourhood system and state space are the same but the energy function is given by

$$H(x) = -\frac{1}{kT}\left[J \sum_{\langle s,t \rangle} x_s x_t - mB \sum_s x_s \right].$$

The German physicist E. ISING (1925; the *I* pronounced like in *ea*gle and not like in *i*ce) tried to explain theoretically certain empirical facts about ferromagnets by means of this model; it was proposed by Ising's doctoral supervisor W. LENZ in 1920. The lattice is thought of as a crystal lattice, $x_s = \pm 1$ means, that there is a small dipole or spin at the lattice point s which is directed either upwards or downwards. Ising considered only one-dimensional (but infinite) lattices and argued by analogy for higher dimension (unfortunately these conclusions were wrong).

The first term represents the interaction energy of the spins. Only neighbouring spins interact and hence the model is not suited for long-range interactions. J is a matter constant. If $J > 0$ then spins with the same direction contribute low energy and hence high probability. Thus the spins tend to have the same direction and we have a *ferromagnet*. For $J < 0$ one has an *antiferromagnet*. The constant $T > 0$ represents absolute temperature and k is the 'Boltzmann factor'. At low temperature (or for large J) there is strong interaction and there are collective phenomena; at high temperature there is weak coupling and the spins act almost independently. The second sum represents a constant external field with intensity B. The constant $m > 0$ depends again on the material. This term becomes minimal if all spins are parallel to the external field. Besides in physics, similar models were also adopted in various fields like biology, economics or sociology. We used it for smoothing.

The increasing strength of coupling with increasing parameter β can be illustrated by sampling from the Ising field at various values of β. The samples in Fig. 3.1 were taken (from left to right) for values $\beta = 0.1, 0.45, 0.47$ and 4.0 on a 56×56 lattice; there is no external field. They range from almost random to 'nearly constant'.

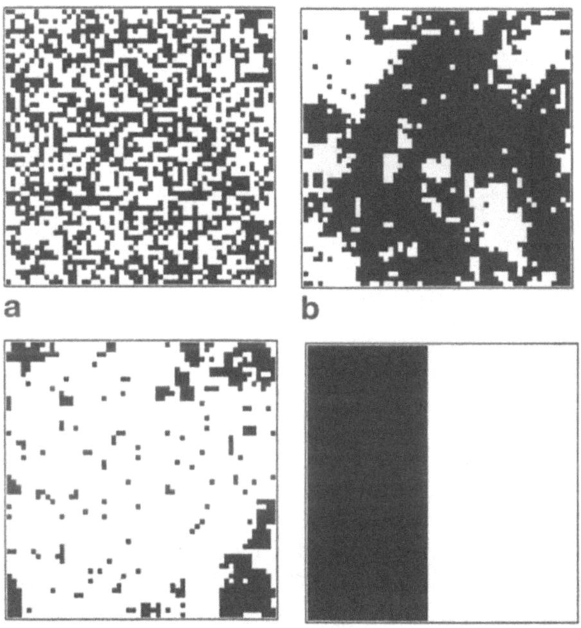

a b c d

Fig. 3.1. Typical configurations of an Ising field at various temperatures

The natural generalization to more than two states is

$$H(x) = -\beta \sum_{\langle s,t \rangle} 1_{\{x_s = x_t\}}.$$

It is called the **Potts model**.

(b) More generally, each term in the sum may be weighted individually, i.e.

$$H(x) = \sum_{\langle s,t \rangle} a_{st} x_s x_t + \sum_s a_s x_s$$

where $x_s = \pm 1$. If $a_{st} = 1$ then $x_s = x_t$ is favourable and, conversely, $a_{st} = -1$ encourages $x_s = -x_t$. For the following pictures, we set all a_s to 0 and almost all a_{st} to $+1$ like in the Ising model but some to -1 (the reader may guess which !). The samples from the associated Gibbs field were taken at the same parameter values as in Fig. 3.1. With increasing β the samples contain larger and larger portions of the image in Fig. 2.3(a) or of its inverse much like the

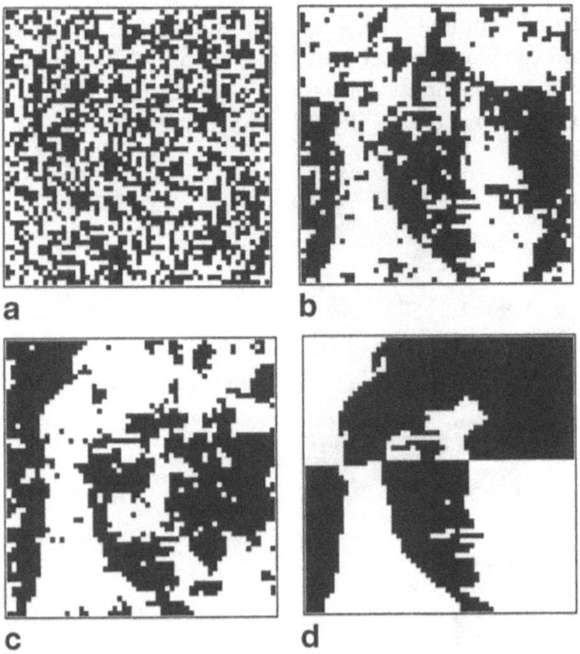

Fig. 3.2. a,b,c,d

samples in 3.1 contain larger and larger patches of black and white. Fig. 3.2 may look nicer than 3.1 but it does not tell us more about Gibbs fields.

(c) Nearest neighbour binary models are lattice models with the same neighbourhood structure as before but with values in $\{0,1\}$:

$$H(x) = \sum_{\langle s,t\rangle} b_{st}x_sx_t + \sum_s b_sx_s,\ x_s \in \{0,1\}\,.$$

In the 'autologistic model', $b_{st} = b_h$ for horizontal and $b_{st} = b_v$ for vertical bonds; sometimes the general form is also called autologistic. In the isotropic case $b_{st} = a$ and $b_s = b$; it looks like an Ising model and in fact, the models in (b) and the nearest neighbour binary models are equivalent by the transformation $\{0,1\} \longrightarrow \{-1,1\}$, $x_s \longmapsto 2x_s - 1$.

Plainly, models of the form (b) or (c) can be defined on any finite undirected graph with a set S of nodes and $\langle s,t\rangle$ if and only if there is a bond between s and t in the graph. Such models play a particularly important role in neural networks (cf. KAMP and HASLER (1990)). In imaging, these and related models are used for description, synthesis and classification of binary textures (cf. Chapter 15). Generalizations (cf. the Potts model) apply to textures with more than two colours.

(d) Spin glass models do not fit into this framework but they are natural generalizations. The coefficients a_{st} and a_s are themselves random variables. In the physical context they model the 'random environment' in which the particles with states x_s live. Spin glasses become more and more popular in the Neural Network community, cf. the work of VAN HEMMEN and others.

If a Markov field is given by a potential then the local characteristics may easily be calculated. For us this is the main reason to introduce potentials.

Proposition 3.2.1. *Let the random field Π be given by some neighbour potential U for the neighbourhood system ∂, i.e.*

$$\Pi(x) = \frac{\exp\left(-\sum_{C\in\mathbf{C}} U_C(x)\right)}{\sum_y \exp\left(-\sum_{C\in\mathbf{C}} U_C(y)\right)}$$

where $\mathbf{C}$ denotes the set of cliques of ∂. Then the local characteristics are given by

$$\Pi\left(X_s = x_s,\ s \in A \,|\, X_s = x_s,\ s \in S\backslash A\right) = \\ = \frac{\exp\left(-\sum_{C\in\mathbf{C},\, C\cap A\neq\emptyset} U_C(x)\right)}{\sum_{y_A\in\mathbf{X}_A} \exp\left(-\sum_{C\in\mathbf{C},\, C\cap A\neq\emptyset} U_C\left(y_A x_{S\backslash A}\right)\right)}.$$

(For a general potential, replace $\mathbf{C}$ on the right-hand side by the power set of S.) Moreover,

$$\Pi\left(X_s = x_s,\ s \in A \,|\, X_s = x_s,\ s \in S\backslash A\right) = \\ = \Pi\left(X_s = x_s,\ s \in A \,|\, X_s = x_s,\ s \in \partial(A)\right)$$

for every subset A of S. In particular, Π is a Markov field w.r.t. ∂.

Proof. By assumption,

$$\begin{aligned} \Pi\left(X_A = x_A \,|\, X_{S\backslash A} = x_{S\backslash A}\right) &= \frac{\Pi\left(X = x_A x_{S\backslash A}\right)}{\Pi\left(X_{S\backslash A} = x_{S\backslash A}\right)} \\ &= \frac{\exp\left(-\sum_{C\in\mathbf{C}} U_C\left(x_A x_{S\backslash A}\right)\right)}{\sum_{y_A\in\mathbf{X}_A} \exp\left(-\sum_{C\in\mathbf{C}} U_C\left(y_A x_{S\backslash A}\right)\right)}. \end{aligned}$$

Divide now the set of cliques into two classes:

$$\mathbf{C} = \mathbf{C}_1 \cup \mathbf{C}_2 = \{C \in \mathbf{C} : C \cap A \neq \emptyset\} \cup \{C \in \mathbf{C} : C \cap A = \emptyset\}.$$

Letting $R = S\backslash(A \cup \partial A)$ where $\partial A = \cup_{s \in A}\partial(s)\backslash A$ and introducing a reference element $o \in \mathbf{X}$,

$$U_C\left(z_A z_{\partial A} z_R\right) = U_C\left(o_A z_{\partial A} z_R\right) \quad \text{if} \quad C \in \boldsymbol{C}_2,$$

and similarly,

$$U_C\left(z_A z_{\partial A} z_R\right) = U_C\left(z_A z_{\partial A} o_R\right) \quad \text{if} \quad C \in \boldsymbol{C}_1.$$

Rewrite the sum as

$$\sum_{C \in \mathcal{C}} \cdots = \sum_{C \in \boldsymbol{C}_1} \cdots + \sum_{C \in \boldsymbol{C}_2} \cdots,$$

and use the multiplicativity of exponentials to check that in the above fraction the terms for cliques in $\boldsymbol{C}_2$ cancel out. Let $x_{\partial A}$ denote the restriction of $x_{S\backslash A}$ to ∂A. Then

$$\Pi\left(X_A = x_A \left| X_{S\backslash A} = x_{S\backslash A}\right.\right) = \frac{\exp\left(-\sum_{C \in \boldsymbol{C}_1} U_C\left(x_A x_{\partial A} o_R\right)\right)}{\sum_{y_A \in \mathbf{X}_A} \exp\left(-\sum_{C \in \boldsymbol{C}_1} U_C\left(y_A x_{\partial A} o_R\right)\right)}$$

which is the desired form since U_C does not depend on the configurations on R.

The last expression equals

$$\begin{aligned}
&= \frac{\exp\left(-\sum_{C \in \boldsymbol{C}_1} U_C\left(x_A x_{\partial A} o_R\right)\right) \cdot \sum_{y_R} \exp\left(-\sum_{C \in \boldsymbol{C}_2} U_C\left(o_A x_{\partial A} y_R\right)\right)}{\sum_{y_A} \exp\left(-\sum_{C \in \boldsymbol{C}_1} U_C\left(y_A x_{\partial A} o_R\right)\right) \cdot \sum_{y_R} \exp\left(-\sum_{C \in \boldsymbol{C}_2} U_C\left(o_A x_{\partial A} y_R\right)\right)} \\
&= \frac{\sum_{y_R} \exp\left(-\sum_{C \in \boldsymbol{C}_1} U_C\left(x_A x_{\partial A} y_R\right)\right) \cdot \exp\left(-\sum_{C \in \boldsymbol{C}_2} U_C\left(x_A x_{\partial A} y_R\right)\right)}{\sum_{y_A}\sum_{y_R} \exp\left(-\sum_{C \in \boldsymbol{C}_1} U_C\left(y_A x_{\partial A} y_R\right)\right) \cdot \exp\left(-\sum_{C \in \boldsymbol{C}_2} U_C\left(y_A x_{\partial A} y_R\right)\right)} \\
&= \Pi\left(X_A = x_A \left| X_{\partial A} = x_{\partial A}\right.\right).
\end{aligned}$$

Specializing to sets of the form $A = \{s\}$ shows that Π is a Markov field for ∂. This completes the proof. □

3.3 More on Potentials

The following results are not needed for the next chapters. They will be used in later chapters and may be skipped in a first reading. On the other hand, they are recommended as valuable exercises on random fields.

For technical reasons, we fix in each component $\mathbf{X}_t$ a reference element o_t and set $o = (o_t)_{t\in S}$. For a configuration x and a subset A of S we denote by ${}^Ax$ the configuration which coincides with x on A and with o off A.

Theorem 3.3.1. *Every random field Π is a Gibbs field for some potential. We may choose the potential V with $V_\emptyset = 0$ and which for $A \neq \emptyset$ is given by*

$$V_A(x) = -\sum_{B\subset A}(-1)^{|A-B|}\ln\left(\Pi({}^Bx)\right). \tag{3.1}$$

For all $A \subset S$ and every $a \in A$,

$$V_A(x) = -\sum_{B\subset A}(-1)^{|A-B|}\ln\left(\Pi\left(X_a = {}^Bx_a\,\middle|X_s = {}^Bx_s,\ s\neq a\right)\right). \tag{3.2}$$

For the potential V one has $V_A(x) = 0$ whenever $x_a = o_a$ for some $a \in A$.

Remark 3.3.1. If a potential V fulfills $V_A(x) = 0$ whenever $x_a = o_a$ for some $a \in A$ then it is called **normalized**. We shall prove that V from the theorem is the *only normalized* potential for Π (cf. Theorem 3.3.3 below). The proof below will show that the vacuum o has probability $\Pi(o) = \left(\sum_z \exp\left(-H_V(z)\right)\right)^{-1} = Z^{-1}$ which is equivalent to $H_V(o) = 0$. This explains why a normalized potential is also called a vacuum potential and the reference configuration o is called the vacuum (in physics, the 'real vacuum' is the natural choice for o). If Π is given in the Gibbsian form by any potential then it is related to the normalized potential by the formula in Theorem 3.3.3.

Example 3.3.1. Let $x_s \in \{0,1\}$, $V_{\{s\}}(x) = b_s x_s$, $V_{\{s,t\}}(x) = b_{st}x_s x_t$ and $V_A \equiv 0$ whenever $|A| \geq 3$. Then V is a normalized potential. Such potentials are of interest in texture modelling and neural networks.

For the proof of Theorem 3.3.1 we need the Moebius inversion formula, which is of independent interest.

Lemma 3.3.1. *Let S be a finite set and Φ and Ψ real-valued functions on the power set of S. Then*

$$\Phi(A) = \sum_{B\subset A}(-1)^{|A-B|}\Psi(B) \quad \textit{for every} \quad A\subset S$$

if and only if

$$\Psi(A) = \sum_{B\subset A}\Phi(B) \quad \textit{for every} \quad A\subset S.$$

Proof (of the lemma). For the above theorem we need that the first condition implies the second one. We rewrite the right-hand side of the second formula as

$$\begin{aligned}\sum_{B\subset A}\Phi(B) &= \sum_{B\subset A}\sum_{D\subset B}(-1)^{|B-D|}\Psi(D)\\ &= \sum_{D\subset A,\, C\subset A\backslash D}(-1)^{|C|}\Psi(D)\\ &= \sum_{D\subset A}\Psi(D)\sum_{C\subset A\backslash D}(-1)^{|C|}=\Psi(A).\end{aligned}$$

Let us comment on the last equation. We note first that the inner sum equals 1 if $A\backslash D=\emptyset$. If $A\backslash D\neq\emptyset$, then we have setting $n=|A\backslash D|$,

$$\begin{aligned}\sum_{C\subset A\backslash D}(-1)^{|C|} &= \sum_{k=0}^{n}|\{C\subset A\backslash D:|C|=k\}|\,(-1)^k\\ &= \sum_{k=0}^{n}\binom{n}{k}(-1)^k=(1-1)^n=0.\end{aligned}$$

Thus the equation is clear.

For the converse implication assume that the second condition holds. Then the same arguments show

$$\begin{aligned}\sum_{B\subset A}(-1)^{|A-B|}\Psi(B) &= \sum_{D\subset B\subset A}(-1)^{|A-B|}\Phi(D)\\ &= \sum_{D\subset A}\Phi(D)\sum_{C\subset A\backslash D}(-1)^{|C|}=\Phi(A)\end{aligned}$$

which proves the lemma. □

Now we can prove the theorem. We shall write $B+a$ for $B\cup\{a\}$.

Proof (of Theorem 3.3.1). We use the Möbius inversion for

$$\Phi(B)=-V_B(x),\ \Psi(B)=\ln\left(\frac{\Pi\left({}^Bx\right)}{\Pi(o)}\right).$$

Suppose $A\neq\emptyset$. Then $\sum_{B\subset A}(-1)^{|A-B|}=0$ (cf. the last proof) and hence

$$\begin{aligned}\Phi(A) &= -V_A(x)\\ &= \sum_{B\subset A}(-1)^{|A-B|}\ln\left(\Pi\left({}^Bx\right)\right)-\ln\left(\Pi(o)\right)\sum_{B\subset A}(-1)^{|A-B|}\\ &= \sum_{B\subset A}(-1)^{|A-B|}\Psi(B)\,.\end{aligned}$$

Furthermore,

$$\Phi(\emptyset) = -V_\emptyset(x) = 0 = \ln\left(\frac{\Pi\left({}^\emptyset x\right)}{\Pi(o)}\right) = \Psi(\emptyset).$$

Hence the assumptions of the lemma are fulfilled. We conlude

$$\ln\left(\frac{\Pi(x)}{\Pi(o)}\right) = \Psi(S) = \sum_{B\subset S} \Phi(B) = -\sum_{B\subset S} V_B(x) = -H_V(x)$$

and thus

$$\Pi(x) = \Pi(o)\exp\left(-H_V(x)\right).$$

Since Π is a probability distribution, $\Pi(o)^{-1} = Z$ where Z is the normalization constant in (3.2). This proves the first part of the theorem.

For $a \in A$ the formula (refformula for V) becomes:

$$V_A(x) = -\sum_{B\subset A-a} (-1)^{|A-B|}\left[\ln\left(\Pi\left({}^B x\right)\right) - \ln\left(\Pi\left({}^{B+a}x\right)\right)\right] \tag{3.3}$$

and this shows that $V_A(x) = 0$ if $x_a = o_a$.

Now the local characteristics enter the game; for $B \subset A\backslash\{a\}$ we have

$$\frac{\Pi\left(X_a = {}^B x_a \,|X_s = {}^B x_s,\ s \neq a\right)}{\Pi\left(X_a = {}^{B+a}x_a \,|X_s = {}^{B+a}x_s,\ s \neq a\right)} = \frac{\Pi\left({}^B x\right)}{\Pi\left({}^{B+a}x\right)}. \tag{3.4}$$

In fact, the denominators of both conditional probabilities on the left-hand side coincide since only x_s for $x \neq a$ appear. Plugging this relation into (3.3) yields (3.3.1). This completes the proof. □

By (3.3.1),

Corollary 3.3.1. *A random field is uniquely determined by the local characteristics for singletons.*

A random field can now be represented as a Gibbs field for a suitable potential. A Markov field is even a neighbour Gibbs field for the original neighbourhood system. Given $A \subset S$ the set ∂A of neighbours is the set $\bigcup_{s\in A}\partial(s)\backslash A$.

Theorem 3.3.2. *Let a neighbourhood system ∂ on S be given. Then the following holds:*
(a) A random field is a Markov field for ∂ if and only if it is a neighbour Gibbs field for ∂.
(b) For a Markov random field Π with neighbourhood system ∂,

$$\begin{aligned}\Pi\left(X_s = x_s,\ s\in A\,|X_s = x_s,\ s\in S\backslash A\right) &=\\ = \ \Pi\left(X_s = x_s,\ s\in A\,|X_s = x_s,\ s\in \partial(A)\right)&\end{aligned}$$

for every subset A of S .

In western literature, this theorem is frequently referred to as the Hammersley-Clifford theorem or the equivalence theorem. One early version is HAMMERSLEY and CLIFFORD (1968), but there are several independent papers in the early 70's on this topic; cf. the literature in GRIMMETT (1975), AVERINTSEV (1978) and GEORGII (1988). The proof using Moebius inversion is due to G.R. GRIMMETT (1975).

Proof (of the theorem). A neighbour Gibbs field for ∂ is a Markov field for ∂ by proposition 3.2.1. This is one implication of (a). The same proposition covers assertion (b) for neighbour Gibbs fields.

To complete the proof of the theorem we must check the remaining implication of (a). Let Π be Markovian w.r.t ∂ and let V be a potential for Π in the form (3.3.1). We must show that V_A vanishes whenever A is not a clique. To this end, suppose that A is not a clique. Then there is $a \in A$ and $b \in A \backslash \partial(a)$. Using (3.3), we rewrite the sum in (3.3.1) in the form

$$\begin{aligned} V_A(x) &= -\sum_{B \subset A \backslash \{a,b\}} (-1)^{|A-B|} \\ &\quad \times \ln \left(\frac{\Pi\left(X_a = {}^B x_a \,\middle|\, X_s = {}^B x_s,\ s \neq a\right)}{\Pi\left(X_a = {}^{B+b} x_a \,\middle|\, X_s = {}^{B+b} x_s,\ s \neq a\right)} \right. \\ &\quad \left. \times \frac{\Pi\left(X_a = {}^{B+a+b} x_a \,\middle|\, X_s = {}^{B+a+b} x_s,\ s \neq a\right)}{\Pi\left(X_a = {}^{B+a} x_a \,\middle|\, X_s = {}^{B+a} x_s,\ s \neq a\right)} \right). \end{aligned}$$

Consider the first fraction in the last line: Since $a \neq b$ we have $\{X_a = {}^B x_a\} = \{X_a = {}^{B+b} x_a\}$; moreover, since $b \notin \partial(a)$, the numerator and the denominator coincide by the very definition of a Markov random field. The same argument applies to the second fraction and hence the argument of the logarithm is 1 and the sum vanishes. This completes the proof of the remaining implication of (a) and thus the proof of the theorem. □

We add some more information about potentials.

Theorem 3.3.3. *The potential V given by (3.3.1) is the unique normalized potential for the Gibbs field Π. A potential U for Π is related to V by*

$$V_A(x) = \sum_{B \subset A \subset D \subset S} (-1)^{|A-B|} U_D\left({}^B x\right).$$

This shows for instance that normalization of pair potentials gives pair potentials.

Proof. Let U and W be normalized potentials for Π. Since two energy functions for Π differ by a constant only and since $H_U(o) = 0 = H_W(o)$ the two energy functions coincide. Let now any $x \in \mathbf{X}$ be given. For every $s \in S$, we have

$$U_{\{s\}}(x) = U_{\{s\}}({}^{s}x) = H_U({}^{s}x) = H_W({}^{s}x) = W_{\{s\}}({}^{s}x) = W_{\{s\}}(x).$$

Furthermore, for each pair $s, t \in S$, $s \neq t$,

$$U_{\{s,t\}}(x) = U_{\{s,t\}}\left({}^{\{s,t\}}x\right) = H_U\left({}^{\{s,t\}}x\right) - U_{\{s\}}\left({}^{\{s,t\}}x\right) - U_{\{t\}}\left({}^{\{s,t\}}x\right).$$

The same holds for W. Since $H_U\left({}^{\{s,t\}}x\right) = H_W\left({}^{\{s,t\}}x\right)$ and $U_{\{s\}}\left({}^{\{s,t\}}x\right) = U_{\{s\}}\left({}^{\{s,t\}}x\right)$ we conclude that $U_A = W_A$ whenever $|A| = 2$. Proceding by induction over $|A|$ shows that $U = W$.

Let now U be any potential for Π. Then for $B \subset S$ and $a \in S$,

$$\ln \frac{\Pi\left({}^{B}x\right)}{\Pi\left({}^{B+a}x\right)} = \sum_{D\subset S} \left(U_D\left({}^{A}x\right) - U_D\left({}^{A+a}x\right)\right).$$

Choose now $A \subset S$ and $a \in A$. Then

$$\begin{aligned}
V_A(x) &= \sum_{B\subset A-a} (-1)^{|A-B|} \ln \frac{\Pi\left({}^{B}x\right)}{\Pi\left({}^{B+a}x\right)} \\
&= \sum_{D\subset S}\sum_{B\subset A-a} (-1)^{|A-B|} U_D\left({}^{B}x\right) - U_D\left({}^{B+a}x\right) \\
&= \sum_{D\subset S}\sum_{B\subset A} (-1)^{|A-B|} U_D\left({}^{B}x\right) \\
&= \sum_{D\subset S}\sum_{B'\subset D\cap A} (-1)^{|A-B'|} U_D\left({}^{B'}x\right) \sum_{B''\subset A-D} (-1)^{|(A-D)-B''|}.
\end{aligned}$$

The first equality is (3.3.1), then the above equality is plugged in. Observing $U_D\left({}^{B}x\right) = U_D\left({}^{B\cap D}x\right)$ gives the next identity. The last term vanishes except for $A\backslash D = \emptyset$, i.e. $A \subset D$. This proves the desired identity. □

Corollary 3.3.2. *Two potentials U and U' determine the same Gibbs field if and only if*

$$\sum_{B\subset A\subset D\subset S} (-1)^{|A-B|} \left(U_D\left({}^{B}x\right) - U'_D\left({}^{B}x\right)\right) = 0$$

for every $A \neq \emptyset$.

Proof. By uniqueness of normalized potentials, two potentials determine the same Gibbs field if and only if they have the same normalized potential. By the explicit representation in the theorem this is equivalent to the above identities. □

The short survey by D. Griffeath (1976) essentially covers the previous material. Random fields for countable index sets S are introduced as well. S.D. Kindermann and J.L. Snell (1980) informally introduce to the physical ideas behind. French readers may consult Prum (1986); there is also an English version Prum and Fort (1991). Presently, the most comprehensive treatment is Georgii (1988).

Part II

The Gibbs Sampler and Simulated Annealing

For the previously introduced models estimates of the true scene were defined as means or modes of posterior distributions, i.e. Gibbs fields on extremely large discrete spaces. They usually are analytically intractable.

A host of algorithms for 'hard' and 'very hard' optimization problems are provided by combinatorial optimization and one might wonder if they cannot be applied or adapted at least to MAP estimation. In fact, there are many examples. Ford-Fulkerson algorithms were applied to the restoration of binary images (GREIG, PORTEOUS and SEHEULT (1986); the exact GNC algorithm was developed for piecewise smoothing (BLAKE and ZISSERMAN (1987), cf. Example 2.3.1); for a Gaussian prior and Gaussian noise, HUNT (1977) successfully applied coordinatewise steepest descent to restoration (though severe computational problems had to be overcome); etc. On the other hand, their range of applications usually is rather limited. For example, multicolour problems cannot be dealt with by the Ford-Fulkerson algorithm and any attempt to incorporate edge sites will in general render the network method inapplicable. Similarly, the GNC algorithm applies to a very special restoration model and white Gaussian noise only. Also, most algorithms from 'classical' optimization are especially tailored for various versions of standard problems like the travelling salesman problem, the graph colouring problem etc.. Hopefully, specialists from combinatorial optimization will contribute to imaging in the future; but in the past there was not too much interplay between the fields.

Given the present state of the art, one wants to play around with various models and hence needs flexible algorithms to investigate the Gibbs fields in question. Dynamic Monte Carlo methods recently received considerable interest in various fields like Discrete Optimization and Neural Networks and they became a useful and popular method in modern image analysis too. In the next chapters, a special version, called the Gibbs sampler is introduced and studied in some detail. We start with the Gibbs sampler and not with the more common Metropolis type algorithms since it is formally easier to analyze. Analysis of the Metropolis algorithms follows the same lines and is postponed to the next part of the text.

4. Markov Chains: Limit Theorems

All algorithms to be developed have three properties in common: (i) A given configuration is updated in subsequent steps. (ii) Updating in the nth step is performed according to some probabilistic rule. (iii) This rule depends only on the number of the step and on the current configuration. The state of such a system evolves according to some random dynamics which have no memory. Markov chains are appropriate models for such random dynamics (in discrete time).

In this chapter, some abstract limit theorems are derived which later can easily be specialized to prove convergence of various dynamic Monte Carlo methods.

4.1 Preliminaries

The following definitions and remarks address those readers who are not familiar with the basic elements of stochastic processes (with finite state spaces and discrete time). Probabilists will not like this section and those who have met Markov chains should skip it. On the other hand, the author learned in many lectures that students from other fields than mathematics often are grateful for some 'stupid' remarks like those to follow.

We are already acquainted with random transitions, since the observations were random functions of the images. The following definition generalizes this concept.

Definition 4.1.1. *Let X be a finite set called* **state space**. *A family*

$$(P(x, \cdot))_{x \in \mathbf{X}}$$

of probability distributions is called a **transition probabability** *or a* **Markov kernel**.

A Markov kernel P can be represented by a matrix – which will be denoted by P as well – where $P(x, y)$ is the element in the x-th row and the y-th coloumn, i.e. a $|\mathbf{X}| \times |\mathbf{X}|$ square matrix with probability vectors in the rows.

If ν is a probability distribution on $\mathbf{X}$ then $\nu(x)P(x, y)$ is the probability to pick x at random from ν and then to pick y at random from $P(x, \cdot)$. The probability of starting anywhere and arriving at y is

$$\nu P(y) = \sum_x \nu(x) P(x,y).$$

Since summation over all y gives 1, νP is a new probability distribution on $\mathbf{X}$. For instance, $\varepsilon_x P(y) = P(x,y)$ for the Dirac distribution ε_x in x (i.e. $\varepsilon(x) = 1$). If we start at x, apply P and then another Markov kernel Q we get y with probability

$$PQ(x,y) = \sum_z P(x,z) Q(z,y).$$

The composition PQ of P and Q is again a Markov kernel as summation over y shows. Note that νP and PQ correspond to multiplication of matrices (if ν is represented by a $1 \times |\mathbf{X}|$ matrix or a row vector). Given ν and kernels P_i one defines recursively $\nu P_1 \dots P_n = (\nu P_1 \dots P_{n-1}) P_n$. All the rules of matrix multiplication apply to the composition of kernels. In particular, composition of kernels is associative.

Definition 4.1.2. *An* **(inhomogeneous) Markov chain** *on the finite space* $\mathbf{X}$ *is given by an initial distribution* ν *and Markov kernels* $P_1, P_2, \dots$ *on* $\mathbf{X}$. *If* $P_i = P$ *for all* i *then the chain is called* **homogeneous**.

Given a Markov chain, the probability that at times $0, \dots, n$ the states are $x_0, x_1, \dots, x_n$ is $\nu(x_0) P_1(x_0, x_1) \dots P_n(x_{n-1}, x_n)$. This defines a probability distribution $\mathsf{P}^{(n)}$ on the space $\mathbf{X}^{\{0,\dots,n\}}$ of such sequences of length $n+1$. These distributions are consistent, i.e. $\mathsf{P}^{(n+1)}$ induces $\mathsf{P}^{(n)}$ by

$$\mathsf{P}^{(n)}((x_0, \dots, x_n)) = \sum_{x_{n+1}} \mathsf{P}^{(n+1)}((x_0, \dots, x_n, x_{n+1})).$$

An infinite sequence $(x_0, \dots x_n, \dots)$ of states is called a **path** (of the Markov chain). The set of all paths is $\mathbf{X}^{\mathsf{N}_0}$. Because of consistency, one can define the probability of those sets of paths, which depend on a finite number of time indices only: Let $A \subset \mathbf{X}^{\mathsf{N}_0}$ be a (finite cylinder) set $A = B \times \mathbf{X}^{\{n+1,\dots\}}$ with $B \subset \mathbf{X}^{\{0,\dots,n\}}$. Then $\mathsf{P}(A) = \mathsf{P}^{(n)}(B)$ is called the probability of A (w.r.t. the given chain).

Remark 4.1.1. The concept of probability was extended from the subsets of a finite set to a class of subsets of an infinite space. It does not contain sets of paths which depend on an infinite number of times, for example defined by a property like 'the path visits state 1 infinitely often'. For applications using such sets the above concept is too narrow. The extension to a probability distribution on a sufficiently large class of sets involves some measure theory. It can be found in almost any introduction to probability theory above the elementary level (e.g. BILLINGSLEY (1979)). For the development of the algorithms in the next chapters this extension is not necessary. It will be needed only for some more advanced considerations in later chapters.

Markov chains can also be introduced via sequences of random variables ξ_i fulfilling the **Markov property**

$$\mathsf{P}(\xi_n = x_n | \xi_0 = x_0, \ldots, \xi_{n-1} = x_{n-1}) = \mathsf{P}(\xi_n = x_n | \xi_{n-1} = x_{n-1})$$

for all $n \geq 1$ and $x_0, \ldots, x_n \in \mathbf{X}$. To obtain Markov chains in the above sense let $\nu(x) = \mathsf{P}(\xi_0 = x)$ be the initial distribution and let the transition probabilities be given by the conditional probablities

$$P_n(x, y) = \mathsf{P}(\xi_n = y | \xi_{n-1} = x).$$

Conversely, given the initial distribution and the transition probabilities the random variables ξ_i can be defined as the projections of $\mathbf{X}^{\mathsf{N}_0}$ onto the coordinates, i.e. the maps

$$\xi_n : \mathbf{X}^{\{0,\ldots\}} \longrightarrow \mathbf{X}, (x_i)_{i \geq 0} \longmapsto x_n.$$

Example 4.1.1. Let us compute the probabilities of some special events for the chain (ξ_i) of projections. In the following computations all denominators are assumed to be strictly positive.

(a) The distribution of the chain in the n-th step is

$$\begin{aligned} \nu_n(x) &= \mathsf{P}(\xi_n = x) = \sum_{x_0, \ldots, x_{n-1}} \mathsf{P}((x_0, \ldots, x_{n-1}, x)) \\ &= \sum_{x_0, \ldots, x_{n-1}} \nu(x_0) P_1(x_0, x_1) \cdot \ldots \cdot P_n(x_{n-1}, x) = \nu P_1 \ldots P_n(x). \end{aligned}$$

ν_n is called (the n-th) **one-dimensional marginal distribution** of the process.

(b) For $m < n$, the **two-dimensional marginals** are given by

$$\begin{aligned} &\nu_{mn}(x, y) = \mathsf{P}(\xi_m = x, \xi_n = y) \\ &= \sum_{x_0, \ldots, x_{m-1}} \sum_{x_{m+1}, \ldots x_{n-1}} \mathsf{P}((x_0, \ldots, x_{m-1}, x, x_{m+1}, \ldots, x_{n-1}, y)) \\ &= \nu P_1 \ldots P_m(x) P_{m+1} \ldots P_n(x, y). \end{aligned}$$

(c) Defining a Markov process via transition probabilities and via the projections ξ_i is consistent:

$$\begin{aligned} \mathsf{P}(\xi_n = y | \xi_{n-1} = x) &= \frac{\mathsf{P}(\xi_{n-1} = x, \xi_n = y)}{\mathsf{P}(\xi_{n-1} = x)} = \frac{\nu_{n-1,n}(x, y)}{\nu_{n-1}(x)} \\ &= \frac{\nu P_1 \ldots P_{n-1}(x) P_n(x, y)}{\nu P_1 \ldots P_{n-1}(x)} = P_n(x, y). \end{aligned}$$

It is now easy to check the Markov property of the projections:

$$
\begin{aligned}
&\mathsf{P}(\xi_n = y|\xi_0 = x_0, \ldots, \xi_{n-1} = x) \\
&= \frac{\mathsf{P}(\xi_0 = x_0, \ldots, \xi_{n-1} = x, \xi_n = y)}{\sum_z \mathsf{P}(\xi_0 = x_0, \ldots, \xi_{n-1} = x, \xi_n = z)} \\
&= \frac{\nu(x_0)P_1(x_0, x_1) \ldots P_{n-1}(x_{n-1}, x)P_n(x, y)}{\sum_z \nu(x_0)P_1(x_0, x_1) \ldots P_{n-1}(x_{n-1}, x)P_n(x, z)} \\
&= P_n(x, y) = \mathsf{P}(\xi_n = y|\xi_{n-1} = x).
\end{aligned}
$$

Expressions like those in (a) and (b) can be derived also for the higher dimensional marginal distributions $\mathsf{P}(\xi_{n_1} = x_1, \ldots, \xi_{n_k} = x_k)$. We shall sometimes call P the **law** of the Markov chain $(\xi_n)_{n\geq 0}$. Given P the expectation $\mathsf{E}(f)$ is defined in the usual way for those functions f on $\mathbf{X}^{\mathbb{N}_0}$ which depend on a finite number of time indices only. More precisely, if there is $k \geq 0$ such that for all $(x_n)_{n\geq 0}$, $f((x_n)_{n\geq 0}) = f(x_1, \ldots, x_k)$ then

$$
\mathsf{E}(f) = \sum_{x_0, \ldots, x_k} f(x_0, \ldots, x_k)\mathsf{P}((x_0, \ldots, x_k)).
$$

Example 4.1.2. Let $x \in \mathbf{X}$ be fixed. Then $h((x_i)_{i\geq 0}) = \sum_{i=0}^{n} 1_{\{\xi_i = x\}}$ is the number of visits of the path (x_i) in x up to time n. The expected number of visits is

$$
\mathsf{E}(h) = \sum_{y_0, \ldots, y_n} h(y_0, \ldots, y_n)\mathsf{P}((y_0, \ldots, y_n)) = \sum_{i=0}^{n} \nu_i(x).
$$

We will be interested in the limiting behaviour of Markov chains. Two concepts of convergence will be used: Let ξ and $\xi_0, \xi_1, \ldots$ be random variables. We shall say that (ξ_i) converges to ξ

(a) **in probability** if for every $\varepsilon > 0$,

$$
\mathsf{P}(|\xi_i - \xi| > \varepsilon) \longrightarrow 0, \ i \to \infty;
$$

(b) **in L^2**, if

$$
\mathsf{E}((\xi_i - \xi)^2) \longrightarrow 0, \ i \to \infty.
$$

For every nonnegative random variable η, Markov's inequality states that

$$
\mathsf{P}(\eta \geq \varepsilon) \leq \frac{\mathsf{E}(\eta^2)}{\varepsilon^2}.
$$

By this inequality,

$$
\mathsf{P}(|\xi_i - \xi| > \varepsilon) \leq \frac{\mathsf{E}((\xi_i - \xi)^2)}{\varepsilon^2}
$$

and hence L^2 -convergence implies convergence in probability. For bounded functions the two concepts are equivalent.

Let us finally note that a Markov chain with strictly positive initial distribution and transition probabilities induces a (finite) Markov field in a natural way: on each time interval $I = \{0, \ldots, n\}$ define a neighbourhood system by $\partial(k) = \{k-1, k+1\} \cap I$. Then for $k \in I \backslash \{0\}$,

$$\begin{aligned}
\mathsf{P}(\xi_k | \xi_i, 0 \leq i \leq n, i \neq k) &= \frac{\mathsf{P}(\xi_i = x_i, 0 \leq i \leq n)}{\mathsf{P}(\xi_i, 0 \leq i \leq n, i \neq k)} \\
&= \frac{\nu(x_0) P_1(x_0, x_1) \ldots P_{k-1}(x_{k-2}, x_{k-1}) P_k(x_{k-1}, x_k)}{\sum_z \nu(x_0) P_1(x_0, x_1) \ldots P_{k-1}(x_{k-2}, x_{k-1}) P_k(x_{k-1}, z)} \\
&\quad \frac{P_{k+1}(x_k, x_{k+1}) \ldots P_n(x_{n-1}, x_n)}{P_{k+1}(z, x_{k+1}) \ldots P_n(x_{n-1}, x_n)} \\
&= \frac{\nu_{k-1}(x_{k-1}) P_k(x_{k-1}, x_k) P_{k+1}(x_k, x_{k+1})}{\sum_z \nu_{k-1}(x_{k-1}) P_k(x_{k-1}, z) P_{k+1}(z, x_{k+1})} \\
&= \frac{\mathsf{P}(\xi_{k-1} = x_{k-1}, \xi_k = x_k, \xi_{k+1} = x_{k+1})}{\mathsf{P}(\xi_{k-1} = x_{k-1}, \xi_{k+1} = x_{k+1})} \\
&= \mathsf{P}(\xi_k = x_k | \xi_{k-1} = x_{k-1}, \xi_{k+1} = x_{k+1})
\end{aligned}$$

and similarly,

$$\mathsf{P}(\xi_0 = x_0 | \xi_i = x_i, 1 \leq i \leq n) = \mathsf{P}(\xi_0 = x_0 | \xi_1 = x_1).$$

This is the spatial Markov property we met in Chapter 3.

Markov chains are introduced at an elementary level in KEMENEY and SNELL (1960). Those who prefer a more formal (matrix-theoretic) treatment may consult SENETA (1981).

4.2 The Contraction Coefficient

To prove the basic limit theorems for homogeneous and inhomogeneous Markov chains, the classical contraction method is adopted, a remarkably simple and transparent argument. The proofs are given explicitely for finite state spaces. Adopting the proper definition of total variation and replacing some of the 'max' by 'l.u.b.' essentially yields the corresponding results for more general spaces.

The special structure of the configuration space $\mathbf{X}$ presently is not needed. Hence $\mathbf{X}$ is merely assumed to be a finite set.

For distributions μ and ν on $\mathbf{X}$, the norm of **total variation** of the difference $\mu - \nu$ is given by

$$\|\mu - \nu\| = \sum_x |\mu(x) - \nu(x)|.$$

Note that this simply is the L^1-norm of the difference. The following equivalent descriptions are useful.

Lemma 4.2.1. *Let μ and ν be probability distributions on $\mathbf{X}$. Then*

$$\begin{aligned}\|\mu-\nu\| &= 2\sum_x(\mu(x)-\nu(x))^+\\ &= 2(1-\sum_x\mu(x)\wedge\nu(x))\\ &= \max\left\{\left|\sum_x h(x)(\mu(x)-\nu(x))\right| : |h|\le 1\right\}.\end{aligned}$$

For a vector $\rho=(\rho(x))_{x\in\mathbf{X}}$ the positive part ρ^+ equals $\rho(x)$ if $\rho(x)>0$ and vanishes otherwise. The negative part ρ^- is $(-\rho)^+$. The symbol $a\wedge b$ denotes the minimum of real numbers a and b.

If $\mathbf{X}$ is not finite a definition of total variation is obtained replacing the sum in the last expression by the integral $\int h\,d(\mu-\nu)$ and the maximum by the least upper bound.

Remark 4.2.1. For probability distributions μ and ν the triangle inequality yields $\|\mu-\nu\|\le 2$. From the second identity in the lemma one reads off that equality holds if and only if μ and ν have disjoint support (the **support** of a distribution ν is the set where it is strictly positive; two distributions with disjoint support are called **orthogonal**).

Proof (of Lemma 4.2.1). Plainly,

$$\begin{aligned}\|\mu-\nu\| &= \sum_x(\mu(x)-\nu(x))^+ + \sum_x(\mu(x)-\nu(x))^-\\ &= \sum_{x:\mu(x)\ge\nu(x)}(\mu(x)-\nu(x)) + \sum_{x:\mu(x)<\nu(x)}(\nu(x)-\mu(x)).\end{aligned}$$

The difference of the sums vanishes since μ and ν are probability distributions and hence the sums are equal. This yields

$$\|\mu-\nu\|/2=\sum_x(\mu(x)-\nu(x))^+$$

and hence the first identity. Furthermore,

$$\begin{aligned}\|\mu-\nu\|/2 &= \sum_{x:\mu(x)\ge\nu(x)}\mu(x) - \sum_{x:\mu(x)\ge\nu(x)}\nu(x)\\ &= \sum_x\mu(x) - \sum_{x:\mu(x)<\nu(x)}\mu(x) - \sum_{x:\mu(x)\ge\nu(x)}\nu(x)\\ &= 1-\sum_x\mu(x)\wedge\nu(x)\end{aligned}$$

which proves the second identity. Finally, the inequality

$$\begin{aligned}\|\mu - \nu\| &= \sum_x |\mu(x) - \nu(x)| \\ &\geq \max\left\{\left|\sum_x h(x)(\mu(x) - \nu(x))\right| : |h| \leq 1\right\}\end{aligned}$$

is obvious. To check equality plug in $h(x) = \mathrm{sgn}(\mu(x) - \nu(x))$. □

The **contraction coefficient** of a Markov kernel P is defined by

$$c(P) = (1/2)\max_{x,y} \|P(x,\cdot) - P(y,\cdot)\|.$$

The notion of a contraction coefficient can be considerably generalized, cf. SENETA (1981), 4.3.

Remark 4.2.2. By the last remark, $c(P) \leq 1$ and equality holds if and only if at least two of the distributions $P(x,\cdot)$ have disjoint support. Plainly, $c(P) = 0$ if and only if all $P(x,\cdot)$ are equal. Hence the contraction coefficient is a rough measure for orthogonality of the distributions $P(x,\cdot)$.

The name 'contraction coefficient' is justified by the next inequality. This and the following one are nearly all what is needed to prove the ergodic theorems below.

Lemma 4.2.2. *Let μ and ν be probability distributions and P and Q be Markov kernels on* $\mathbf{X}$. *Then*

$$\begin{aligned}\|\mu P - \nu P\| &\leq c(P)\|\mu - \nu\|, \\ c(PQ) &\leq c(P)c(Q).\end{aligned}$$

In particular,

$$\begin{aligned}\|\mu P - \nu P\| &\leq \|\mu - \nu\|, \\ \|\mu P - \nu P\| &\leq 2c(P).\end{aligned}$$

Proof. Let us start with the first inequality. For a real function f on $\mathbf{X}$ let

$$d = (\max_x f(x) + \min_x f(x))/2.$$

Then

$$\max_x |f(x) - d| = (1/2)\max_{x,y} |f(x) - f(y)|.$$

Writing $\mu(f)$ for $\sum_x f(x)\mu(x)$, we conclude

$$\begin{aligned}|\mu(f) - \nu(f)| &= |\mu(f-d) - \nu(f-d)| \leq \max_x |f(x) - d| \cdot \|\mu - \nu\| \\ &= (1/2)\max_{x,y} |f(x) - f(y)| \cdot \|\mu - \nu\|. \qquad (4.1)\end{aligned}$$

For a function h on $\mathbf{X}$, the function Ph is defined by

$$Ph(x) = \sum_y h(y)P(x,y).$$

Plugging in Ph for f yields

$$\begin{aligned}
\|\mu P - \nu P\| &= \max\{|(\mu P)h - (\nu P)h| : |h| \le 1\} \\
&= \max\{|\mu(Ph) - \nu(Ph)| : |h| \le 1\} \\
&\le \max\left\{(1/2)\max_{x,y}|Ph(x) - Ph(y)| : |h| \le 1\right\}\|\mu - \nu\| \\
&= (1/2)\max_{x,y}\max\{|Ph(x) - Ph(y)| : |h| \le 1\}\|\mu - \nu\| \\
&= c(P)\|\mu - \nu\|
\end{aligned}$$

and hence the first inequality. The second one follows from

$$\begin{aligned}
c(PQ) &= (1/2)\max_{x,y}\|PQ(x.\cdot) - PQ(y,\cdot)\| \\
&= (1/2)\max_{x,y}\|P(x,\cdot)Q - P(y,\cdot)Q\| \\
&\le c(P)c(Q).
\end{aligned}$$

The other inequalities follow from the first two since $c(P) \le 1$ and $\|\mu - \nu\| \le 2$. This completes the proof. □

Remark 4.2.3. An immediate consequence is **asymptotic loss of memory** or **weak ergodicity** of Markov chains:

Let P_n, $n \ge 1$, be Markov kernels and μ and ν two initial distributions. Then $c(P_1 \ldots P_n) \to 0$ implies

$$\|\mu P_1 \ldots P_n - \nu P_1 \ldots P_n\| \longrightarrow 0.$$

Markov chains will converge quickly if the contraction coefficient is small. Therefore the following estimate is useful.

Lemma 4.2.3. *For every Markov kernel Q on a finite space $\mathbf{X}$,*

$$c(Q) \le 1 - |\mathbf{X}|\min\{Q(x,y) : x,y \in \mathbf{X}\} \le 1 - \min\{Q(x,y) : x,y \in \mathbf{X}\}.$$

In particular, if Q is strictly positive then $c(Q) < 1$.

Proof. By Lemma 4.2.1,

$$\|\mu - \nu\|/2 = 1 - \sum_x \mu(x) \wedge \nu(x)$$

for probability distributions μ and ν. Hence

$$c(Q) = 1 - \min\left\{\sum_z Q(x,z) \wedge Q(y,z) : x,y \in \mathbf{X}\right\}$$

which implies the first two inequalities. The rest is an immediate consequence. □

4.3 Homogeneous Markov Chains

A Markov chain is called **homogeneous** if all its transition probabilities are equal. We prove convergence of marginals and a law of large numbers for homogeneous Markov chains.

Lemma 4.3.1. *For each Markov kernel P on a finite state space the sequence $(c(P^n))_{n\geq 0}$ decreases. If P has a strictly positive power P^τ then the sequence decreases to* 0.

Markov kernels with a strictly positive power are called **primitive**. A homogeneous chain with primitive Markov kernel eventually reaches each state with positive probability from any state. This property is called **irreducibility** (a characterization of primitive Markov kernels more common in probability theory is to say that they are irreducible and aperiodic, cf. SENETA (1981)).

Proof (of Lemma 4.3.1). By Lemma 4.2.2,

$$c(P^{n+1}) \leq c(P)c(P^n) \leq c(P^n).$$

If $Q = P^\tau$ then

$$c(P^n) \leq (Q^k P^{n-\tau k}) \leq c(Q)^k$$

for $n \geq \tau$ and the greatest number k with $\tau k \leq n$. If Q is strictly positive then $c(Q) < 1$ by Lemma 4.2.3 and $c(P^n)$ tends to zero as n tends to infinity. This proves the assertion. □

Let μ be a probability distribution on $\mathbf{X}$. If $\mu P = \mu$ then $\mu P^n = \mu$ for every $n \geq 0$ and hence such distributions are natural candidates for limit distributions of homogeneous Markov chains. A distribution μ satisfying $\mu P = \mu$ is called **invariant** or **stationary** for P. The limit theorem reads:

Theorem 4.3.1. *A primitive Markov kernel P on a finite space has a unique invariant distribution μ and*

$$\nu P^n \longrightarrow \mu \quad as \quad n \to \infty$$

uniformly in all distributions ν.

Proof. Existence and uniqueness of the invariant distribution is part of the Perron-Frobenius theorem (Appendix B). By Lemma 4.3.1, the sequence $(c(P^n))$ decreases to zero and the theorem follows from

$$\|\nu P^n - \mu\| = \|\nu P^n - \mu P^n\| \leq \|\nu - \mu\| c(P^n) \leq 2 \cdot c(P^n). \tag{4.2}$$

□

Homogeneous Markov chains with primitive kernel even obey the law of large numbers. For an initial distribution ν and a Markov kernel P let $(\xi_i)_{i\geq 0}$ be a corresponding sequence of random variables (cf. Section 4.1). The expectation $\sum_x f(x)\mu(x)$ of a function f on $\mathbf{X}$ w.r.t. a distribution μ will be denoted by $\mathsf{E}_\mu(f)$.

Theorem 4.3.2 (Law of Large Numbers). *Let $\mathbf{X}$ be a finite space and let P be a primitive Markov kernel on $\mathbf{X}$ with invariant distribution μ. Then for every initial distribution ν and every function f on $\mathbf{X}$,*

$$\frac{1}{n}\sum_{i=1}^{n} f(\xi_i) \longrightarrow \mathsf{E}_\mu(f)$$

in $L^2(\mathsf{P}_\nu)$. Moreover, for every $\varepsilon > 0$,

$$\mathsf{P}\left(\left|\frac{1}{n}\sum_{i=1}^{n} f(\xi_i) - \mathsf{E}_\mu(f)\right| > \varepsilon\right) \leq \frac{13\|f\|^2}{(1-c(P))n\varepsilon^2}$$

where $\|f\| = \sum_x |f(x)|$.

For identically distributed independent random variables ξ_i the Markov kernel $(P(x,y))$ does not depend on x, hence the rows of the matrix coincide and $c(P) = 0$. In this case the theorem boils down to the usual weak law of large numbers.

Proof. Choose $x \in \mathbf{X}$ and let $f = 1_{\{x\}}$. By elementary calculations,

$$\begin{aligned}
&\mathsf{E}\left(\left(\frac{1}{n}\sum_{i=1}^{n} f(\xi_i) - \mathsf{E}_\mu(f)\right)^2\right) \\
= \; &\mathsf{E}\left(\left(\frac{1}{n}\sum_{i=1}^{n} 1_{\{\xi_i = x\}} - \mu(x)\right)^2\right) \\
= \; &\frac{1}{n^2}\sum_{i,j=1}^{n} \mathsf{E}((1_{\{\xi_i=x\}} - \mu(x))(1_{\{\xi_j=x\}} - \mu(x))) \\
= \; &\frac{1}{n^2}\sum_{i,j=1}^{n} ((\nu_{ij}(x,x) - \mu(x)^2) - (\mu(x)\nu_j(x) - \mu(x)^2) \\
&-(\mu(x)\nu_i(x) - \mu(x)^2)).
\end{aligned}$$

There are three means to be estimated. The first one is most difficult. Since $\mu P = \mu$, for $i, k > 0$ and $x, y \in \mathbf{X}$ the following rough estimates hold:

$$\begin{aligned}
&|\nu P^i(x)\varepsilon_x P^k(y) - \mu(x)\mu(y)| \\
\leq\ & |\nu P^i(x)\varepsilon_x P^k(y) - \mu P^i(x)\varepsilon_x P^k(y)| \\
&+ |\mu(x)\varepsilon_x P^k(y) - \mu(x)\mu P^k(y)| \\
\leq\ & \|(\nu - \mu)P^i\| + \|(\varepsilon_x - \mu)P^k\| \\
\leq\ & 2\cdot(c(P)^i + c(P)^k).
\end{aligned}$$

Using the explicit expression

$$\sum_{i=1}^{n} a^i = a\cdot\frac{1-a^n}{1-a}, \qquad 0<a<1,$$

for the finite geometric series, one computes

$$\begin{aligned}
&\frac{1}{n^2}\sum_{i=1}^{n-1}\sum_{j>i}|\nu_{ij}(x,y) - \mu(x)\mu(y)| \\
\leq\ & 2\left(\frac{c(P)}{1-c(P)}\frac{1}{n}(1-c(P)^{n-1}) + \frac{c(P)}{1-c(P)}\frac{n-1}{n^2}(1-c(P)^n)\right) \\
\leq\ & \frac{4}{1-c(P)}\frac{1}{n}.
\end{aligned}$$

The same estimate holds for the mean over pairs (i,j) of indices with $j<i$. For convenience of notation set $\nu_{ii}(x,x) = \nu P^i(x)$ and $\nu_{ii}(x,y) = 0$ if $x \neq y$. The sum over the corresponding terms is bounded by n and hence

$$\frac{1}{n^2}\sum_{i=1}^{n}\sum_{j=1}^{n}|\nu_{ij}(x,y) - \mu(x)\mu(y)| \leq \frac{9}{1-c(P)}\frac{1}{n}.$$

By (4.2) the second and third mean can be estimated:

$$\begin{aligned}
&\frac{1}{n^2}\sum_{i=1}^{n}\sum_{j=1}^{n}|\mu(x)\nu_j(y) - \mu(x)\mu(y)| \\
=\ & \mu(x)\frac{c(P)}{1-c(P)}\frac{2}{n}(1-c(P)^n) \leq \frac{2}{1-c(P)}\frac{1}{n}.
\end{aligned}$$

Hence the above expectation is bounded by $(13/n)(1-c(P))^{-1}$. For general f, the triangle inequality gives a bound $(c/n)(1-c(P))^{-1}$ with $c = 13\|f\|^2$, $\|f\| = \sum_x |f(x)|$. This proves the first part of the theorem. The second one follows form Markov's inequality. □

Remark 4.3.1. [continuous state space] With a little extra work the above program (and also the extension to inhomogeneous chains in the next section) can be carried out on abstract measurable spaces. MADSON and ISAAKSON (1973) give proofs for the special case

$$P(x,dy) = f_x(y)\,d\nu(x)$$

with densities f_x w.r.t. a σ-finite measure ν. In particular, they cover the important case of densities w.r.t. Lebesgue measure on $\mathbf{X}= \mathsf{R}^d$. They also indicate the extension to the case where densities do not exist. This type of extension is carried out in M. IOSIFESCU (1972). Some remarks on the limits of the contraction technique can be found in Remark 5.1.2.

4.4 Inhomogeneous Markov Chains

Let us now turn to inhomogeneous Markov chains. We first note a simple observation.

Lemma 4.4.1. *If μ_n, $n \geq 1$, are probability distributions on $\mathbf{X}$ such that $\sum_n \|\mu_{n+1} - \mu_n\| < \infty$ then there is a probability distribution μ_∞ such that $\mu_n \to \mu_\infty$ (in $\|\cdot\|$) as $n \to \infty$.*

Since $\mathbf{X}$ is finite, pointwise convergence and convergence in the L^1-norm $\|\cdot\|$ coincide.

Proof. For $m < n$,

$$\|\mu_n - \mu_m\| \leq \sum_{k \geq m} \|\mu_{k+1} - \mu_k\|$$

which tends to zero as m tends to infinity. Thus (μ_n) is a Cauchy sequence in the compact space $\{\mu \in \mathsf{R}^{\mathbf{X}} : \mu \geq 0, \sum_x \mu(x) = 1\}$ and hence has a limit μ_∞ in this set. □

The limit theorem for inhomogeneous Markov chains reads:

Theorem 4.4.1. *Let P_n, $n \geq 1$, be Markov kernels and assume that each P_n has an invariant probability distribution μ_n. Assume further that the following conditions are satisfied*

$$\sum_n \|\mu_n - \mu_{n+1}\| < \infty, \tag{4.3}$$

$$\lim_{n\to\infty} c(P_i \dots P_n) = 0 \quad \text{for every} \quad i \geq 1. \tag{4.4}$$

Then $\mu_\infty = \lim_{n\to\infty} \mu_n$ exists and uniformly in all initial distributions ν,

$$\nu P_1 \dots P_n \longrightarrow \mu_\infty \quad \text{for} \quad n \to \infty.$$

Proof. The existence of the limit μ_∞ was proved in the preceding lemma. Let now $i \geq 1$ and $k \geq 1$. Use $\mu_n P_n = \mu_n$ for

$$\begin{aligned}
&\mu_\infty P_i \ldots P_{i+k} - \mu_\infty \\
= \;& (\mu_\infty - \mu_i) P_i \ldots P_{i+k} + \mu_i P_{i+1} \ldots P_{i+k} - \mu_\infty \\
= \;& (\mu_\infty - \mu_i) P_i \ldots P_{i+k} + \sum_{j=1}^{k} (\mu_{i-1+j} - \mu_{i+j}) P_{i+j} \ldots P_{i+k} \\
& + \mu_{i+k} - \mu_\infty .
\end{aligned}$$

For $i \geq N$ this implies

$$\|\mu_\infty P_i \ldots P_{i+k} - \mu_\infty\| \leq 2 \cdot \sup_{n \geq N} \|\mu_\infty - \mu_n\| + \sum_{n \geq N} \|\mu_n - \mu_{n+1}\|. \tag{4.5}$$

We used Lemma 4.2.2 and that the contraction coefficient is bounded by 1. By condition (4.3) and since μ_∞ exists, for large N the expression on the right hand becomes small. Fix now a large N. For $2 \leq N \leq i \leq n$ we may continue with

$$\begin{aligned}
&\|\nu P_1 \ldots P_n - \mu_\infty\| \\
= \;& \|(\nu P_1 \ldots P_{i-1} - \mu_\infty) P_i \ldots P_n + \mu_\infty P_i \ldots P_n - \mu_\infty\| \qquad (4.6)\\
\leq \;& 2 \cdot c(P_i \ldots P_n) + \|\mu_\infty P_i \ldots P_n - \mu_\infty\|
\end{aligned}$$

For large n, the first term becomes small by (4.4). This proves the result. □

The proof shows that convergence of inhomogeneous chains basically is asymptotic loss of memory plus convergence of the invariant distributions.

The theorem frequently is referred to as DOBRUSHIN's theorem (DOBRUSHIN (1956). There are various closely related approaches and it can even be traced back to MARKOV (cf. SENETA (1973) and (1981), pp. 144-145). The contraction technique is exploited systematically in ISAACSON and MADSON (1976).

There are some simple but useful criteria for the conditions in the theorem.

Lemma 4.4.2. *For probability distributions μ_n, $n \geq 1$, condition (4.3) is fulfilled if each of the sequences $(\mu_n(x))_{n \geq 1}$ de- or increases eventually.*

Proof. By Lemma 4.2.1,

$$0 \leq \sum_n \|\mu_{n+1} - \mu_n\| = 2 \sum_x \sum_n (\mu_{n+1}(x) - \mu_n(x))^+ .$$

By monotony, there is n_0 such that either $(\mu_{n+1}(x) - \mu_n(x))^+ = 0$ for all $n \geq n_0$ and thus $\sum_{n \geq n_0} (\mu_{n+1}(x) - \mu_n(x))^+ = 0$ or $(\mu_{n+1}(x) - \mu_n(x))^+ = \mu_{n+1}(x) - \mu_n(x)$, and thus

$$\sum_{n=n_0}^{N} (\mu_{n+1}(x) - \mu_n(x))^+ = \mu_{N+1}(x) - \mu_{n_0}(x) \leq 1$$

for all large N. This implies that the double sum is finite and hence condition (4.3) holds. □

Lemma 4.4.3. *Condition (4.4) is implied by*

$$\prod_{k\geq i} c(P_k) = 0 \quad \textit{for every} \quad i \geq 1. \tag{4.7}$$

or by

$$c(P_n) > 0 \quad \textit{for every } n \textit{ and } \quad \prod_{k\geq 1} c(P_k) = 0. \tag{4.8}$$

Proof. Condition (4.7) implies (4.4) by the second rule in Lemma 4.2.2 and obviously (4.8) implies (4.7). □

This can be used to check convergence of a given inhomogeneous Markov chain in the following way: The time axis is subdivided into 'epochs' $(\tau(k-1), \tau(k)]$ over which the transitions

$$Q_k = P_{\tau(k-1)+1} \cdots P_{\tau(k)}$$

are strictly positive (and hence also the minimum in the above estimate). Given a time i and a large n there are some epochs inbetween and

$$\begin{aligned} & c(P_i \ldots P_n) \\ \leq\ & c(P_i \ldots P_{\tau(p-1)}) c(Q_p \ldots Q_r) c(P_{\tau(r)+1} \cdots P_n) \\ \leq\ & c(Q_p) \ldots c(Q_r) \\ \leq\ & \prod_{k=p}^{r} \left(1 - |\mathbf{X}| \min_{x,y} Q_k(x,y)\right). \end{aligned}$$

In order to ensure convergence, the factors (which are strictly smaller than 1) have to be small enough to let the product converge to zero, i.e. the numbers $\min_{x,y} Q_k(x,y)$ should not decrease too fast.

The following comments concern condition (4.4).

Example 4.4.1. It is easy to see that condition (4.4) cannot be dropped: for each n let $P_n = I$ where I is the unit matrix. Then $c(P_n) = 1$, every probability disribution ρ is invariant w.r.t. P_n and (4.3) holds for $\mu_n = \rho$. On the other hand $\nu P_1 \ldots P_n \to \nu$ for every ν. One can modify this example such that the μ_n are the *unique* invariant distributions for the P_n. Let

$$P_n = \begin{pmatrix} 1-a_n & a_n \\ a_n & 1-a_n \end{pmatrix}$$

with small positive numbers a_n. For these Markov kernels the uniform distribution $\mu = (1/2, 1/2)$ is the unique invariant distribution. The contraction coefficients are $c(P_n) = |1 - 2a_n|$. There are a_n such that

$$\prod_{n\geq 1} c(P_n) = \prod_{n\geq 1} (1 - 2a_n) \geq \frac{3}{4}.$$

(or which amounts to the same $\sum_n \ln(1-2a_n) \geq \ln(3/4)$). Let now $\nu = (1,0)$ be the initial distribution. Then the one-dimensional marginals $\nu_n = (\nu_n(1), \nu_n(2)) = \nu P_1 \ldots P_n$ of the chain fulfill

$$\nu_n(1) \geq (1-a_1)(1-a_2)\ldots(1-a_n) \geq (3/4) \quad \text{for each} \quad n$$

and hence do not converge to μ.

Similarly, conditions (4.4), (4.7) or (4.8) cannot be replaced by

$$c(P_1 \ldots P_n) \to 0$$

or

$$\prod_k c(P_k) = 0,$$

respectively. In the example, $\nu_1 = (1-a_1, a_1)$. If P_1 is replaced by

$$P_1 = \begin{pmatrix} 1-a_1 & a_1 \\ 1-a_1 & a_1 \end{pmatrix},$$

then $\nu P_1 = (1-a_1, a_1)$ for every initial distribution ν. Convergence of this chain is the same as before but $\prod_k c(P_k) = 0$ since $c(P_1) = 0$.

The Remarks 4.3.1 on continuous state spaces hold for inhomogeneous chains as well.

5. Sampling and Annealing

In this chapter, the Gibbs sampler is established and a basic version of the annealing algorithm is derived. This is sufficient for many applications in imaging like the computation of MMS or MPM estimators. The reader may (and is encouraged to) perform own computer experiments with these algorithms. He or she may get some ideas from the appendix which provides the necessary tools.

In the following, the underlying space $\mathbf{X}$ is a finite product of finite state spaces $\mathbf{X}_s$, $s \in S$, with a finite set S of sites.

5.1 Sampling

Sampling from a Gibbs field

$$\Pi(x) = Z^{-1}\exp(-H(x))$$

is the basis of MMS estimation. Direct sampling from such a discrete distribution (cf. Appendix A) is impossible since the underlying space $\mathbf{X}$ is too large (its cardinality typically being of order $10^{100.000}$); in particular, the partition function is computationally intractable. Therefore, static Monte Carlo methods are replaced by dynamic ones, i.e. by the simulation of computationally feasible Markov chains with limit distribution Π. Theorem 4.3.1 tells us that we should look for a strictly positive Markov kernel P for which Π is invariant. One natural construction is based on the local characteristics of Π. For every $I \subset S$ a Markov kernel on $\mathbf{X}$ is defined by

$$\Pi_I(x,y) = \begin{cases} Z_I^{-1}\exp(-H(y_I x_{S\setminus I})) & \text{if } y_{S\setminus I} = x_{S\setminus I} \\ 0 & \text{otherwise} \end{cases} \tag{5.1}$$

$$Z_I = \sum_{z_I}\exp(-H(z_I x_{S\setminus I})).$$

These Markov kernels will again be called the **local characteristics** of Π. They are merely artificial extensions of the local characteristics introduced in Chapter 3 to all of $\mathbf{X}$. Sampling from $\Pi_I(x,\cdot)$ changes x at most on I. Note that the local characteristics can be evaluated in reasonable time if they depend on a relatively small number of neighbours (cf. the examples in Chapter 3).

The Gibbs field Π is stationary (or invariant) for Π_I. The following result is stronger but easier to prove.

Lemma 5.1.1. *The Gibbs field Π and its local characteristics Π_I fulfill the detailed balance equation, i.e. for all $x, y \in \mathbf{X}$ and $I \subset S$,*

$$\Pi(x)\Pi_I(x,y) = \Pi(y)\Pi_I(y,x).$$

This concept can be formulated for arbitrary distributions μ and transition probabilities P; they are said to fulfill the **detailed balance equation** if

$$\mu(x)P(x,y) = \mu(y)P(y,x)$$

for all x and y. Basically, this means that the homogeneous Markov chain with initial distribution μ and transition kernel P is reversible in time (this concept will be discussed in an own chapter). Therefore P is called **reversible** w.r.t. μ.

Remark 5.1.1. Reversibility holds if and only if P induces a selfadjoint operator on the space of real functions on $\mathbf{X}$ endowed with the inner product $\langle f,g\rangle_\mu = \sum_x f(x)g(x)\mu(x)$ by $Pf(x) = \sum_y f(y)P(x,y)$. In fact,

$$\begin{aligned}\langle Pf,g\rangle_\mu &= \sum_x \left(\sum_y P(x,y)f(y)\right) g(x)\mu(x) \\ &= \sum_y f(y) \left(\sum_x P(y,x)g(x)\right) \mu(y) = \langle f, Pg\rangle_\mu.\end{aligned}$$

For the converse, plug in suitable f and g.

Proof (of Lemma 5.1.1). Both sides of the identity vanish unless $y_{S\backslash I} = x_{S\backslash I}$. Since $x = x_I y_{S\backslash I}$ and $y = y_I x_{S\backslash I}$ one has the identity

$$\begin{aligned}&\exp(-H(x))\frac{\exp(-H(y_I x_{S\backslash I}))}{\sum_{z_I}\exp(-H(z_I x_{S\backslash I}))} \\ =\ &\exp(-H(y))\frac{\exp(-H(x_I y_{S\backslash I}))}{\sum_{z_I}\exp(-H(z_I y_{S\backslash I}))}\end{aligned}$$

which implies detailed balance. □

Stationarity follows easily.

Theorem 5.1.1. *If μ and P fulfill the detailed balance equation then μ is invariant for P. In particular, Gibbs fields are invariant for their local characteristics.*

Proof. Summation of both sides of the detailed balance equation over x yields the result. □

An enumeration $S = \{s_1, \ldots, s_\sigma\}$ of S will be called a **visiting scheme**. Given a visiting scheme, we shall write $S = \{1, \ldots, \sigma\}$ to simplify notation. A Markov kernel is defined by

$$P(x, y) = \Pi_{\{1\}} \ldots \Pi_{\{\sigma\}}(x, y). \tag{5.2}$$

Note that (5.2) is the composition of matrices and not a multiplication of real numbers. The homogeneous Markov chain with transition probability P induces the following algorithm: an initial configuration x is chosen or picked at random according to some initial distribution ν. In the first step, x is updated at site 1 by sampling from the single-site characteristic $\Pi_{\{1\}}(x, \cdot x_{S\setminus\{1\}})$. This yields a new configuration $y = y_1 x_{S\setminus\{1\}}$ which in turn is updated at site 2. This way all the sites in S are sequentially updated. This will be called a **sweep**. The first sweep results in a sample from νP. Running the chain for many sweeps produces a sample from $\nu P \ldots P$. Since Gibbs fields are invariant w.r.t. local characteristics and hence for the composition P of local characteristics too, one can hope that after a large number of sweeps one ends up in a sample from a distribution close to Π. This is made precise by the following result.

Theorem 5.1.2. *For every $x \in \mathbf{X}$,*

$$\lim_{n\to\infty} \nu P^n(x) = \Pi(x)$$

uniformly in all initial distributions ν.

Whereas the marginal probability distributions converge the sequence of configurations generated by subsequent updating will in general never settle down. This finds an explanation in the law of large numbers below.

Convergence was first studied analytically in D. GEMAN and S. GEMAN (1984). These authors called the algorithm the **Gibbs sampler** since it samples from the local characteristics of a Gibbs field. Frequently, it is referred to as stochastic relaxation, although this term is also used for other (stochastic) algorithms which update site by site.

Proof (of Theorem 5.1.2). The Gibbs field $\mu = \Pi$ is invariant for its local characteristics by Theorem 5.1.1 and hence also for P. Moreover, $P(x, y)$ is strictly positive since in each $s \in S$ the probability to pick y_s is strictly positive. Thus the theorem is a special case of Theorem 4.3.1. □

There were no restrictions on the visiting scheme, except that it proposed sites in a strictly prescribed order. The sites may as well be chosen at random:

Let G be some probability distribution on S. Replace the local characteristics (5.1) in (5.2) by kernels

$$\tilde{\Pi}(x,y) = \begin{cases} G(s)\Pi_{\{s\}}(x,y) & \text{if } y_{S\backslash\{s\}} = x_{S\backslash\{s\}} \text{ for some } s \in S \\ 0 & \text{otherwise} \end{cases} \tag{5.3}$$

and let $\tilde{P} = \tilde{\Pi}^{\sigma}$. G is called the **proposal** or **exploration distribution**. Frequently G is the uniform distribution on S.

Theorem 5.1.3. *Suppose that G is strictly positive. Then*

$$\lim_{n\to\infty} \nu\tilde{P}^n(x) = \Pi(x)$$

for every $x \in \mathbf{X}$.

Irreducibility of G is also sufficient. Since we want to keep the introductory discussion simple, this concept will be introduced later.

Proof. Since G is strictly positive, detailed balance holds for Π and $\tilde{P}$ and hence Π is invariant for $\tilde{P}$. Again, $\tilde{P}$ is strictly positive and convergence follows from Theorem 4.3.1. □

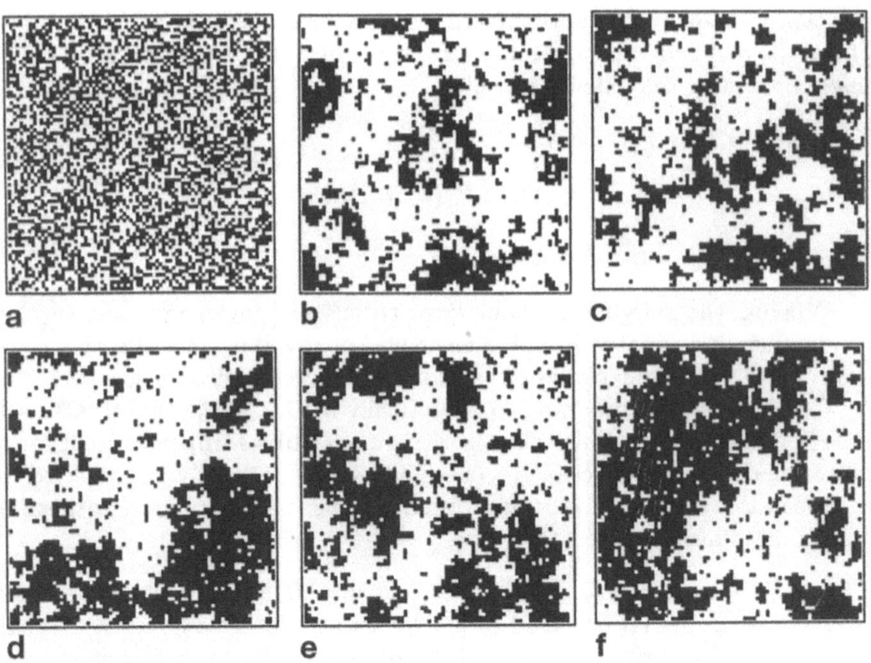

Fig. 5.1. Sampling at high temperature

Sampling from a Gibbs field yields 'typical' configurations. If, for instance, the regularity conditions for some sort of texture are formulated by means of an energy function then such textures can be synthesised by sampling from the associated Gibbs field. Such samples can then be used to test the quality of the model (cf. Chapter 12). Simple examples are shown in Chapter 3. Figs. 5.1 and 5.2 show states of the algorithm after various numbers of steps and for different parameters in the energy function. We chose the simple Ising model $H^{\beta}(x) = \beta \sum_{\langle s,t \rangle} x_s x_t$ on a 80×80-square lattice. In Fig. 5.1, we sampled from the Ising field at inverse temperature $\beta = 0.43$. Fig. (a) shows the pepper and salt initial configuration and (b)–(f) show the result after 400, 800, 1200, 1600 and 2000 sweeps. A raster scanning-visiting scheme was adopted, i.e. the sites were updated line by line from left to right (there are better visiting schemes). Similarly, Fig. 5.2 illustrates sampling at inverse temperature $\beta = 4.5$. Note that for high β the samples are considerably smoother than for low β. This observation is fundamental for the optimization method developed in the next section.

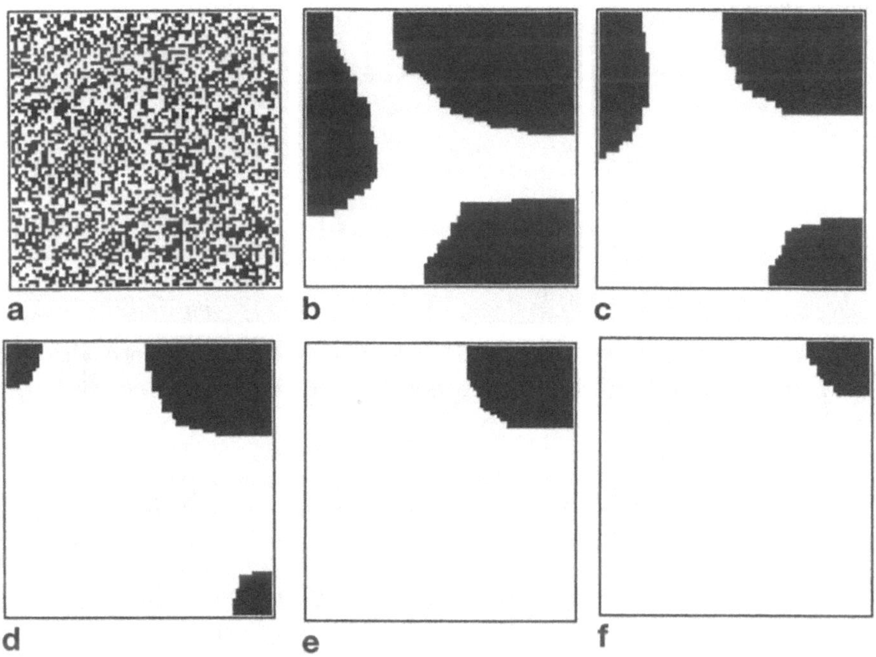

Fig. 5.2. Sampling at low temperature

Now we turn to the computation of MMS estimates, i.e. the expectations of posterior distributions. In a more abstract formulation, expectations of Gibbs distributions have to be computed or at least approximated. Recall that in general analytic approaches will fail even if the Gibbs distribution is known. In statistics, the standard approximation method exploits some law of large numbers. A typical version reads: Given independent random variables ξ_i with common law μ, the expectation $\mathsf{E}_{\mu}(f)$ of a function f on $\mathbf{X}$

w.r.t. μ can be approximated by the means in time $(1/n)\sum_{i=0}^{n-1} f(\xi_i)$ with high probability. Sampling independently for many times from Π by the Gibbs sampler is computationally too expensive and hence such a law of large numbers is not useful. Fortunately, the Gibbs sampler itself obeys the law of large numbers. The following notation will be adopted:

$$\delta_s = \sup\{|H(x) - H(y)| : x_{S\setminus\{s\}} = y_{S\setminus\{s\}}\}$$

is the **oscillation** of H at site s and

$$\Delta = \max\{\delta_s : s \in S\}$$

is the **maximal local oscillation** of H. Finally, (ξ_i) denotes a sequence of random variables the law of which is induced by the Markov chain in question.

Theorem 5.1.4. *Let the law of (ξ_i) be induced by (5.2) or (5.3). Then for every function f on $\mathbf{X}$,*

$$\frac{1}{n}\sum_{i=0}^{n-1} f(\xi_i) \longrightarrow \mathsf{E}_\Pi(f)$$

in L^2 and in probability. For every $\varepsilon > 0$,

$$\mathsf{P}\left(\left|\frac{1}{n}\sum_{i=0}^{n-1} f(\xi_i) - \mathsf{E}_\Pi(f)\right| > \varepsilon\right) \leq \frac{c}{n\varepsilon^2} e^{\sigma\Delta}$$

where $c = 13\|f\|^2$ for (5.2) and $c = 13\|f\|^2 \min_S G(s)^{-\sigma}$ for (5.3).

Proof. The Markov kernel P in (5.2) is strictly positive and hence Theorem 4.3.2 applies and yields L^2 convergence. For the law of large numbers, the contraction coefficient is estimated:

Given $x \in \mathbf{X}$, let z_s be a local minimizer in s, i.e.

$$H(z_s x_{S\setminus\{s\}}) = m_s = \min\{H(v_s x_{S\setminus\{s\}}) : v_s \in \mathbf{X}_s\}.$$

Then

$$\Pi_{\{s\}}(x, y_s x_{S\setminus\{s\}}) = \frac{\exp\left(-\left(H(y_s x_{S\setminus\{s\}}) - m_s\right)\right)}{\sum_{v_s\in\mathbf{X}_s} \exp\left(-\left(H(v_s x_{S\setminus\{s\}}) - m_s\right)\right)} \geq |\mathbf{X}|^{-1}\mathrm{e}^{-\delta_s}$$

and thus

$$\min_{x,y} P(x,y) \geq \prod_{s=1}^{\sigma} \left(|\mathbf{X}_s| e^{-\delta_s}\right) \leq |\mathbf{X}|^{-1}\mathrm{e}^{-\Delta\sigma}.$$

By the general estimate in Lemma 4.2.3,

$$c(P) \leq 1 - |\mathbf{X}| \cdot \min_{x,y} P(x,y) \leq 1 - \mathrm{e}^{-\Delta\sigma}. \tag{5.4}$$

This yields the law of large numbers for (5.2).

The proof for (5.3) requires some minor modifications which are left to the reader. □

Convergence holds even almost surely.

By the law of large numbers the expected value $\mathsf{E}(f)$ can be approximated by means of the values $f(x_1), f(x_2), \ldots, f(x_n)$ where x_k is the configuration of the Gibbs sampler after the k-th sweep. If the states are real numbers or vectors the means in time approximate the expected state. In particular, if Π is the posterior given data y then the expectation is the minimum mean squares estimate (cf. Chapter 1). The law of large numbers hence allows to compute approximations of MMSEs.

Sampling from Π amounts to the synthesis of typical configurations or 'patterns'. Thus *analysis* and *inference* is based on pattern *synthesis* or, in the words of U. GRENANDER, the above method realizes the maxim 'pattern analysis = pattern synthesis' (GRENANDER (1983), p. 61 and 71). We did not yet prove that this maxim holds for MAP estimators but we shall shortly see that it is true.

The law of large numbers implies that the algorithm cannot terminate with positive probability. In fact, in each state it spends a fraction of time proportional the probability of the state. To be more precise, let for each $x \in \mathbf{X}$,

$$A_{x,n} = \frac{1}{n} \sum_{i=0}^{n-1} 1_{\{x\}}(\xi_i)$$

be the relative frequency of visits in x in the first $n-1$ steps. Since $\mathsf{E}_\Pi(1_{\{x\}}) = \Pi(x)$, the theorem implies

Proposition 5.1.1. *Under the assumptions of Theorem 5.1.4, $A_{x,n} \longrightarrow \Pi(x)$ in probability.*

In particular, the Gibbs sampler visits each state infinitely often.

A final remark concerns the applicability of the contraction technique to continuous state spaces.

Remark 5.1.2. We mentioned in Remark 4.3.1 that the results extend to continuous state spaces. The problem is to verify the assumptions. Sometimes it is easy: Assume, for example, that all $\mathbf{X}_s$ are compact subsets of R^d with positive Lebesgue measure and let the Markov kernel be given by $P(x, dy) = f_x(y)\,dy$ with densities f_x. If the function $(x, y) \mapsto f_x(y)$ is continuous and strictly positive then it is bounded away from 0 by some real number $a > 0$ and by the continuous analogues of the Lemmata 4.2.1 through 4.2.3,

$$c(P) \leq 1 - a \int_{\mathbf{X}} dx < 1.$$

By compactness, P has an invariant distribution which by the argument in Theorem 5.1.2 for every initial distribution ν is the limit of νP^n in the norm of total variation.

For unbounded state space the theorems hold as well, but the estimate 4.2.3 usually is useless. If, for example, $\mathbf{X}$ is a subset of R^d with infinite

Lebesgue measure then $\inf_y f(y) = 0$ for every Lebesgue density f. Hence the contraction technique cannot be used e.g. in the important case of (compound) Gaussian fields. The following example shows this more clearly.

Let for simplicity $|S| = 1$ and $\mathbf{X} = \mathrm{R}$. A homogeneous Markov chain is defined by the Gaussian kernels

$$P(x, dy) = \frac{1}{\sqrt{2\pi(1-\rho^2)}} \exp\left(-\frac{(y-\rho x)^2}{2(1-\rho^2)}\right) dy,$$

$0 < \rho < 1$. This is the transition probability for the autoregressive sequence

$$\xi_n = \rho \xi_{n-1} + \eta_n$$

with a (Gaussian) white noise sequence (η_n) of mean 0 and variance $1 - \rho^2$ (similar processes play a role in texture synthesis which will be discussed later). It is not difficult to see that

$$\nu P^n(dy) \longrightarrow \frac{1}{\sqrt{2\pi}} \mathrm{e}^{-y^2/2}\, dy,$$

for every initial distribution ν, i.e. the marginals converge to the standard normal distribution. On the other hand, $c(P^n) = 1$ for every n. In fact, a straightforward induction shows that

$$P^n(x, dy) = \frac{1}{\sqrt{2\pi(1-\rho^{2n})}} \exp\left(-\frac{(y-\rho^n x)^2}{2(1-\rho^{2n})}\right)$$

and

$$\begin{aligned} c(P^n) &= 1 - \frac{1}{2} \int \sup_{x,x'} \frac{1}{\sqrt{2\pi(1-\rho^{2n})}} \\ &\quad \times \left| \exp\left(-\frac{(y-\rho^n x)^2}{2(1-\rho^{2n})}\right) - \exp\left(-\frac{(y-\rho^n x')^2}{2(1-\rho^{2n})}\right) \right| dy = 1. \end{aligned}$$

Hence Theorem 4.3.1 does not apply in this case. A solution can be obtained for example using Ljapunov functions (LASOTA and MACKEY (1985)).

5.2 Simulated Annealing

The computation of MAP estimators for Gibbs fields amounts to the minimization of energy functions. Surprisingly, a simple modification of the Gibbs sampler yields an algorithm which – at least theoretically – finds minima on the image spaces.

Let a function H on $\mathbf{X}$ be given. The function βH will for large β have the same minima as H but the minima are much deeper. Let us investigate what this means for the associated Gibbs fields.

Given an energy function H and a real number β, the Gibbs field for **inverse temperature** β is defined by

$$\Pi^{\beta}(x) = (Z^{\beta})^{-1}\exp(-\beta H(x)), Z^{\beta} = \sum_{z}\exp(-\beta H(z)).$$

Let M denote the set of (global) minimizers of H.

Proposition 5.2.1. *Let Π be a Gibbs field with energy function H. Then*

$$\lim_{\beta\to\infty}\Pi^{\beta}(x) = \begin{cases} \frac{1}{|M|} & \text{if } x \in M \\ 0 & \text{otherwise} \end{cases}.$$

For $x \in M$, the function $\beta \to \Pi^{\beta}(x)$ increases, and for $x \notin M$, it decreases eventually.

This is the first key observation: The Gibbs fields for inverse temperature β converge to the uniform distribution on global minimizers of H as β tends to infinity. Sampling from this distribution yields minima of H and sampling from Π^{β} at high β approximately yields minima.

Proof. Let m denote the minimal value of H. Then

$$\begin{aligned}\Pi^{\beta}(x) &= \frac{\exp(-\beta H(x))}{\sum_z \exp(-\beta H(z))} \\ &= \frac{\exp(-\beta(H(x)-m))}{\sum_{z:H(z)=m}\exp(-\beta(H(z)-m)) + \sum_{z:H(z)>m}\exp(-\beta(H(z)-m))}.\end{aligned}$$

If x or z is a minimum then the respective exponent vanishes whatever β may be and the exponential equals 1. The other exponents are strictly negative and their exponentials decrease to 0 as β tends to infinity. Hence the expression increases monotonically to $|M|^{-1}$ if x is a minimum and tends to 0 otherwise. Let now $x \notin M$ and set $a(y) = H(y) - H(x)$. Rewrite $\Pi^{\beta}(x)$ in the form

$$\left(|\{y : H(y) = H(x)\}| + \sum_{a(y)<0}\exp(-\beta a(y))) + \sum_{a(y)>0}\exp(-\beta a(y)))\right)^{-1}.$$

It is sufficient to show that the denominator eventually increases. Differentiation w.r.t β results in

$$\sum_{y:a(y)<0}(-a(y))\exp(-\beta a(y)) + \sum_{y:a(y)>0}(-a(y)\exp(-\beta a(y)).$$

The second term tends to zero and the first term to infinity as $\beta \nearrow \infty$. Hence the derivative eventually becomes positive which shows that $\beta \mapsto \Pi^{\beta}(x)$ decreases eventually. □

Remark 5.2.1. If $\beta \to 0$ the Gibbs fields Π^β converge to the uniform distribution on all of $\mathbf{X}$. In fact, in the sum

$$\tilde{Z}^\beta(x) = \sum_y \exp(-\beta(H(y) - H(x)))$$

each exponential converges to 1. Hence $\Pi^\beta(x) = \tilde{Z}^\beta(x)^{-1}$ converges to $|\mathbf{X}|^{-1}$. We conclude that for low β the states in different sites are almost independent.

Let now H be fixed. In the last section we learned that the Gibbs sampler for each Π^β converges. The limits in turn converge to the uniform distribution on the minima of H. Sampling from the latter yields minima. Hence it is natural to ask if increasing β in each step of the Gibbs sampler gives an algorithm which minimizes H. Basically, the answer is 'yes'. On the other hand, an arbitrary diagonal sequence from a sequence of convergent sequences with convergent limits in general does not converge to the limit of limits. Hence we must be careful.

Again, we choose a visiting scheme and write $S = \{1, \ldots, \sigma\}$. A **cooling schedule** is an increasing sequence of positive numbers $\beta(n)$. For every $n \geq 1$ a Markov kernel is defined by

$$P_n(x,y) = \Pi_{\{1\}}^{\beta(n)} \ldots \Pi_{\{\sigma\}}^{\beta(n)}(x,y)$$

where $\Pi_{\{k\}}^{\beta(n)}$ is the single-site local characteristic of $\Pi^{\beta(n)}$ in k. Given an initial distribution these kernels define an inhomogeneous Markov chain. The associated algorithm randomly picks an initial configuration and performs one sweep with the Gibbs sampler at temperature $\beta(1)$. For the next sweep inverse temperature is increased to $\beta(2)$ and so on.

Theorem 5.2.1. *Let $(\beta(n))_{n\geq 1}$ be a cooling schedule increasing to infinity such that eventually,*

$$\beta(n) \leq \frac{1}{\sigma\Delta} \ln n$$

where $\Delta = \max\{\delta_s : s \in S\}$. Then

$$\lim_{n\to\infty} \nu P_1 \ldots P_n(x) = \begin{cases} |M|^{-1} & \text{if } x \in M \\ 0 & \text{otherwise} \end{cases}$$

uniformly in all initial distributions ν.

The theorem is due to S. and D. GEMAN (1984). The proof below is based on DOBRUSHIN's contraction argument.

The following simple observation will be used.

Lemma 5.2.1. *Let $0 \leq a_n \leq b_n \leq 1$ for real sequences (a_n) and (b_n). Then $\sum_n a_n = \infty$ implies $\prod_n (1 - b_n) = 0$.*

Proof. The inequality

$$\ln x \leq x - 1 \quad \text{for} \quad x \geq 0$$

implies

$$\ln(1 - b_n) \leq \ln(1 - a_n) \leq -a_n.$$

By divergence of the sum, we have

$$\sum_n \ln(1 - b_n) = -\infty,$$

which is equivalent to

$$\prod_n (1 - b_n) = 0. \qquad \square$$

Proof (of the theorem). If there are $\beta(n)$ such that the assumptions of Theorem 4.4.1 hold for P_n and $\mu_n = \Pi^{\beta(n)}$ then the result follows from this theorem and Proposition 5.2.1

The Gibbs fields μ_n are invariant for the kernels P_n by Theorem 5.1.1. Since $(\beta(n))$ increases the sequences $(\mu_n(x))$, $x \in \mathbf{X}$, de- or increase eventually by Proposition 5.2.1 and hence (4.3) holds by Lemma 4.4.2. By (5.4),

$$c(P_n) \leq 1 - \mathrm{e}^{-\beta(\mathrm{n})\Delta\sigma}.$$

This allows to derive a sufficient condition for (4.7), i.e. $\prod_{k \geq i} c(P_k) = 0$ for all i. By Lemma 5.2.1, this holds if $\exp(-\beta(n)\Delta\sigma) \geq a_n$ for $a_n \in [0, 1]$ with divergent infinite sum. A natural choice is $a_n = n^{-1}$ and hence

$$\beta(n) \leq \frac{1}{\sigma\Delta} \ln n$$

for eventually all n is sufficient. This completes the proof. $\square$

Note that the logarithmic cooling schedule is somewhat arbitrary, since the crucial condition is

$$\sum_n \exp(-\beta(n)\Delta\sigma) = \infty.$$

For instance, inverse temperature may be kept constant for a while, then increased a bit and so on. Such piecewise constant schedules are frequently adopted in practice.

The result holds as well for the random visiting schemes in (5.3). Here $P_n = \left(\tilde{\Pi}^{\beta(n)}\right)^{\sigma}$ and

$$c(P_n) \leq 1 - \gamma \mathrm{e}^{-\beta(\mathrm{n})\Delta\sigma}$$

with $\gamma = \min_s G(s)^{\sigma}$. If G is strictly positive, then $\gamma > 0$ and

$$\gamma \exp(-\beta(n)\Delta\sigma) \geq \gamma n^{-1}.$$

Since $(\gamma n^{-1})_n$ has divergent infinite sum, the theorem is proved.

Note, that in contrast to many descent algorithms simulated annealing yields global minima and does not get trapped in local minima. In the present context, it is natural to call $x \in \mathbf{X}$ a **local minimum** if $H(y) > H(x)$ for every y which differs from X in precisely one site.

Remark 5.2.2. The algorithms were inspired by statistical physics. Large physical systems tend to states of minimal energy - called ground states - if cooled down carefully. These ground states usually are highly ordered like ice crystals or ferromagnets. The emphasis is on 'carefully'. For example if melted silicate is cooled too quickly one gets a metastable material called glass and not crystals which are the ground states.

Similarly, minima of the energy are found by the above algorithm only if β increases at most logarithmically. Otherwise it will be trapped in 'local minima'. This explains why the term 'annealing' is used instead of 'freezing'. The former means controlled cooling.

The parameter β was called inverse temperature, since it corresponds to the factor $(kT)^{-1}$ in physics where T is absolute temperature (cf. Chapter 3).

J. BRETAGNOLLE constructed an example which shows that the constant $(\Delta\sigma)^{-1}$ cannot be increased arbitrarily (cf. PRUM (1986), p. 181). On the other hand, better constants can be obtained exploiting knowledge about the energy landscape. Best constants for the closely related Metropolis annealing are given in Section 8.3.

A more general version will be developed in the next chapters. In particular, we shall see that it is not necessary to keep the temperature constant over the sweeps.

Remark 5.2.3. For continuous state spaces cf. Remark 5.1.2. A proof for the Gaussian case using Ljapunov functions can be found in JENG and WOODS (1990). HAARIO and SAKSMAN (1991) study (Metropolis) annealing in the general setting where the finite set $\mathbf{X}$ (equipped with the uniform distribution) is replaced by an arbitrary probability space $(\mathbf{X}, \mathcal{F}, m)$ and H is a bounded $\mathcal{F}$-measurable function. In particular, they show that one has to be careful generalizing Proposition 5.2.1: $\|\Pi^{\beta} - m|_M\| \to 0$ as $\beta \nearrow \infty$ if and only if $m(M) > 0$ ($m|_M$ denotes the restriction of m to M). A weak result holds if $m(M) = 0$.

Under the above cooling schedule, the Markov chain spends more and more time in minima of H. For the set M of minimizers of H let

$$A_n = \frac{1}{n} \sum_{i=0}^{n-1} 1_M(\xi_i)$$

be the fraction of time which the algorithm spends in the minima up to time $n-1$.

Corollary 5.2.1. *Under the assumptions of the theorem, A_n converges to 1 in probability.*

Proof. Plainly,

$$\mathsf{E}(A_n) = \frac{1}{n}\sum_{i=0}^{n-1} \mathsf{E}\left(1_M(\xi_i)\right) = \frac{1}{n}\sum_{i=0}^{n-1} \nu_i(M) \longrightarrow 1$$

as $n \to \infty$. Since $A_n \leq 1$, $\mathsf{P}(A_n \geq 1-\varepsilon) \to 1$ for every $\varepsilon > 0$. □

Hence the chain visits minima again and again.

Remark 5.2.4. We shall prove later that (for a slightly slower annealing schedule) the chain visits *each single* minimum again and again. In particular, it eventually leaves each minimum after a visit (at least if there are several global minima). Even if the energy levels are recorded at each step one cannot decide if the algorithm left a local or a global minimizer. Hence the algorithm *visits* global minima but *does not detect them* and thus there is no obvious criterion when to stop the algorithm. By the same reason, almost sure convergence cannot be expected in general.

Similarly, the probability to be in a minimum increases to 1.

Corollary 5.2.2. *Under the assumptions of the theorem,*

$$\mathsf{P}(H(\xi_n) = \min_x H(x)) \longrightarrow 1 \quad \textit{as} \quad n \to \infty.$$

Proof. Assume that H is not constant. Let $m = \min_x H(x)$. By the theorem,

$$\mathsf{E}(H(\xi_n) - m) = \sum_x (H(x) - m)\nu_n(x) \longrightarrow 0,$$

where ν_n denotes the law of ξ_n. Since $H(x) - m \geq 0$, for every $\varepsilon > 0$,

$$\mathsf{P}(H(\xi_n) - m \geq \varepsilon) \longrightarrow 0 \quad \text{as} \quad n \to \infty.$$

Let m' be the value of H strictly greater than but next to m. Choosing $\varepsilon = (m' - m)/2$ yields the result. □

5.3 Discussion

Keeping track of the constants in the proofs yields rough estimates for the speed of convergence.

For the homogeneous case the estimate (4.2) yields:

$$\|\nu P^n - \Pi\| \leq 2\rho^n$$

where $\rho = 1 - \exp(-\Delta\sigma)$ ($\geq c(P)$). If H is not constant then $\rho < 1$ and the Gibbs sampler converges with geometric rate.

For the inhomogeneous algorithm (4.5) and (4.6) imply the inequality

$$\begin{aligned} &\|\nu P_1 \dots P_n - \mu_\infty\| \qquad\qquad (5.5) \\ \leq\ & 2\prod_{k=1}^{n} c(P_k) + 2\max_{n\geq 1}\|\mu_\infty - \mu_n\| + \sum_{k=1}^{n}\|\mu_{k+1} - \mu_k\|. \end{aligned}$$

All three terms have to be estimated. Let us assume

$$\beta(k) = \frac{1}{\Delta\sigma}\ln k.$$

Then $c(P_k) \leq 1 - k^{-1}$ and hence

$$\prod_{k=i}^{n} c(P_k) \leq \prod_{k=i}^{n}(1 - k^{-1}) \leq \exp\left(-\sum_{k=i}^{n} k^{-1}\right) \leq \frac{i}{n}.$$

The second inequality holds because of $(1 - a) \leq \exp(-a)$ and the last one since

$$\begin{aligned} \ln(ni^{-1}) \leq \ln(n+1) - \ln i &= \sum_{k=i}^{n}(\ln(k+1) - \ln k) \\ = \sum_{k=i}^{n}\ln(1 + k^{-1}) &\leq \sum_{k=i}^{n} k^{-1}. \end{aligned}$$

For the rest we may and shall assume that the minimal value of H is 0. Let $\tilde{m}$ denote the value of H next to the best. Since convergence eventually is monotone the maximum in (5.5) eventually becomes $\|\mu_\infty - \mu_i\|$. If x is not minimal then

$$\exp(-\beta(i)H(x)) \leq \exp(-(\Delta\sigma)^{-1}\ln(i\tilde{m})) = i^{-\tilde{m}/(\Delta\sigma)}$$

and

$$|\mu_i(x) - \mu_\infty(x)| = \frac{\exp(-\beta(i)H(x))}{|M| + \sum^* \exp(-\beta(i)H(z))} \leq \frac{1}{|M|} i^{-\tilde{m}/(\Delta\sigma)}$$

(as before, $|M|$ is the number of global minima and $\sum^*$ extends over the non-minimal configurations z). For minimal x, the distance fulfills the inequality

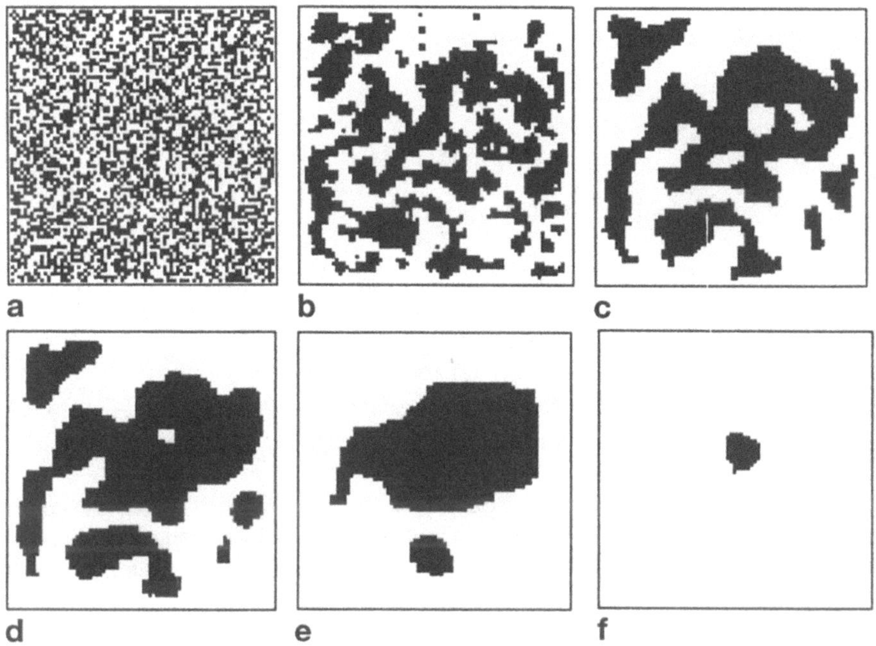

Fig. 5.3. Sampling from the Ising model

$$
\begin{aligned}
|\mu_i(x) - \mu_\infty(x)| &= \left| \frac{1}{|M| + \sum^* \exp(\beta(i)H(z))} - \frac{1}{|M|} \right| \\
&\leq \frac{\sum^*}{|M|^2} \leq \left(\frac{|\mathbf{X}| - |M|}{|M|^2} \right) i^{-\tilde{m}/(\Delta\sigma)}.
\end{aligned}
$$

Writing $f(n) = O(g(n))$ if $|f(n)| \leq c|g(n)|$, the last two inequalities read

$$\|\mu_i - \mu_\infty\| = O\left(i^{-\tilde{m}/(\Delta\sigma)}\right).$$

Finally, for large i the sum

$$\sum_{k=i}^{n} (\mu_{k+1}(x) - \mu_k(x))^+$$

either vanishes – if x is not minimal – or it is dominated by

$$
\begin{aligned}
|\mu_{n+1}(x) - \mu_i(x)| &\leq \|\mu_{n+1} - \mu_\infty\| + \|\mu_i - \mu_\infty\| \\
&\leq 2\|\mu_i - \mu_\infty\| = O\left(i^{-\tilde{m}/(\Delta\sigma)}\right).
\end{aligned}
$$

Hence a bound for the expressions in (5.5) is given by

$$\frac{i}{n} + \text{const}\, i^{-\alpha}, \quad \alpha = \frac{\tilde{m}}{\Delta\sigma}.$$

This becomes optimal for

$$i = (\alpha \cdot const)^{\frac{1}{\alpha+1}} n^{\frac{1}{\alpha+1}}$$

and since $\frac{\alpha}{\alpha+1} = \frac{\tilde{m}}{\tilde{m}+\Delta\sigma}$ we conclude

$$\|\nu P_1 \dots P_n - \mu_\infty\| = O\left(n^{-\tilde{m}/(\tilde{m}+\Delta\sigma)}\right).$$

Figure 5.3 illustrates the performance for the Ising model $H(x) = -\sum_{\langle s,t\rangle} x_s x_t$ on an 80×80 square lattice. Annealing was started with the random configuration (a). The configurations after 5, 15, 25, 100 and 550 sweeps of raster scanning are shown in Figs. (b)–(f). An optimum was reached after about 600 sweeps.

The Ising model is ill-famed for very slow convergence (cf. KINDERMANN and SNELL (1980)). This is caused by vast plateaus in the energy landscape and a lot of shallow local minima (a local minimum is a configuration the energy of which cannot be decreased changing the state in a single site). Although global minima seem to be quite different from local minima for the human observer, their energy is not much lower. Consider for instance the local minimum of size $n \times n$ in Fig. 5.4(a).

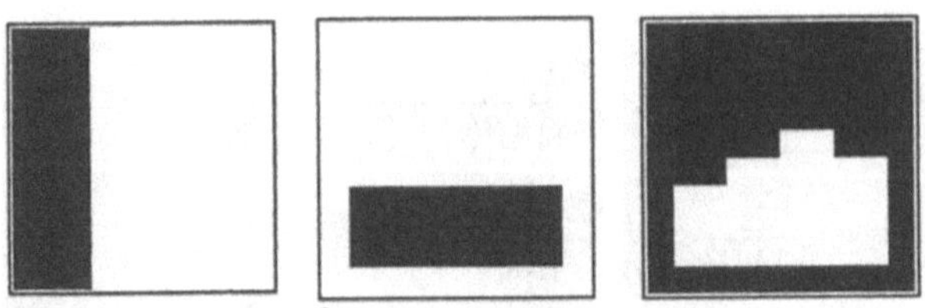

Fig. 5.4. Local minima of the Ising energy function

Its energy is $h = -2n(n-1) + 2n$. Let us follow the course of energy if we peel off the rightmost black coloumn. Flipping the uppermost pixel, two terms in the energy function of value 1 are replaced by two terms of value -1 and a -1 is replaced by a 1. This results in a gross increase of energy by 2. Flipping successively the next pixels does not change the energy until flipping the lowest pixel lowers the energy by 2 and we have again the energy h. The same happens if we peel off the next coloumns until we arrive at the left coloumn. Flipping the upper pixel does not change the energy (since -1 and 1 are replaced by 1 and -1). Flipping the next pixel lowers the energy by 2 each time and the last pixel contributes a decrease by 4 (the final energy is

$$h - (n-2)2 - 4 = -2n(n-1) + 2n - 2n + 4 - 4 = -2n(n-1)$$

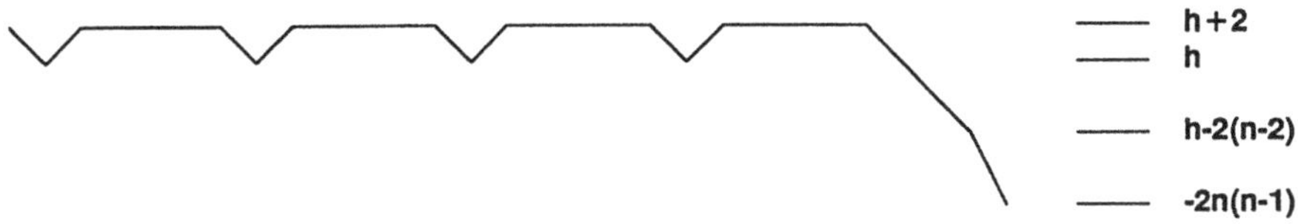

Fig. 5.5. Energy plateaus and local minima

which in fact is the energy of the white picture). The course of the energy is displayed in Fig. 5.5. The length of the plateaus is $n-2$ and increases linearly with the size of the picture. Simulated annealing has to travel across a flat country-side before it reaches a global minimum. Other local minima are shown in Fig. 5.4(b) and (c). Although this is an extreme example, similar effects can appear in nearly all applications. For Metropolis annealing, which is very similar to the algorithm developed here, the evolution of the n-step probabilities for a function with many minima (but in low dimension) is illustrated in the Figures 8.4–9.

Various steps are taken to arrive at faster algorithms. Let us mention some.

- Fast cooling. The logarithmic increase of inverse temperature and the small multiplicative constant may cause very slow convergence (on a small computer this may range from annoying to agonizing). So faster cooling schedules are adopted like $\beta(n) = n$ or $\beta(n) = \alpha^n$ for example with $\alpha = 1.01$ or $\alpha = 1.05$ (sometimes without mentioning, like in RIPLEY (1988)). Even $\beta(n) = \infty$ is a popular choice. This may give suboptimal results sufficient for practical purposes. Convergence to an optimum, on the other hand, is no longer guaranteed. We shall comment on fast cooling in the next chapter.
- Fast visiting schemes. The way one runs through S affects the finite time behaviour of annealing. For instance, if S is a finite square lattice then a 'chequer board' enumeration usually is preferable to raster scanning. Various random visiting schemes are adopted as well. There are only few papers in which visiting schemes are studied systematically (cf. AMIT and GRENANDER (1989)). For the Metropolis algorithm some remarks can be found in Chapter 8.
- Updating sets of sites. The number of steps is reduced updating sets of sites simultaneously i.e. using the local characteristics for sets instead of singletons. On the other hand, computation time increases for each single step. Nevertheless, this may pay off in special cases. This method is studied in Chapter 7.
- Special algorithms. In general, the Gibbs sampler is not recommendable if the number of states is large. A popular alternative is the Metropolis sampler which will be discussed in Chapter 8. Sometimes approximations, for example Gaussian, or variants of basic algorithms provide faster convergence. For instance for the Ising model, SWENDSON and WANG (1987)

proposed an algorithm which changes whole clusters of sites simultaneously and thus improves speed considerably (cf. Section 10.1.2).

- Partially synchroneous updating. An obvious way of speeding up is partially parallel implementation. Suppose that H is given by a neighbour potential. Suppose further that S is partitioned into disjoint totally disconnected sets $S_1, \ldots, S_r$, i.e. the S_j do not contain any neighbours. Then the sites in each S_j are conditionally independent and updating the sites in S simultaneously does not affect convergence of the algorithm. For instance in the Ising model, S can be divided into two totally disconnected sets and partially parallel implementation theoretically reduces the computation time of sequential implementation by a factor $2/|S|$. In the near future, parallel computers will be available at low cost (as compared to bigger sequential machines) and partially parallel algorithms will become more and more relevant.
- Synchroneous updating. Simultaneous application of the single-site local characteristics (instead of the sequential one), technically is one of the most appealing methods. In general, such algorithms neither sample from the desired distribution nor give minima of the objective function in question. Presently there is a lot of research on such problems, cf. AZENCOTT (1992a). Synchroneous algorithms will be studied in some detail in Chapter 10.
- Adapting models. Models frequently are chosen to keep computation time within reasonable limits. Such a procedure must carefully be commented in order to prevent misinterpretations.

6. Cooling Schedules

Annealing with the theoretical cooling schedule may work very slowly. Therefore, in practice faster cooling schedules are adopted. We shall compare the results of such algorithms with exact MAP estimations.

6.1 The ICM Algorithm

To get a feeling what happens for fast cooling, consider the extreme case of infinite inverse temperature. Fix a configuration $x \in \mathbf{X}$ and an index set $I \subset S$. The local characteristic for Π^β on I has the form

$$\Pi_I^\beta(x,y) = \begin{cases} (Z_I^\beta)^{-1}\exp(-\beta H(y_I x_{S\backslash I})) & \text{if } y_{S\backslash I} = x_{S\backslash I}, \\ 0 & \text{otherwise,} \end{cases}$$

$$Z_I^\beta = \sum_{z_I} \exp(-\beta H(z_I x_{S\backslash I})).$$

Denote by $N_I(x)$ the set of I-neighbours of x, i.e. those configurations which coincide with x off I. Let $M_I(x)$ be the set of I-neighbours which minimize H when x runs through $N_I(x)$. Like in Lemma 5.2.1,

$$\Pi_I^\beta(x, y_I x_{S\backslash I}) \longrightarrow \begin{cases} |M_I(x)|^{-1} & \text{if } y_I x_{S\backslash I} \in M_I(x) \\ 0 & \text{otherwise} \end{cases}, \quad \beta \to \infty.$$

In the visiting schemes considered previously, the sets I were singletons $\{s\}$. Sampling from $\Pi_{\{s\}}^\beta$ at $\beta = \infty$ can be described as follows: Given $x \in \mathbf{X}$, pick $y_s \in \mathbf{X}_s$ uniformly at random from the set

$$\{y_s : H(y_s x_{S\backslash\{s\}}) = \min\{H(z_s x_{S\backslash\{s\}}) : z_s \in \mathbf{X}_s)\}\}$$

and choose $y_s x_{S\backslash\{s\}}$ as the new configuration.

Sampling from the limit distribution hence gives a s-neighbour of minimal energy and sequential updating boils down to a coordinatewise 'greedy' algorithm. Call $y \in \cup_s N_s(x)$ a neighbour of x. The greedy algorithm gets trapped in basins of configurations which do not have neighbours of lower energy, i.e. in **local minima**.

The greedy algorithm usually terminates in a local minimum next to the initial configuration after few sweeps. The result sensitively depends on the initial configuration and on the visiting scheme. Despite of its obvious drawbacks, 'zero temperature sampling' is a popular method since it is fast and easy to implement.

Though coordinatewise maximal descent is common in combinatorial optimization, in the statistical community, it is frequently ascribed to J. BESAG (1983) (it was independently described in J. KITTLER und J. FÖGLEIN (1984)) who called it 'the method of iterated conditional modes' or, shorter, the **ICM-method**. In fact, updating in s results in a maximum of the single-site conditional probability, i.e. in a **conditional mode**. BESAG's motivation came from estimation rather than optimization. He and others do not mainly view zero temperature sampling as an extreme case of annealing but as an estimator in its own right (besides MAP, MPM and other estimators). We feel that this estimator is difficult to analyse in a general context, since it strongly depends on the special form of the Gibbs field in question, the initial configuration and the visiting scheme.

In Fig. 6.2, convergence to local minima of the ICM algorithm is illustrated and contrasted with the performance of annealing in Fig. 6.1. We use the simple Ising model like in the last chapter. Both algorithms are started with a configuration originally black on the left third and white on the rest and degraded by independently flipping the colours (Figs. 6.1(a) and 6.2(a)). Figs. (b)–(f) show the configurations of annealing and steepest descent, respectively, after m=5, 15, 25, 100 and 400 sweeps. Note the large number of steps between the similar configurations in Figs. 6.2(e) and (f). The arguments in Section 5.3 suggest that the greedy algorithm is rather inefficient near plateaus in the energy landscape and there we are.

Remark 6.1.1. It is our concern here, to *compare algorithms*, more precisely, their ability to minimize a function (in the examples $H(x) = -\alpha \sum_{\langle s,t \rangle} x_s x_t$, $\alpha > 0$). We are not discussing 'restoration' of an image from the data in the Figs. (a) (as a cursory glance at Fig. 6.2 might suggest).

Better results are obtained with better initial configurations. To find them one can run annealing for a while or use some classical method. For instance, for data y and configurations x living on the same lattice S (like in restoration), BESAG (1986), 2.5, suggests to choose the initial configuration $x^{(0)}$ for the ICM algorithm according to a conventional maximum likelihood method, which at each site s chooses a maximizer $x_s^{(0)}$ of $\mathsf{P}(x_s|y_s)$ (many commercial systems use the configuration found this way as the final output; cf. Section 12.4.3).

Remark 6.1.2. A correctly implemented annealing algorithm can degenerate to a greedy algorithm at high inverse temperature because of the following effect:

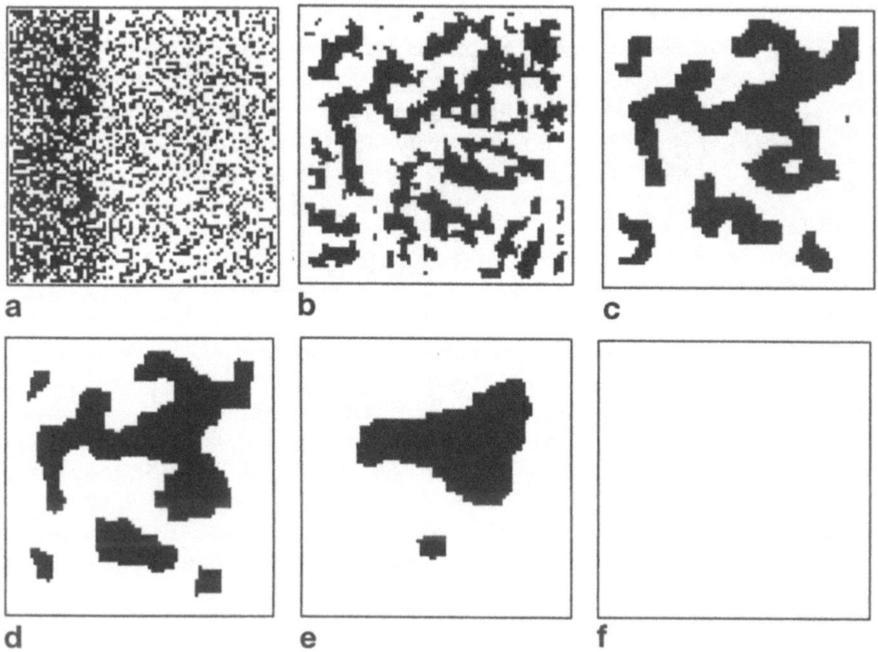

Fig. 6.1. Various steps of SA

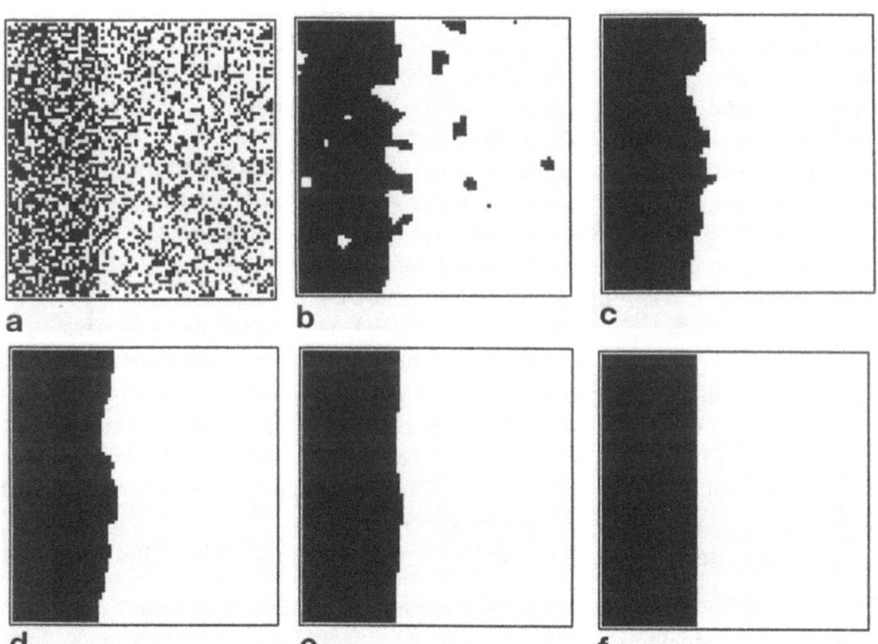

Fig. 6.2. Various steps of ICM

Let $x \in \mathbf{X}$, $s \in S$ and β be given and set $p^{\beta}(g) = \Pi^{\beta}_{\{s\}}(gx_{S\backslash\{s\}})$. Assume that a random number generator (cf. Appendix A) picks a number *rnd* uniformly at random from $R = \{1, \ldots, maxrand\} \subset \mathsf{N}$. The interval $(0, maxrand] \subset \mathsf{R}$ is partitioned into subintervals I_g – one for each grey value – of length $p^{\beta}(g) \cdot maxrand$, respectively, and h with $rnd \in I_h$ is taken as the new grey value in s. Let M_s be the set of all grey values maximizing p^{β}. Since $p^{\beta}(g)$ decreases to 0 for each $g \notin M_s$, for large β,

$$\sum_{g \notin M_s} p^{\beta}(g) \cdot maxrand < 1.$$

If the I_g are ordered according to their length then

$$\left(\bigcup_{g \notin M_s} I_g \right) \cap R = \emptyset$$

and one always gets a $g \in M_s$.

6.2 Exact MAPE Versus Fast Cooling

Annealing with the theoretic cooling schedule and the coordinatewise greedy algorithm are extreme cases in the variety of intermediate schedules. A popular choice, for example, are **exponential cooling** schedules $\beta(n) = A\rho^n$, $A > 0$ and $\rho > 1$ but close to 1. Too little is known about their performance (for some recent results due to O. Catoni cf. Azencott (1992), Chapter 3). They are difficult to analyze for several reasons. The outcomes depend on the initial configuration, on the visiting scheme and on the number of sweeps. Moreover, in general the exact estimate (say the MAP estimate) is not known and it is hard to say what the estimator and the outcome of an algorithm have in common. Experiments by Greig, Porteous and Seheult (1986) and (1989) shed some light on these questions.

The authors adopt the prior model $\Pi(x) = Z^{-1} \exp(\alpha \cdot v(x))$ with $x_s \in \{0, 1\}$ where $v(x)$ is the number of neighbour pairs with like colours (for the neighbourhood system comprising the eight adjacencies of each pixel except for the boundary modifications). They compare exact MAP estimates with the outcome of annealing under various cooling schedules. The algorithms are applied to the posterior for Gaussian and channel noise and then the error rates and other relevant quantities are contrasted.

To compute exact MAP estimates the Ford-Fulkerson algorithm is adopted.

Example 6.2.1 (Ford-Fulkerson Algorithm). To binary scenes and Ising type priors the classical Ford-Fulkerson algorithm from linear optimization applies. Though limited in application, this method is extremely useful for testing other – for example stochastic – algorithms which in general are suboptimal only.

Consider binary images $x \in \{-1,1\}^S$ on a finite lattice with prior

$$H(x) = -\sum_{\langle s,t\rangle} b_{st}[x_s x_t].$$

Notation is simplified by transformation into the function

$$H(x) = -\sum_{\langle s,t\rangle} b_{st}\left[x_s x_t + (1-x_s)(1-x_t)\right].$$

where $x_s \in \{0,1\}$. In fact, in both expressions the terms in square brackets have value 1 if $x_s = x_t$ and values -1 and 0, respectively, if $x_s \neq x_t$, and hence they are equivalent. For channel noise, the observation y is governed by the law

$$P(x,y) = \prod_s p(1,y_s)^{x_s} p(0,y_s)^{1-x_s}$$

and the posterior distribution is proportional to

$$\exp\left(\sum_s \lambda_s x_s + \sum_{\langle s,t\rangle} b_{st}\left[x_s x_t (1-x_s)(1-x_t)\right]\right)$$

where $\lambda_s = \ln(p(1,y_s)/p(0,y_s))$. The MAP estimate is computed by minimization of the posterior energy function

$$H(x|y) = -\sum_s \lambda_s x_s - \sum_{\langle s,t\rangle} b_{st}[x_s x_t + (1-x_s)(1-x_t)].$$

This optimization problem can be transformed into the problem of finding minimal cuts in networks:

The network is a graph with $|S|+2$ nodes – one node for each pixel and two additional nodes ρ and σ called source and sink. An arrow is drawn from the source ρ to each pixel s for which $\lambda_s > 0$. One may think of such an arrow as a pipe-line through which a liquid can flow from ρ to s; its capacity, i.e. the maximal possible flow from ρ to s is $c_{\rho s} = \lambda_s$. Similarly, there are arrows from pixels s with $\lambda_s < 0$ to the sink σ with capacity $c_{s\sigma} = -\lambda_s$. To complete the graph, one draws arrows between pairs s,t of neighbouring pixels with capacity $c_{st} = b_{st}$ (into each direction). Given a binary image x, the colours define a partition of the nodes into the two sets

$$\begin{aligned}\{\rho\}\cup\{s\in S : x_s = 1\} &= \{\rho\}\cup B(x),\\ \{s\in S : x_s = 0\}\cup\{\sigma\} &= W(x)\cup\{\sigma\}.\end{aligned}$$

Conversely, from such a partition the image can be reconstructed: black pixels are on the source-side, i.e. in $B(x)$, and white pixels are on the sink-side, i.e. in $W(x)$. The maximal possible flow from $\{\rho\}\cup B$ to $W\cup\{\sigma\}$ is

$$C(x) = \sum_{s \to t} c_{st}$$

where summation extends over $s \in \{\rho\} \cup B$ and $t \in W \cup \{\sigma\}$ for which there is an arrow from s to t. Evaluation of the function C gives

$$\begin{aligned} C(x) &= \sum_{t \in W, \lambda_s > 0} c_{\rho t} + \sum_{s \in B, \lambda_s < 0} c_{s\sigma} + \sum_{s \in B, t \in W} c_{st} \\ &= \sum_{s \in S} (1 - x_s)(\lambda_s \vee 0) + \sum_{s \in S} x_s(-\lambda_s \vee 0) + \sum_{\langle s,t \rangle} b_{st}(x_s - x_t)^2 \end{aligned}$$

where $a \vee b$ denotes the maximum of the real numbers a and b. Since $a \vee 0 - (-a) \vee 0 = a$ and $x_s^2 = x_s$,

$$\begin{aligned} C(x) &= -\sum_s \lambda_s x_s + \sum_s \lambda_s \\ &\quad + \left(\sum_{\langle s,t \rangle} b_{st}(x_s^2 + x_t^2 - 2x_s x_t) - \sum_{\langle s,t \rangle} b_{st} \right) + \sum_{\langle s,t \rangle} b_{st} \\ &= \sum_s \lambda_s x_s - \sum_{\langle s,t \rangle} b_{st}(x_s x_t + (1 - x_s)(1 - x_t)) + c \\ &= H(x|y) + c \end{aligned}$$

where the constant c does not depend on x. Hence we are done if we find minimizers of C, i.e. minimizing partitions $\rho \cup B(x)$, $W(x) \cup \{\sigma\}$. There are efficient algorithms for the exact computation of such 'cuts' with minimal value $C(x)$. The basic version is due to FORD and FULKERSON (1962) (cf. also most introductions to operations research). The DMKM-algorithm is a considerable improvement (DINIC (1970), MALHORTA, KUMAR and MAHESHWARI (1978); a detailed analysis can be found in MEHLHORN (1984)).

Although extremely useful for theoretical reasons, this approach is rather limited in application. Any attempt to incorporate edge sites like in Chapter 2 will in general render the network method inapplicable. Similarly, the multicolour problem cannot be dealt with by this method. For large images, the computational load is remarkable.

GREIG, PORTEOUS and SEHEULT (1986), (1989) contrast the outcomes of the following algorithms:

- the (exact) Ford Fulkerson algorithm,
- annealing with logarithmic schedules of the form $\beta(k) = C \cdot \ln(1+k)$ where k ranges from 1 to K, for several values of C and K,
- geometric schedules of the form $\beta(k)^{-1} = A\rho^{k-1}$ with $A = 2(\ln 2)^{-1}$ and K chosen such that the final inverse temperature is greater than 100,
- the ICM method for 8 iterations.

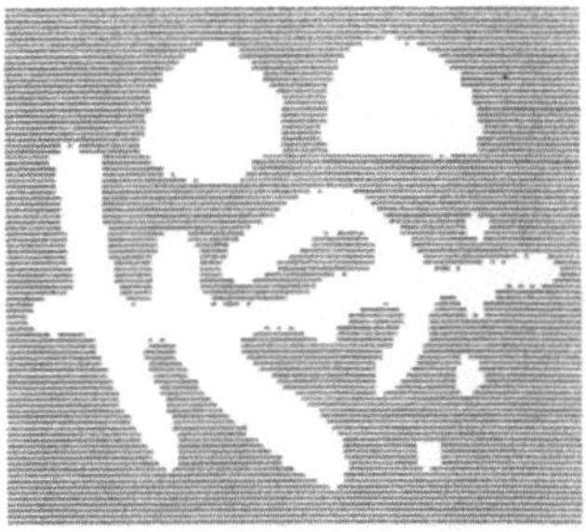

Fig. 6.3. True two-colour scene: 88 × 100; from BESAG (1986), by courtesy of A.H. SEHEULT, Durham, and The Royal Statistical Society, London

Two synthetic binary scenes are used. The first one shows some white islands in a black sea on a 88 × 100 lattice. It is displayed in Fig. 6.3.

Records are created by adding independent Gaussian noise of mean zero and with variance 0.9105 leading to a 30% expected misclassification rate for the maximum likelihood classifier. The misclassification rates are summarized in Table 6.1.

Table 6.1

α	MAP	annealing						ICM
		logarithmic			geometric			
		$C=$ 0.5	$C=$ 0.5	$C=$ 0.25	$\rho=$ 0.95	$\rho=$ 0.99	$\rho=$ 0.995	
		$K=$ 5000	$K=$ 750	$K=$ 5000	$K=$ 112	$K=$ 565	$K=$ 1131	
0.3	5.5	6.1	6.3	8.1	5.7	5.6	5.4	7.6
0.5	6.7	6.0	5.8	7.0	5.6	5.6	5.8	6.4
0.7	9.5	7.7	7.3	8.5	6.6	7.1	7.7	7.0
0.9	16.8	9.7	9.5	11.4	8.0	9.7	9.2	7.7
1.1	27.1	12.2	11.7	14.2	9.5	10.8	12.1	8.3

The first coloumn confirms our intuition that smoothing by an Ising prior does not restore a degraded image, and once more illustrates the sensitive dependence of MAP estimates on the smoothing parameter α. The error rate generally is a U-shaped function of α for all estimators. For logarithmic schedules, the misclassification rates for slower cooling are closer to the rates of the exact estimates. For weak coupling the rates are comparable while for large α they are far apart: this corresponds to the fact that equilibriums are reached faster at high than at low temperature. Increasing the number of sweeps improves the results (and gives worse 'restorations'). Nevertheless, the rates are far from the exact ones and 5000 sweeps are not enough, at least for strong coupling. In this case, geometric schedules are much too fast and, plainly, ICM then is not a good method to compute MAP estimates (and thus – following BESAG – should be considered as an own estimator).

Further examples are displayed in Fig. 6.4(a)–(f). Exact MAP estimates in the left coloumn are contrasted with the 750th iteration of annealing for

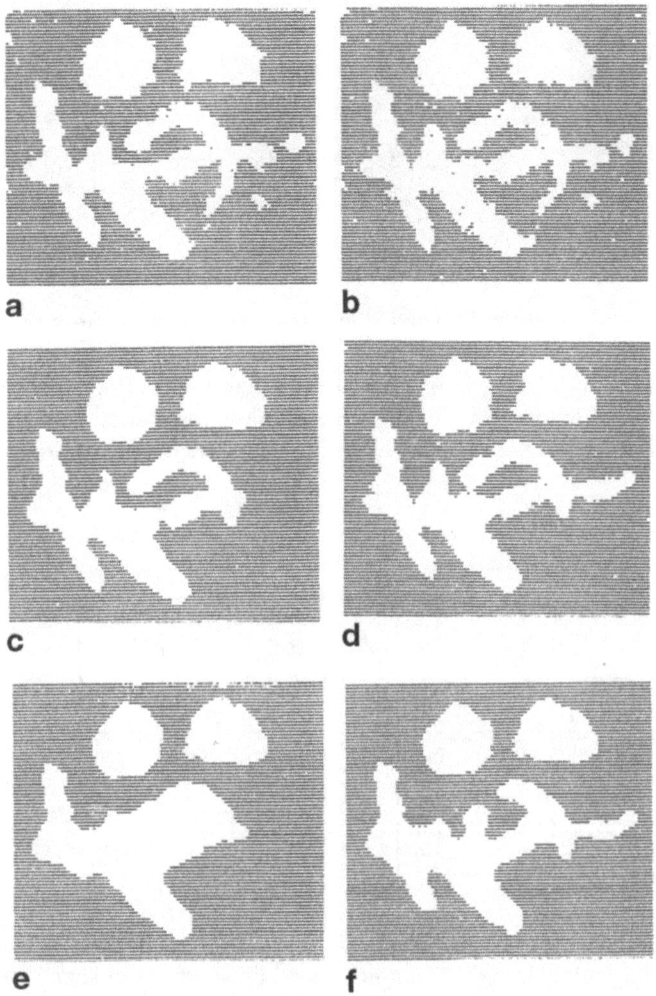

Fig. 6.4. (**a**) MAP estimate: $\alpha = 1/3$, 5% error rate; (**b**) simulated annealing: $\alpha = 1/3$, 5.5% error rate; (**c**) MAP estimate: $\alpha = 1/2$, 6.4% error rate; (**d**) simulated annealing: $\alpha = 1/2$, 5.8% error rate; (**e**) MAP estimate: $\alpha = 2/3$, 10.2% error rate; (**f**) simulated annealing: $\alpha = 2/3$, 7.6% error rate. From BESAG (1986), by courtesy of A.H. SEHEULT, Durham, and The Royal Statistical Society, London

inverse temperature schedule $\beta(n) = (\ln(1+n))/2$ in the right coloumn. The different values of α are given in the caption. For further comments cf. GREIG, PORTEOUS and SEHEULT (1986), pp. 282–284.

The second scene is a bold letter 'A' on a 64×64-lattice and the records are created by applying a binary channel with 25% error rate (i.e. flip probability 1/4). The results in Table 6.2 support the above conclusions. Some of the corresponding image estimates are displayed in Fig. 6.5.

Table 6.2

α	MAP	annealing				ICM
		logarithmic		geometric		
		$C=$ 0.5	$\rho=$ 0.95	$\rho=$ 0.99	$\rho=$ 0.995	
		$K=$ 750	$K=$ 112	$K=$ 565	$K=$ 1131	
0.3	5.2	6.6	5.3	5.3	5.4	6.9
0.7	9.6	7.9	7.2	7.2	7.2	6.4
1.1	22.8	10.4	9.1	10.6	11.1	6.3

Fig. 6.3 is taken from BESAG (1986), p. 277, Fig. 6.4 from p. 283 in the same reference, and Fig. 6.5 from GREIG, PORTEOUS and SEHEULT (1989), p. 274. The author is indebted to A.H. SEHEULT, University of Durham, and to the ROYAL STATISTICAL SOCIETY, London, for kind permission to reprint these Figures.

In the last example, a standard algorithm was applied to a problem in imaging. Conversely, the following algorithm is specially tailored for a problem in image restoration. The idea of gradient descent is pushed through for special functions with many local minima. We give a rough sketch of this method.

Example 6.2.2 (The GNC Algorithm). A model for edge preserving restoration of noisy pictures was discussed in Chapter 2. We shall continue with notation from Example 2.3.1. For quadratic disparity function Ψ, fixed penalty α for each break and additive white Gaussian noise the posterior energy is

$$\begin{aligned} H(x,b) &= H_1(x,b) + H_2(b) + D(x) \\ &= \lambda^2 \sum_{\langle s,t\rangle} (x_s - x_t)^2 (1 - b_{\langle st\rangle}) + \alpha \sum_{\langle s,t\rangle} b_{\langle s,t\rangle} + \sum_s (y_s - x_s)^2. \end{aligned}$$

The GNC-algorithm (graduated non-convexity) approximates global minima of *this special* H by local minima of suitable approximating functions (BLAKE (1983), BLAKE and ZISSERMAN (1987)).

The variables x_s take real values and hence the GNC algorithm does not lend itself to discrete-valued problems. In a preliminary step, the binary line process is eliminated. Since D does not depend on b one has

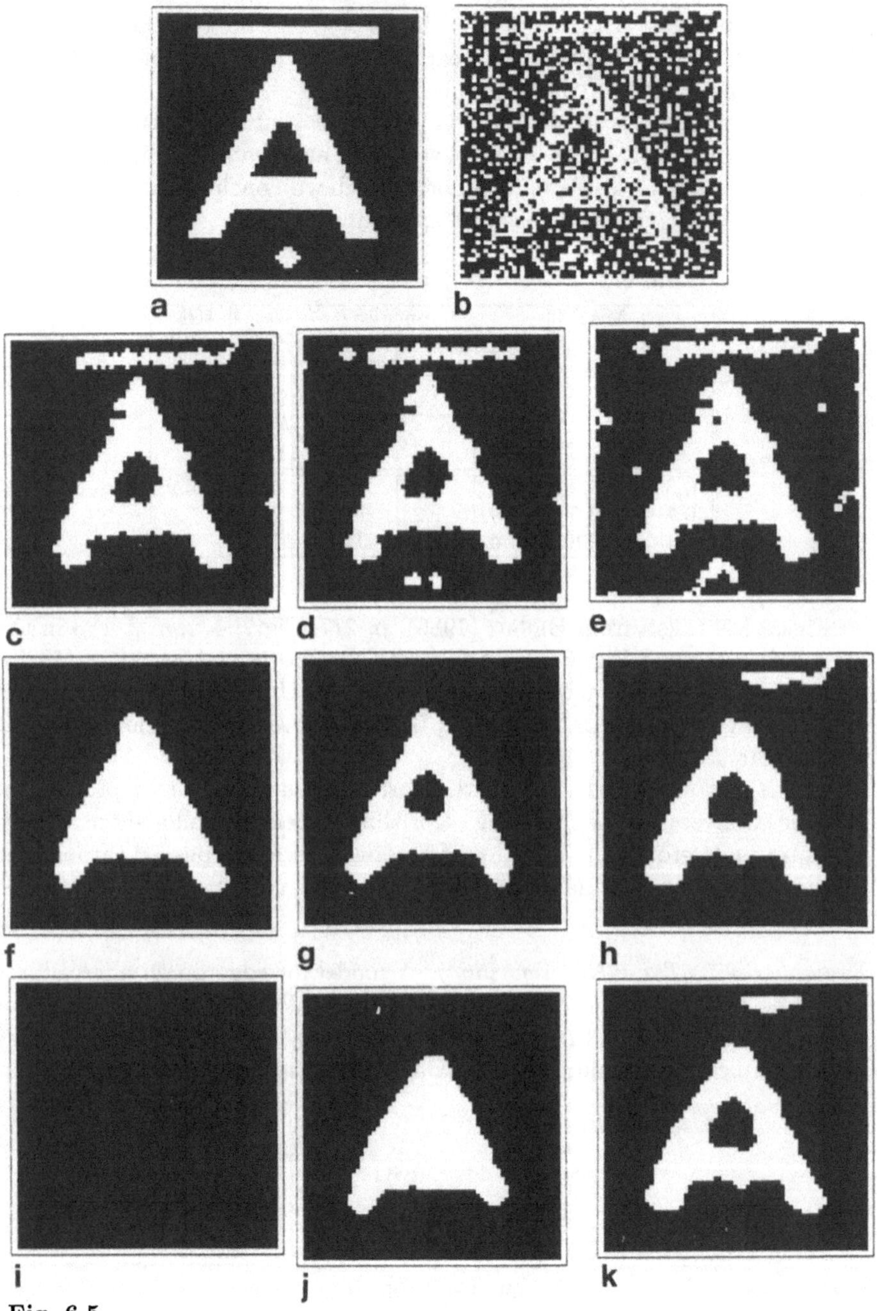

Fig. 6.5.

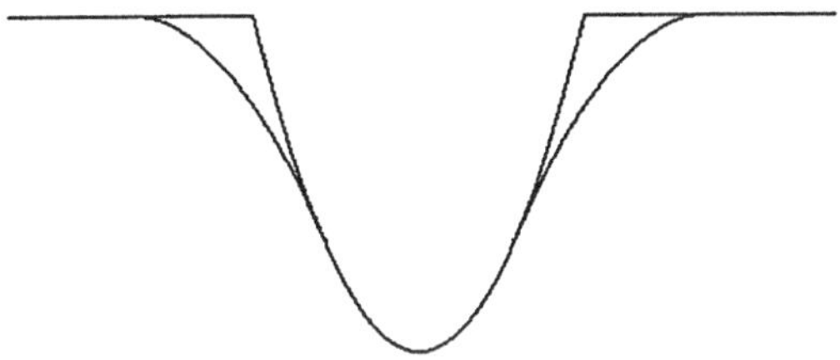

Fig. 6.6.

$$\min_{x,b} H(x,b) = \min_{x} \left(D(x) + \min_{b} \sum_{\langle s,t \rangle} h(x_s - x_t, b_{\langle s,t \rangle}) \right)$$

where

$$h(\Delta, l) = \lambda^2 \Delta^2 (1 - l) + \alpha \cdot l.$$

Hence for each x one may first minimize the terms in the sum separately in $b_{\langle s,t \rangle}$ to get the minimum over b and then minimize in x. For the first step let

$$g(\Delta) = \min_{l \in \{0,1\}} h(\Delta, l).$$

Since $h(\Delta, 1) = \alpha$ and $h(\Delta, 0) = \lambda^2 \Delta^2$, $g(\Delta)$ equals $\lambda^2 \Delta^2$ if $\lambda^2 \Delta^2 \leq \alpha$, i.e. if $|\Delta| \leq \sqrt{\alpha}\lambda^{-1}$, and the constant α otherwise. This way, the problem is reduced to the minimization of

$$G(x) = D(x) + \sum_{\langle s,t \rangle} g(x_s - x_t).$$

The function g is approximated from below by the following functions:

$$g^{(p)} = \begin{cases} \lambda^2 \Delta^2 & \text{if } |\Delta| \leq (p) \\ \alpha - (c(p)/2)\left(|\Delta| - r(p)\right)^2 & \text{if } q(p) \leq |\Delta| \leq r(p) \\ \alpha & \text{if } |\Delta| \geq r(p) \end{cases}$$

Figure 6.5 (**a**) True 64 × 64 binary scene; (**b**) true scene corrupted by a binary channel with 25% error rate; (**c**) exact MAP estimate ($\alpha = 0.3$); (**d**) simulated annealing estimate with geometric schedule $A\rho^{k-1}$ ($k = 1, \ldots, K$), with $A = 2/\ln 2$, $\rho = 0.99$ and $K = 565$ ($\alpha = 0.3$); (**e**) ICM estimate ($\alpha = 0.3$); (**f**) exact MAP estimate ($\alpha = 0.7$); (**g**) simulated annealing estimate with geometric schedule $A\rho^{k-1}$ ($k = 1, \ldots, K$), with $A = 2/\ln 2$, $p = 0.99$ and $K = 565$ ($\alpha = 0.7$); (**h**) ICM estimate ($\alpha = 0.7$); (**i**) exact MAP estimate ($\alpha = 1.1$); (**j**) simulated annealing estimate with geometric schedule $A\rho^{k-1}$ ($k = 1, \ldots, K$), with $A = 2/\ln 2$; $\rho = 0.99$ and $K = 565$ ($\alpha = 1.1$); (**k**) ICM estimate ($\alpha = 1.1$). From GREIG, PORTEOUS and SEHEULT (1989), by courtesy of A.H. SEHEULT, Durham, and The Royal Statistical Society, London where

$$c(p) = cp^{-1}, \ r(p)^2 = \alpha(2c(p)^{-1} + \lambda^2), \ q(p) = \alpha\lambda^{-2}r(p)^{-1}$$

and c is some constant (cf. Fig. 6.6).

Plainly, the sequence $\left(g^{(p)}\right)$ increases pointwise to g as p decreases to 0. Hence the sequence of functions

$$G^{(p)}(x) = D(x) + \sum_{\langle s,t\rangle} g^{(p)}(x_s - x_t)$$

increases to G. There is a constant c such that $G^{(1)}$ is strictly convex and hence has a unique minimum $x^{(1)}$. Starting from this minimum, local minima $x^{(p)}$ of the $G^{(p)}$ are tracked continuously as p varies from 1 to 0. Under reasonable hypothesis, the net $(x^{(p)})$ converges to a global minimum of G. In practice, a discrete sequence $(p(n))_n$ is used and each $G^{(p(n))}$ is minimized by some descent algorithm using the local minimum $x^{(p(n))}$ of $G^{(p(n-1))}$ as the starting point. For a discussion, proofs and applications we refer to the detailed treatment by A. BLAKE and A. ZISSERMAN (1987). For those interested in restoration or optimization, this book is a must.

There are also several studies comparing simulated annealing and the GNC algorithm for restoration. The latter applies to real-valued problems only. KASHKO (1987) shows that GNC requires about the same computational effort to solve a real-valued reconstruction problem in two dimensions (cf. Example 2.3.1) as annealing does to perform a similar Boolean-valued reconstruction. For a special one-dimensional reconstruction, BLAKE (1989) compares GNC to several types of annealing like the Gibbsian version and two Metropolis algorithms. Plainly, the specially tailored GNC algorithm wins. This underlines the demand to construct fast exact algorithms as soon as a (Bayesian) method is developed to a degree where it applies in practice to a well-defined class of problems.

Fig. 6.7 symbolically displays what can be expected from the various algorithms.

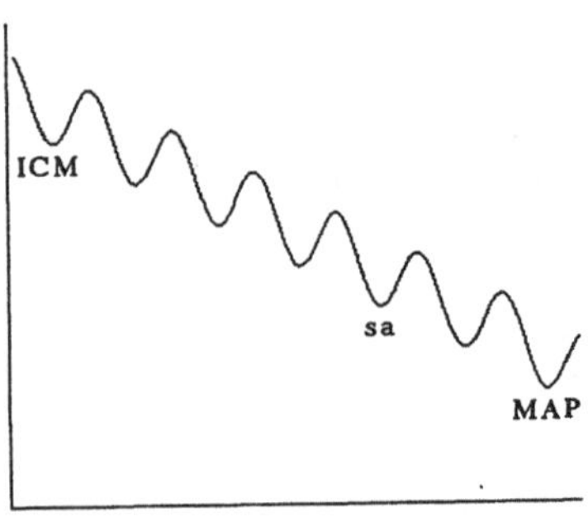

Fig. 6.7.

Here 'sa' means simulated annealing for realistic constants and cooling schedules. MAP is reached for the theoretical schedules only. In fact, a celebrated result by HAJEK (1988) provides a necessary condition for $\mathsf{P}(\xi_n \text{ minimal}) \to 1$ (cf. Theorem 8.3.1). It is violated by exponential schedules as soon as H has a proper local minimum.

6.3 Finite Time Annealing

This introduction is no manual for the intended or practical annealer. Nevertheless let us shortly comment on the notion of 'finite time annealing'. This is important, since resources are limited and there is a bounded amount of available CPU time.

It is not obvious that the theoretical (logarithmic) cooling schedule is optimal w.r.t. natural performance criteria if computation time is limited to a number N of sweeps. In most papers, the temperature parameters are carefully tuned to obtain good results. On the other hand, there are only few general results. Most research is done for Metropolis type algorithms (Chapter 8)) which are closely related to the Gibbs sampler. Heuristics on the actual choice of schedules can be found in LAARHOVEN and AARTS (1987) and SIARRY and DREYFUS (1989).

For example, HOFFMANN and SALAMAN (1990) find a schedule for a function on three points where one peak has to be overpassed. The schedule with optimal mean final energy coincides in the limit $N \to \infty$ with the optimal theoretic schedule found by HAJEK (1988). For the set M of global minimizers, CATONI (in AZENCOTT (1992a)) shows that the rate

$$\mathsf{P}(\xi_N \notin M) \sim (c/n)^{\alpha} \tag{6.1}$$

computed in Section 5.3 (with the best possible α) can be obtained by exponential schedules $A\rho_N^n$ with A independent of N and $\rho_N = (c \ln N)^{-1/N}$. AZENCOTT (p. 5 of the reference) concludes that 'suitably adjusted exponential cooling schedules are to be preferred to logarithmic cooling schedules'.

All the mentioned schedules increase. HAJEK and SASAKI (1989) construct a family of problems for which any monotone schedule is not optimal. In summary, finite time annealing is an intricate matter and this explains why this section is so short. Let us quote literally from HAJEK and SASAKI (1989)

> [] '... it is unclear how to efficiently find an optimal temperature sequence ... for a problem instance. It may be that computing such a sequence may be far more difficult than to solve the problem instance.'

Notwithstanding these misgivings, something *can* be said. For example, one can ask how to spend the available N sweeps wisely. AZENCOTT (1992b) asks if it is better to anneal for N sweeps or to run annealing L times independently with $K < N/2$ sweeps. Plainly K and L must fulfill

$$\frac{N}{L} < K \leq \frac{N}{L}.$$

Each of the L independent versions is carried through with the same cooling schedule. At the end there are L independent terminal configurations $\{\xi_{K,1}, \ldots, \xi_{K,L}\}$. A configuration Ξ with the least energy finally is selected. The computing time does not exceed N but the error probability is

$$\mathsf{P}(\Xi \notin M) = \prod_{1 \leq p \leq K} \mathsf{P}(\xi_{K,p} \notin M).$$

Running annealing for N sweeps follows the rate $(c/N)^{\alpha}$ in (6.1) while distributed annealing has the rate $(c/K)^{\alpha L} \sim ((cL)/N)^{\alpha L}$ which is a great improvement of the exponent (at the cost of an increased constant).

For more details cf. AZENCOTT (1992b).

There is also the possibility to adopt adaptive schedules which exploit their past experience with the energy landscape. Such random cooling schedules have been proposed by many authors but they are still in the state of heuristics and speculation.

7. Sampling and Annealing Revisited

The results from Chapter 5 will be generalized in several respects:

(i) Single-site visiting schemes are replaced by schemes selecting subsets of sites.
(ii) The functions $H_n = \beta(n)H$ or $H_n = H$ are replaced by more general functions.

The latter include functions of the type $H_n = \beta(n)(H + \lambda(n)V)$ or $H_n = H + \lambda(n)V$ with functions $V \geq 0$. Letting $\lambda(n)$ tend to infinity, higher and higher energy barriers are set up on the set $\{V > 0\}$ and the algorithms finally spend most of their time on $\{V = 0\}$. This amounts to the minimization of H or sampling from Π^H on the set $\{V = 0\}$, respectively. Via the function V, constraints can be introduced in addition to the weak ones formulated in terms of H. This is useful and appropriate if expectations about certain constraints are precise and rigid.

Moreover, a law of large numbers for simulated annealing is proved which allows deeper insight into the behaviour of the algorithm.

7.1 A Law of Large Numbers for Inhomogeneous Markov Chains

In this chapter a law of large numbers for inhomogeneous Markov chains is derived. It generalizes the corresponding result 4.3.2 for homogeneous chains.

7.1.1 The Law of Large Numbers

We continue with the notation from Chapter 4. Let P_ν be the probability distribution on $\mathbf{X}^{\mathsf{N}_0}$ generated by the initial distribution ν and the transition kernels P_n and let $\xi = (\xi_n)_{n\geq 0}$ be a sequence of random variables with law P_ν. By ν_{ij} we denote the joint distribution of ξ_i and ξ_j, i.e. $\nu_{ij}(x,y) = \mathsf{P}_\nu(\xi_i = x,\ \xi_j = y)$; we set $\nu_{ii}(x,x) = \nu_i(x)$ and $\nu_{ii}(x,y) = 0$ if $x \neq y$ where ν_i is the distribution of ξ_i.

The proof is based on a slight generalization of the central Theorem 4.4.1.

Theorem 7.1.1. *Let P_n, $n \geq 1$, be Markov kernels and assume that each P_n has an invariant probability distribution μ_n. Assume further that the following conditions are satisfied*

$$\sum_n \|\mu_n - \mu_{n+1}\| < \infty, \tag{7.1}$$

$$\lim_{n \to \infty} c\left(P_n \dots P_{n+k(n)}\right) = 0 \quad \textit{for some sequence } k(n) > 0. \tag{7.2}$$

Then $\mu_\infty = \lim \mu_n$ exists and uniformly in all initial distributions ν,

$$\nu P_1 \dots P_n \longrightarrow \mu_\infty \quad as \quad n \to \infty, \tag{a}$$

$$\nu P_i \dots P_n \longrightarrow \mu_\infty \quad as \quad i \to \infty,\ n \geq i + k(i). \tag{b}$$

Remark 7.1.1. More precisely, in (b) we mean that for every $\varepsilon > 0$ there is i_o such that $\|\nu P_i \dots P_n - \mu_\infty\| < \varepsilon$ for every $i \geq i_o$ and $n \geq i + k(i)$.

Proof (of Theorem 7.1.1). The proof is the same as for Theorem 4.4.1. To be pedantic we replace the last lines by: For $2 \leq N \leq i \leq i + k(i) \leq n$ we may continue with

$$\begin{aligned} &\|\nu P_i \dots P_n - \mu_\infty\| \\ &= \|(\nu - \mu_\infty) P_i \dots P_n + \mu_\infty P_i \dots P_n - \mu_\infty\| \\ &\leq 2c\left(P_i \dots P_{i+k(i)}\right) + \|\mu_\infty P_i \dots P_n - \mu_\infty\| \end{aligned}$$

For large i, the first term becomes small by (7.2). This proves the second statement. The first one follows similarly. □

Remark 7.1.2. Theorem 7.1.1 implies Theorem 4.4.1: Assume that (4.4) holds, i.e. for each $i, c(P_i \dots P_n) \longrightarrow 0$ as $n \to \infty$. Then there are $k(i)$ such that $c\left(P_i \dots P_{i+k(i)+j}\right) \leq c\left(P_i \dots P_{i+k(i)}\right) \leq 2^{-i}$ for all $j \geq 0$. Hence (7.2) holds for this sequence $(k(i))$ and thus part (a) of 7.1.1 .

Lemma 7.1.1. *If the conditions (7.1) and (7.2) in Theorem 7.1.1 are fulfilled then*

$$\nu_{ij}(x,y) \longrightarrow \mu_\infty(x) \cdot \mu_\infty(y) \quad for \quad x, y \in \mathbf{X} \quad as \quad i \to \infty,\ j \geq i + k(i).$$

Proof. For $j > i$, the two-dimensional marginals have the form

$$\nu_{ij}(x,y) = \left(\nu P_1 \dots P_i\right)(x) \cdot \left(\varepsilon_x P_{i+1} \dots P_j\right)(y)$$

where ε_x denotes the point or Dirac measure in x. By 7.1.1(a) there is N such that $\nu_i(x)$ is close to $\mu_\infty(x)$ for every $i \geq N$. Choose now i according to 7.1.1(b). □

For the law of large numbers, Cesaro convergence is essential. As a preparation we prove the following elementary result:

Lemma 7.1.2. *Let $(a_{ij})_{j>i}$ be a bounded family of real numbers. Assume that*

$$a_{ij} \longrightarrow 0 \quad as \quad i \to \infty,\ j \geq i + k(i), \quad where \quad \frac{k(i)}{i} \to 0.$$

Then

$$\frac{1}{n^2} \sum_{i=1}^{n} \sum_{j=i+1}^{n} a_{ij} \longrightarrow 0 \quad as \quad n \to \infty.$$

Proof. Choose $\varepsilon > 0$. By assumption, there is m such that

$$|a_{ij}| < \varepsilon \quad \text{for every} \quad i \geq m, j \geq i + k(i).$$

We need an estimate of the number of those indices for which this fails. Plainly,

$$\begin{aligned} &\{(i,j) : 1 \leq i < j \leq n,\ |a_{ij}| \geq \varepsilon\} \\ &\quad \subset \{(i,j) : 1 \leq i < j \leq n,\ i \leq m \quad \text{or} \quad (j - i \leq k(i))\}. \end{aligned}$$

The cardinality χ of the lower set can be estimated from above by

$$\chi \leq nm + \sum_{i=1}^{n} k(i).$$

Let $c = \max |a_{ij}|$. Then

$$\left| \frac{1}{n^2} \sum_{i=1}^{n} \sum_{j=i+1}^{n} a_{ij} \right| \leq \varepsilon + \frac{m}{n} + c \cdot \frac{1}{n^2} \sum_{i=1}^{n} k(i) \leq \varepsilon + \frac{m}{n} + c \cdot \frac{1}{n} \sum_{i=1}^{n} \frac{k(i)}{i}.$$

The last inequality holds for every $\varepsilon > 0$ and the Cesaro mean of a sequence converging to 0 converges to 0 as well. This proves the result. □

Lemma 7.1.3. *Assume that 7.1.1(a) and (b) hold and, moreover, $\frac{k(i)}{i} \to 0$. Then*

$$\frac{1}{n^2} \sum_{i,j=1}^{n} \nu_{ij}(x,y) \longrightarrow \mu_\infty(x)\mu_\infty(y) \quad for\ all \quad x, y \in \mathbf{X} \quad as \quad n \to \infty.$$

Proof. In the last lemma plug in $a_{ij} = \nu_{ij}(x,y) - \mu_\infty(x) \cdot \mu_\infty(y)$ if $j > i$. By Lemma 7.1.1,

$$\frac{1}{n^2} \sum_{i=1}^{n} \sum_{j=i+1}^{n} (\nu_{ij}(x,y) - \mu_\infty(x)\mu_\infty(y)) \longrightarrow 0 \quad \text{for all} \quad x, y \in \mathbf{X} \quad \text{as} \quad n \to \infty.$$

The mean over the lower triangle and the diagonal converge to 0 as well. This proves the lemma. □

These preparations are sufficient to prove the law of large numbers.

Theorem 7.1.2. *[Law of Large Numbers] Let* $\mathbf{X}$ *be a finite space and let* P_n, $n \geq 1$, *be Markov kernels on* $\mathbf{X}$. *Assume that each* P_n *has an invariant distribution* μ_n *and the conditions*

$$\sum_n \|\mu_n - \mu_{n+1}\| < \infty, \tag{7.5}$$

$$\lim_{i\to\infty} c\left(P_i \ldots P_{i+k(i)}\right) = 0 \quad \text{for } k(i) > 0,\ \frac{k(i)}{i} \to 0. \tag{7.6}$$

Then $\mu_\infty = \lim \mu_n$ *exists and for every initial distribution* ν *and every function* f *on* $\mathbf{X}$,

$$\frac{1}{n}\sum_{i=1}^{n} f(\xi_i) \longrightarrow \mathsf{E}_{\mu_\infty}(f) \quad \text{in} \quad L^2(\mathsf{P}_\nu).$$

In particular, the means in time converge to the mean in space in P_ν-*probability.*

The proof below follows WINKLER (1990).

Proof. Existence of μ_∞ was verified in Theorem 7.1.1. Let E denote expectation w.r.t. P_ν. By linearity, it is sufficient to prove the theorem for functions $f(x) = \mathbf{1}_{\{x\}}$, $x \in \mathbf{X}$. Elementary calculations give

$$\begin{aligned}
&\mathsf{E}\left(\left[\frac{1}{n}\sum_{i=1}^{n} f(\xi_i) - \mathsf{E}_{\mu_\infty}(f)\right]^2\right) \\
&= \mathsf{E}\left(\left[\frac{1}{n}\sum_{i=1}^{n}(\mathbf{1}_{\{\xi_i=x\}} - \mu_\infty(x))\right]^2\right) \\
&= \frac{1}{n^2}\sum_{i,j=1}^{n} \mathsf{E}\left((\mathbf{1}_{\{\xi_i=x\}} - \mu_\infty(x))(\mathbf{1}_{\{\xi_j=x\}} - \mu_\infty(x))\right) \\
&= \frac{1}{n^2}\sum_{i,j=1}^{x} \left(\nu_{ij}(x,x) - \mu_\infty(x)\nu_j(x) - \mu_\infty(x)\nu_i(x) + \mu_\infty(x)\mu_\infty(x)\right).
\end{aligned}$$

By convergence of the one-dimensional marginals and by Lemma 7.1.3 each of the four means converges to $\mu_\infty(x)\mu_\infty(x)$ and hence the Cesaro mean vanishes in the limit. This proves the law of large numbers. □

The following observation simplifies the application of the theorem in the next chapter.

Remark 7.1.3. Let $(\gamma_i)_{i\geq 1}$ be an increasing sequence in the interval $(0,1)$. Then

(a) $i \cdot (1 - \gamma_i) \to \infty$ as $i \to \infty$,

implies

(b) there is a sequence $(k(i))_{i\geq 1}$ of natural numbers such that

$$\prod_{j=i}^{i+k(i)} \gamma_i \to 0 \quad \text{and} \quad \frac{k(i)}{i} \to 0 \quad \text{as} \quad i \to \infty.$$

If a sequence $(\gamma_i)_{i\geq 1}$ satisfies (a) and $c(P_i) \leq \gamma_i$ then

$$c\left(P_i \dots P_{i+k(i)}\right) \leq \prod_{j=i}^{i+k(i)} c(P_j) \leq \prod_{j=i}^{i+k(i)} \gamma_i \to 0.$$

In particular, if there is such a sequence $(\gamma_i)_{i\geq 1}$ then condition (7.6) is fulfilled.

Proof. Suppose that (a) holds. The sequence $\rho(i) = \inf_{k\geq i} k \cdot (1-\gamma_k)$ increases to ∞. Let $k(i)$ be the least integer greater than $i \cdot \rho(i)^{-1/2}$; then

$$i \cdot \rho(i)^{-1/2} \leq k(i) \leq i \cdot \rho(i)^{-1/2} + 1$$

and

$$\frac{k(i)}{i} \leq \rho(i)^{-1/2} + i^{-1} \to 0.$$

Moreover,

$$\begin{aligned}
\left(k(i)+1\right)\left(1-\gamma_{i+k(i)}\right) &\geq \frac{(k(i)+1)\rho(i+k(i))}{i+k(i)} \geq \frac{k(i)\rho(i)}{i+k(i)} \\
&\geq \frac{i\rho(i)^{1/2}}{i+k(i)} = \frac{\rho(i)^{1/2}}{1+\frac{k(i)}{i}} \to \infty.
\end{aligned}$$

This implies

$$\sum_{k=i}^{i+k(i)} (1-\gamma_k) \geq (k(i)+1)\left(1-\gamma_{i+k(i)}\right) \to \infty$$

and hence $\gamma_i \cdot \ldots \cdot \gamma_{i+k(i)} \to 0$. □

Since Theorem 7.1.2 deals with convergence in probability it is a 'weak' law of large numbers. 'Strong' laws provide almost sure convergence. The strong version below can be found in GANTERT (1990). It is based on theorem I.2.23 in IOSIFESCU and THEODORESCU (1969).

Theorem 7.1.3. *Given the setting of Theorem 7.1.2, assume that each P_n has an invariant distribution μ_n, that (7.5) holds and*

$$c_n = \max\{c(P_i) : 1 \leq i \leq n\} < 1.$$

Moreover, assume

$$\sum_{n=1}^{\infty} \frac{1}{2^n (1 - 2c_{2^n})} < \infty.$$

Then $\mu_\infty = \lim \mu_n$ exists and for every initial distribution ν and every function f on $\mathbf{X}$,

$$\frac{1}{n}\sum_{i=1}^{n} f(\xi_i) \to \mathsf{E}_{\mu_\infty}(f) \quad \mathsf{P}_\nu - \textit{almost everywhere.}$$

Note that the set where the means converge does not depend on a finite set of ξ_i only and hence the primitive notion of probability from Chapter 4 is not sufficient. Some measure theory is required and we do not prove the theorem here.

7.1.2 A Counterexample

For the law of large numbers stronger assumptions are required than for convergence of the one-dimensional marginal distributions. This is refleced by lower cooling schedules in annealing. We shall show that these assumptions cannot be dropped in general. It is easy to construct *some* counterexample. For instance, take a Markov chain which fulfills the assumptions of the general convergence Theorem 4.4.1. One may queeze in between the transition kernels sufficiently many identity matrices such that the law of large numbers fails. In annealing, the transition probabilies are strictly positive and the contraction coefficients increase strictly. The following counterexample takes this into account.

Example 7.1.1. The conditions

$$\sum_n \|\mu_n - \mu_{n+1}\| < \infty,$$

$$\prod_{k \geq N} c(P_k) = 0 \quad \text{for every} \quad N \geq 1,$$

imply convergence of the one- and two-dimensional marginal distributions ν_i and ν_{ij} to μ_∞ and $\mu_\infty \otimes \mu_\infty$, respectively. The following elementary example shows that they are not sufficient for the (L^2-version of the) law of large numbers. The reason is that in

$$\nu_{ij}(x, y) = (\nu P_1 \ldots P_i)(x)\,(\varepsilon_x P_{i+1} \ldots P_j)(x)$$

for $i, j \to \infty$ the convergence of the second term may be very slow and destroy Cesaro convergence in the Lemmata 7.1.2 and 7.1.3. The condition $k(i)/i \to 0$ controls the speed of convergence and thus enforces the law of large numbers.

For $x \in \mathbf{X}$ and $f = \mathbf{1}_{\{x\}}$ the theorem implies that

$$\frac{1}{n^2}\sum_{i,j=1}^{n}(\nu_{i,j}(x,x)-\mu_\infty(x)\nu_j(x)-\mu_\infty(x)\nu_i(x)+\mu_\infty(x)\mu_\infty(x)) \to 0, n\to\infty.$$

By convergence of the one-dimensional marginals and since the Cesaro mean of the diagonal vanishes in the limit this is equivalent to

$$\frac{1}{n^2}\sum_{i=1}^{n-1}\sum_{j=i+1}^{n}\nu_{ij}(x,x) = \frac{1}{n^2}\sum_{i=1}^{n-1}\sum_{j=i+1}^{n}\nu_i(x)P_{i,j}(x,x) \to 1/2\mu_\infty(x)^2$$

where $P_{i,j} = P_{i+1}\dots P_j$. Since $\nu_i(x) \to \mu_\infty$ this fails as soon as

$$\liminf_{n\to\infty}\frac{1}{n^2}\sum_{i=1}^{n-1}\sum_{j=i+1}^{n}P_{i,j}(x,x) > \mu_\infty(x)/2. \tag{7.7}$$

Let now $\mathbf{X} = \{0,1\}$ and let the transition kernels be given by

$$P_n = \begin{bmatrix} 1-1/n & 1/n \\ 1/n & 1-1/n \end{bmatrix}.$$

Then $c(P_n) = 1-2/n$, $\mu_n = (1/2,1/2)$ and thus $\mu_\infty = (1/2,1/2)$. In particular, the Markov kernels are strictly positive and the contraction coefficients increase strictly. The sum in (4.3) vanishes and hence is finite; by $\sum 1/n = \infty$ one has $\sum \ln(1-2/n) = -\infty$ which implies $\prod c(P_n) = \prod(1-2/n) = 0$. Hence (4.8) holds and consequently (7.6) is fulfilled.

Elementary calculations will show that for $x = 1$ condition (7.7) holds as well and hence we have a counterexample. More precisely, we shall see that the mean in (7.7) is greater than 1/4:

$$\begin{aligned}\frac{1}{n^2}\sum_{i=1}^{n-1}\sum_{j=i+1}^{n}P_{i,j}(1,1) &= \frac{1}{n^2}\sum_{i=1}^{n-1}\sum_{j=i+1}^{n}(1,0)P_{i+1}\dots P_j\begin{pmatrix}1\\0\end{pmatrix}\\ &= \frac{1}{n^2}\sum_{i=1}^{n-1}\sum_{j=i+1}^{n}\frac{1}{2}\left(\prod_{k=i+1}^{j}\left(1-\frac{2}{k}\right)+1\right)\\ &= \frac{1}{2n^2}\sum_{i=1}^{n-1}\left(i\cdot(i-1)\cdot\left(\frac{1}{i}-\frac{1}{n}\right)+(n-i)\right) \overset{n\to\infty}{\longrightarrow} \frac{1}{4}-\frac{1}{6}+\frac{1}{4}=\frac{1}{3}>\frac{1}{4}.\end{aligned}$$

The second and third identity will be verified below.

The same counter example is given in GANTERT (1990). The reasoning there follows H.-R. KÜNSCH. Our elementary calculations are replaced by an abstract argument based on a $0-1$-law for tail-σ-fields.

In particular, the example shows that the L^2-theorem 1.3 in GIDAS (1985) and the conclusions fail. In part (iii) of this theorem the conditions (1.25) and (1.27) follow from (7.5) and (7.6). Moreover, $P = \lim_{n\to\infty} P_n$ is the unit matrix and hence all requirements in this paper are fulfilled. Part (i) and (ii) in theorem 1.3 of GIDAS (1985) do not hold for similar reasons.

Here are the missing computations: For the second identity, we show

$$(1,0)P_{i+1}\dots P_j\begin{pmatrix}1\\0\end{pmatrix} = \frac{1}{2}\left(\prod_{k=i+1}^{j}\left(1-\frac{2}{k}\right)+1\right).$$

For $j = i+1$ the left-hand side is the upper left element of the matrix P_{i+1}, i.e. $1-\frac{1}{i+1} = \frac{i}{i+1}$. The right-hand side is

$$1/2\left((1-\frac{1}{i+1})+1\right) = 1/2\frac{i+1-2+i+1}{i+1} = \frac{i}{i+1}.$$

For the induction step $j \to j+1$ observe that products of matrices of the form $\left(\begin{smallmatrix}a & b\\ b & a\end{smallmatrix}\right)$ are of the same form:

$$\begin{pmatrix}a & b\\ b & a\end{pmatrix}\cdot\begin{pmatrix}a' & b'\\ b' & a'\end{pmatrix} = \begin{pmatrix}aa'+bb' & ab'+a'b\\ a'b+ab' & aa'+bb'\end{pmatrix} = \begin{pmatrix}c & d\\ d & c\end{pmatrix}$$

Specializing to

$$P_{i+1}\dots P_j = \begin{pmatrix}a & (1-a)\\ (1-a) & a\end{pmatrix},\ P_{j+1} = \begin{pmatrix}1-\frac{1}{j+1} & \frac{1}{j+1}\\ \frac{1}{j+1} & 1-\frac{1}{j+1}\end{pmatrix}$$

yields

$$c = P_{i+1}\dots P_jP_{j+1}(1,1) = a\cdot\left(1-\frac{1}{j+1}\right)+(1-a)\cdot\frac{1}{j+1}.$$

By hypothesis,

$$a = \frac{1}{2}\prod_{k=i+1}^{j}\left(1-\frac{2}{k}\right)+\frac{1}{2}.$$

Hence

$$\begin{aligned}
c &= \left(1-\frac{2}{j+1}\right)\cdot a+\frac{1}{j+1}\\
&= \left(1-\frac{2}{j+1}\right)\frac{1}{2}\prod_{k=i+1}^{j}\left(1-\frac{2}{k}\right)+\frac{1}{2}\left(1-\frac{2}{j+1}\right)+\frac{1}{j+1}\\
&= \frac{1}{2}\left(\prod_{k=i+1}^{j+1}\left(1-\frac{2}{k}\right)+1\right),
\end{aligned}$$

which we had to prove. For the second identity, we show again by induction that

$$\sum_{j=i+1}^{n} \prod_{k=i+1}^{j} \left(1-\frac{2}{k}\right) = i\cdot(i-1)\cdot\left(\frac{1}{i}-\frac{1}{n}\right).$$

Plainly, the identity holds for $i = n-1$. For the step $i+1 \to i$ we compute

$$\begin{aligned}\sum_{j=i+1}^{n} \prod_{k=i+1}^{j} \left(1-\frac{2}{k}\right) &= \left(1-\frac{2}{j+1}\right)\left(1+\sum_{j=i+2}^{n} \prod_{k=i+2}^{j} \left(1-\frac{2}{k}\right)\right)\\ &= \left(1-\frac{2}{j+1}\right)\cdot\left(1+(i+1)i\left(\frac{1}{j+1}-\frac{1}{n}\right)\right)\\ &= i\cdot(i-1)\cdot\left(\frac{1}{i}-\frac{1}{n}\right).\end{aligned}$$

This completes the discussion of the example.

7.2 A General Theorem

In this chapter, a general result from GEMAN and GEMAN (1987), cf. also GEMAN (1990) combined with an extension from WINKLER (1990) is proved. It will be exploited in the next section to derive several versions of Gibbs samplers.

Let S be a set of $\sigma < \infty$ sites, $\mathbf{X}_s$, $s \in S$, finite spaces and $\mathbf{X}$ their Cartesian product. The Gibbs field for the energy function H on $\mathbf{X}$ is given by

$$\Pi^H(x) = \frac{1}{Z^H}\exp(-H(x)),\ Z^H = \sum_{y\in\mathbf{X}}\exp(-H(x)),\ y \in \mathbf{X},$$

and for $I \subset S$ the local characteristic is

$$\Pi_I^H(x,y) = \begin{cases} \frac{1}{Z_I^H}\exp\left(-H(y_I x_{S\setminus I})\right) & \text{if } y_{S\setminus I} = x_{S\setminus I} \\ 0 & \text{otherwise,}\end{cases}$$

$$Z_I^H = \sum_{z_I}\exp\left(-H(z_I x_{S\setminus I})\right),$$

where summation extends over all $z_I \in \prod_{s\in I}\mathbf{X}_s$. In the estimates of local characteristics the oscillation of H on I will be used. It is defined by

$$\delta_I^H = \sup\left\{|H(x)-H(y)| : x_{S\setminus I} = y_{S\setminus I}\right\}.$$

Once more, Markov chains constructed from local characteristics will be considered. The sites will be visited according to some generalized **visiting scheme**, i.e. a sequence $(S_n)_{n\geq 1}$ of nonempty subsets of S. In every step a new energy function H_n will be used. We shall write μ_n for Π^{H_n}, P_n for

$\Pi_{S_n}^{H_n}$, Z_n for $Z_{S_n}^{H_n}$ and δ_n for $\delta_{S_n}^{H_n}$. For instance, the version of annealing from Chapter 5 will be the case $S_n = \{s_n\}$ and $H_n = \beta(n)H$.

The following conditions enforce (4.3) or (7.1):

$$\text{For every } x \in \mathbf{X} \text{ the sequence } (H_n(x))_{n\geq 1} \text{ increases eventually,} \tag{7.8}$$

$$\text{there is } x \in \mathbf{X} \text{ such that the sequence } (H_n(x))_{n\geq 1} \text{ is bounded from above.} \tag{7.9}$$

The Lemmata 7.2.1 and 7.2.2 are borrowed from GEMAN and GEMAN (1987).

Lemma 7.2.1. *The conditions (7.8) and (7.9) imply condition (7.1).*

Proof. Condition (7.9) implies $a = \inf Z_n > 0$. By (7.8), $b = \sup Z_n$ exists. For $x \in \mathbf{X}$ let $h_n = \exp(-H_n(x))$. Then

$$\begin{aligned}
&|\mu_{n+1}(x) - \mu_n(x)| \\
&= \left|\frac{h_{n+1}}{Z_{n+1}} - \frac{h_n}{Z_n}\right| = \frac{1}{Z_n Z_{n+1}} |h_{n+1}Z_n - h_n Z_{n+1}| \\
&\leq \frac{1}{Z_n Z_{n+1}} (h_{n+1}|Z_{n+1} - Z_n| + Z_{n+1}|h_{n+1} - h_n|) \\
&\leq \frac{b}{a^2} (|Z_{n+1} - Z_n| + |h_{n+1} - h_n|) .
\end{aligned}$$

Since the sequences $(h_n)_{n\geq 1}$ and $(Z_n)_{n\geq 1}$ both are strictly positive and decrease eventually by (7.8), the series

$$\sum_n \|\mu_{n+1} - \mu_n\| = \sum_x \sum_n |\mu_{n+1}(x) - \mu_n(x)|$$

converges and (7.5) holds. □

The visiting scheme has to cover S again and again and therefore we require

$$S = \bigcup_{j=\tau(k-1)+1}^{\tau(k)} S_j \quad \text{for every} \quad k \geq 1 \tag{7.10}$$

for some increasing sequence $\tau(k)$, $k \geq 1$, of times; finally, we set $\tau(0) = 0$. We estimate the contraction coefficients of the transitions over epochs $]\tau(k-1), \tau(k))$, i.e. $c(Q_k)$ for the kernels

$$Q_k = P_{\tau(k-1)+1} \cdots P_{\tau(k)}.$$

The maximal oscillation of H over the k-th epoch is

$$\Delta_k = \max\{\delta_j : \tau(k-1) < j \leq \tau(k)\} .$$

Lemma 7.2.2. *If the visiting scheme fulfills condition (8.10) then there is a positive constant c, such that*

$$c(Q_k) \leq 1 - c \cdot e^{-\sigma \Delta_k} \quad \textit{for every} \quad k \geq 1. \tag{7.11}$$

Proof. By Lemma 4.2.3,

$$c(Q_k) \leq 1 - |\mathbf{X}| \cdot \min_{x,y} Q_k(x,y). \tag{7.12}$$

To estimate $c(Q_k)$ we estimate first the numbers $Q_k(x,y)$. Let $j \in]\tau(k-1), \tau(k))$. For every configuration $x \in \mathbf{X}$ choose z_{S_j} such that

$$H_j\left(z_{S_j} x_{S \backslash S_j}\right) = m_j = \min\left\{H_j(y) : y_{S \backslash S_j} = x_{S \backslash S_j}\right\}.$$

Then

$$\begin{aligned} P_j\left(x, y_{S_j} x_{S \backslash S_j}\right) &= \frac{\exp\left(-H_j(y_{S_j} x_{S \backslash S_j}) + H_j(z_{S_j} x_{S \backslash S_j})\right)}{\sum_v \exp\left(-H_j(v x_{S \backslash S_j}) + m_j\right)} \\ &\geq \frac{\exp(-\delta_j)}{|\prod_{j \in S_j} \mathbf{X}_j|} \geq \frac{\exp(-\Delta_k)}{|\mathbf{X}|}. \end{aligned}$$

Now we enumerate the sites according to the last visit of the visiting scheme during the k-th epoch. Let $L_1 = S_{\tau(k)}$, $l_1 = \tau(k)$ and define recursively

$$l_{i+1} = \max\left\{ j \in (\tau(k-1),\, l_i) : S_j \backslash \bigcup_{m \leq i} L_m \neq \emptyset \right\},\ L_{i+1} = S_{l_{i+1}} \backslash \bigcup_{m \leq i} L_m.$$

By (8.10) this defines a partition of S into at most σ nonempty sets $L_1, \ldots, L_\rho$; a site is an element of L_i, if it was visited at l_i for the last time. Finally, set $L_{\rho+1} = \emptyset$. If ν is an initial distribution for the Markov process generated by the P_n (we continue with notation from Chapter 4), we may procede with

$$\begin{aligned} & Q_k(x,y) = \mathsf{P}_\nu\left(\xi(\tau(k)) = y \,|\xi(\tau(k-1)) = x\right) \qquad (7.13) \\ = & \sum_{z \in \mathbf{X}} \mathsf{P}\left(\xi(l_\rho - 1) = z \,|\xi(\tau(k-1)) = x\right) \mathsf{P}\left(\xi(l_i)_s = y_s, s \in L_i,\right. \\ & \left. 1 \leq i \leq \rho \,|\xi(l_\rho - 1)) = z\right) \\ = & \sum_{x \in \mathbf{X}} P_{xz} \prod_{1 \leq i \leq \rho} \mathsf{P}\left(\xi(l_i)_s = y_s, s \in L_i \,|\xi(l_m)_s = y_s, s \in L_m, i < m \leq \rho,\right. \\ & \left. \xi(l_\rho - 1) = z_s, s = L_n, 1 \leq n \leq i\right) \\ = & \sum_{z \in \mathbf{X}} P_{xz} \prod_{1 \leq i \leq \rho} \mathsf{P}\left(\xi(l_i)_s = y_s, s \in L_i \,|\xi(l_i - 1)_s = y_s, s \in L_m, i < m \leq \rho,\right. \\ & \left. \xi(l_i - 1) = z_s, s = L_n, 1 \leq n \leq i\right) \\ \geq & \sum_{z \in \mathbf{X}} P_{xz} \prod_{1 \leq i \leq \rho} \min_{x',y' \in \mathbf{X}} P_{l_i - 1}(x', y') \geq \sum_{z \in \mathbf{X}} P_{xz} \,|\mathbf{X}|^{-\sigma} \cdot \exp(-\sigma \cdot \Delta_k) \\ = & |\mathbf{X}|^{-1} \cdot \exp(-\sigma \cdot \Delta_k). \end{aligned}$$

By (7.12) the inequality (7.11) holds for $c = |\mathbf{X}|^{-\sigma+1}$. This completes the proof. □

The previous abstract results can now be applied to prove the desired limit theorem. As before, P_ν denotes the law of a Markov process $(\xi_i)_{i\geq 0}$ with transition kernels P_n and initial distribution ν.

Theorem 7.2.1. *Let $(S_n)_{n\geq 1}$ be a visiting scheme on S satisfying condition 8.10 and let $(H_n)_{n\geq 1}$ be a sequence of functions on $\mathbf{X}$ fulfilling (7.8) and (7.9). Then:*

(a) If

$$\sum_{k\geq 1} \exp(-\sigma \Delta_k) = \infty, \tag{7.14}$$

then $\mu_\infty = \lim_{n\to\infty} \mu_n$ exists and

$$\nu P_1 \dots P_n \longrightarrow \mu_\infty \quad as \quad n \to \infty$$

uniformly in all initial distributions ν.

(b) Let the epochs be bounded, i.e. $\sup_{k\geq 1}(\tau(k) - \tau(k-1)) < \infty$, and let

$$k \cdot \exp\left(-\sigma \cdot \max_{j\leq k} \Delta_j\right) \to \infty. \tag{7.15}$$

Then $\mu_\infty = \lim \mu_n$ exists. For every initial distribution ν and every function f on $\mathbf{X}$,

$$\frac{1}{n}\sum_{i=1}^{n} f(\xi_i) \to \mathsf{E}_{\mu_\infty}(f) \quad in \quad L^2(\mathsf{P}_\nu) \quad as \quad n \to \infty.$$

In particular, the means in time converge to the means in space in probability.

Proof. The assumptions of Theorem 7.1.1 and 7.1.2, respectively, have to be verified. Invariance $\mu_n = \mu_n P_n$ was proved in Theorem 5.1.1; condition (7.1) is met by Lemma 7.2.1. Furthermore, for $1 \leq i < \tau(p-1)1\tau(r) < n$ the contraction coefficients fulfill:

$$c(P_i \dots P_n) \leq c(P_i \dots P_{\tau(p-1)}c(Q_p \dots Q_r)c(P_{\tau(r)+1} \dots P_n) \leq \prod_{k=p}^{r} c(Q_k). \tag{7.16}$$

(a) Because of this relation and by (7.11) condition (4.7) is implied by

$$\prod_{k\geq p} c(Q_k) \leq \prod_{k\geq p} (1 - c \cdot \exp(-\sigma \Delta_k)) = 0$$

(hence (7.2) holds according to Remark 7.1.1). The equality may be rewritten as

$$\sum_{k\geq p} \ln\left(1 - c \cdot \exp(-\sigma \Delta_k)\right) = -\infty.$$

Since $\ln(1-x) \leq -x$ for $x < 1$ the equality

$$\sum_{k\geq 1} \exp(-\sigma\Delta_k) = \infty$$

implies (4.7) and hence (7.2).

(b) Since the epochs are bounded and by (7.16) there is a sequence $k(i)$ in (7.6) for the kernels P_n if there is such a sequence for the kernels Q_k. We use criterion 7.1.3. The sequence

$$\gamma_k = 1 - c \cdot \exp\left(-\sigma \max_{j\leq k} \Delta_j\right)$$

increases and fulfills $c(Q_k) \leq \gamma_k$. Hence the condition (7.15) means that $k \cdot (1-\gamma_k) \to \infty$. This proves (b) and the proof of the theorem is complete. □

Remark 7.2.1. (a) Part (a) is – up to a minor generalization – the main result in GEMAN and GEMAN (1987) (cf. GEMAN (1990)), part (b) is contained in WINKLER (1990).

(b) If the epochs are shorter than σ or if S is covered in few steps at the end of the epoch then σ can be replaced by the smaller number ρ determined by (7.3).

(c) There is an almost sure version of the law of large numbers. It requires more careful cooling. For the special case in Chapter 5, N. GANTERT (1990) derived from Theorem 7.1.3 sufficient conditions (which mutatis mutandis apply also in the general case):

Let H be a function on $\mathbf{X}$ and let M denote the set of global minima of H. Let (ξ_i) be a Markov chain for the initial distribution ν and the kernels $P_n = \Pi_{\{1\}}^{\beta(n)} \ldots \Pi_{\{\sigma\}}^{\beta(n)}$ (where $1, \ldots \sigma$ is an enumeration of S). Then for every function f on $\mathbf{X}$ the condition

$$\beta(n) \leq 1/2 \cdot \frac{1}{\sigma\Delta} \cdot \ln n$$

implies

$$\frac{1}{n}\sum_{i=1}^{n} f(\xi_i) \to \frac{1}{|M|}\sum_{x\in M} f(x) \quad \text{almost surely.}$$

7.3 Sampling and Annealing under Constraints

Specializing from Theorem 7.2.1, the central convergence Theorem 5.2.1 will be reproved and some useful generalizations will be obtained.

7.3.1 Simulated Annealing

Let H be the energy function to be minimized and choose a cooling schedule $\beta(n)$ increasing to infinity. Set $\gamma = \min\{H(z) : z \in \mathbf{X}\}$ and

$$H_n(x) = \beta(n) \cdot (H(x) - \gamma).$$

For every $x \in \mathbf{X}$, the value $H(x) - \gamma$ is nonnegative, and hence H_n increases in n. On minimizers of H the functions H_n vanish. Hence the sequence $(H_n)_n$ fulfills the conditions (7.8) and (7.9). Since H_n determines the same Gibbs field μ_n as $\beta(n) \cdot H$ the limit distribution μ_∞ is the uniform distribution on the minimizers of H (Proposition 5.2.1). Let now $(S_k)_{k \geq 1}$ be a visiting scheme and

$$\Delta = \max\left\{\delta_{S_j}^H : j \geq 0\right\}$$

(or as a rough estimate the diameter of the range of H). Then the maximal oscillation of H during the k-th epoch fulfills $\Delta_k \leq \beta(\tau(k)) \cdot \Delta$. If the condition

$$\beta(\tau(k)) \leq \frac{1}{\sigma\Delta} \ln k + c \tag{7.17}$$

is fulfilled for all k greater than some k_o and some $c \in \mathsf{R}$ then

$$\sum_{k \geq 1} \exp(-\sigma \Delta_k) \geq \sum_{k \geq k_o} c' \cdot \exp(-\sigma\beta(\tau(k))\Delta) \geq c' \cdot \sum_{k \geq k_o} \frac{1}{k} = \infty$$

where $c' > 0$, and thus condition (7.14) holds.

Remark 7.3.1. In the common case $\tau(k) = k\sigma$ or, more generally, if the epochs are uniformly bounded then we may replace $\tau(k)$ by k.

In summary,

Convergence of Simulated Annealing. Assume that the visiting scheme $(S_k)_{k \geq 1}$ fulfills condition (8.10) and that $(\beta(n))$ is a cooling schedule increasing to infinity and satisfying condition (7.17). Let M be the set of minimizers of H. Then:

$$\nu_n(x) = \nu P_1 \ldots P_n(x) \to \begin{cases} \frac{1}{|M|} & \text{if } x \in M \\ 0 & \text{if } x \in M \end{cases} \quad \text{as} \quad n \to \infty.$$

Specializing to singletons $S_{k+n \cdot \sigma} = \{s_k\}$, $n \geq 0$, where $s_1, \ldots, s_\sigma$ is an enumeration of S yields Theorem 5.2.1. In fact, the transition probabilities P_n there describe transitions over a whole sweep with systematic sweep strategy and hence correspond to the previous Q_n for epochs given by $\tau(n) = n\sigma$. By the above remark the $\tau(n)$ may be replaced by n and Theorem 5.2.1 is reproved.

In experiments, updating whole sets of pixels simultaneously may be favourable to pixel by pixel updating. E.g. GEMAN, GEMAN, GRAFFIGNE and PING DONG (1990) use crosses S_k of five pixels. Therefore general visiting schemes are allowed in the theorem.

For the law of large numbers it is sufficient to require

$$\beta(\tau(k)) \leq \frac{(1-\varepsilon)}{\sigma \cdot \Delta} \cdot \ln k + c \quad \text{for} \quad k \geq k_o \tag{7.18}$$

for some $\varepsilon > 0$, $c \in \mathsf{R}$ and $k_o \geq 1$. Then

$$k \cdot \exp\left(-\sigma \cdot \max_{j \leq k} \Delta_j\right) \geq k \cdot c' \cdot \exp\left(-\sigma \cdot \beta(\tau(k)) \cdot \Delta\right) \geq k^{\varepsilon}$$

for $c' > 0$ and the right-hand side converges to ∞ as $k \to \infty$. Hence (7.18) implies (7.15).

Law of Large Numbers for Simulated Annealing. Assume the hypothesis of the convergence theorem and let the cooling schedule fulfill condition (7.18. Let ξ_i denote the random state of the annealing algorithm at time i. Then

$$\frac{1}{n}\sum_{i=1}^{n} f(\xi_i) \to \frac{1}{|M|}\sum_{x \in M} f(x)$$

for every initial distribution ν and every function f on $\mathbf{X}$ in $L^2(\mathsf{P}_\nu)$ and in probability.

Specializing $f = \mathbf{1}_{\{x\}}$ for minima $x \in M$ yields

Corollary 7.3.1. *Assume the hypothesis of the law of large numbers. Then for a fixed minimum of H the mean number of visits up to time n converges to $\frac{1}{|M|}$ in $L^2(\mathsf{P}_\nu)$ and in probability as $n \to \infty$.*

This is a sharper version of Corollary 5.2.1. It follows by the standard argument that there is an almost surely convergent subsequence and hence with probability one the annealing algorithm visits *each* minimum infinitely often. This sounds pleasant but reveals a drawback of the algorithm. Assume that H has at least two minima. Then the common criterion to stop it if it stays in the same state, is useless – in summary, the algorithm *visits* minima but *does not detect* them.

7.3.2 Simulated Annealing under Constraints

Theorem 7.2.1 covers a considerable extension of simulated annealing.

Sometimes a part of the expectations about the constraints are quite precise and rigid; for instance, there may be forbidden local configurations of labels or boundary elements. This suggests to introduce the **feasible set** $\mathbf{X}^{\mathrm{f}}$ of those configurations with no forbidden local ones and minimize H on this set only. Optimization by annealing under constraints was developed in GEMAN and GEMAN (1987).

Given $\mathbf{X}$ and H specify a feasible subset $\mathbf{X}^{\mathbf{f}}$. Choose then a function V on $\mathbf{X}$ such that

$$V(x) = 0 \quad \text{if} \quad x \in \mathbf{X}^{\mathbf{f}},\ V(x) > 0 \quad \text{if} \quad x \notin \mathbf{X}^{\mathbf{f}}.$$

Besides the cooling schedule $\beta(n)$ choose another sequence $\lambda(n)$ increasing to infinity. Set

$$H_n = \beta(n)\left((H - \kappa) + \lambda(n)V\right),$$

where $\kappa = \min\left\{H(y) : y \in \mathbf{X}^{\mathbf{f}}\right\}$. Similarly as in Proposition 5.2.1, the Gibbs fields $\mu_n = \Pi^n$ for the energy functions H_n converge to the uniform distribution μ_∞ on the minimizers of $H\left|\mathbf{X}^{\mathbf{f}}\right.$ as $\beta(n) \to \infty$ and $\lambda(n) \to \infty$. On such minima H_n vanishes which implies (7.9). The term in large brackets eventually becomes positive and hence (H_n) increases eventually and satisfies (7.8). For a visiting scheme $(S_k)_{k\geq 1}$ let

$$\Gamma = \max\left\{\delta_{S_j}^V : j \geq 0\right\}.$$

Then

$$\Delta_k \leq \beta\left(\tau(k)\right) \cdot \left(\Delta + \lambda(\tau(k))\Gamma\right)$$

and condition (7.14) in Theorem 7.2.1 holds if

$$\sum_n \exp\left(-\sigma \cdot \beta(\tau(n))\left[\Delta + \lambda(\tau(n))\Gamma\right]\right) = \infty.$$

This is implied by

$$\beta\left(\tau(k)\right) \cdot \left(\Delta + \lambda(\tau(k)) \cdot \Gamma\right) \leq \frac{1}{\sigma} \ln k + c. \tag{7.19}$$

Since $\beta(k) \leq \beta(k)\lambda(k)$ for large k a sufficient condition is

$$\beta(\tau(k)) \cdot \lambda(\tau(k)) \leq \alpha \cdot \ln k + \mathit{const}$$

for large k and $\alpha = \left(\sigma \cdot (\Delta + \Gamma)\right)^{-1}$. In summary, the convergence theorem holds in presence of one of these conditions for visiting schemes fulfilling (8.10) and in the limit the marginals of the algorithm converge to the uniform distribution on the minima of H relative to $\mathbf{X}^{\mathbf{f}}$.

Similarly, for the law of large numbers the condition

$$\beta(\tau(k)) \cdot \left(\Delta + \lambda\left(\tau(k)\right) \cdot \Gamma\right) \leq \frac{1-\varepsilon}{\sigma} \ln k + c$$

is sufficient. All conclusions in Section 7.3.1 keep valid under this condition if 'minimum of H on $\mathbf{X}$' is replaced by 'minimum of $H\left|\mathbf{X}^{\mathbf{f}}\right.$'.

This algorithm sets up higher and higher potential barriers on the forbidden area. If these regions would completely be blocked off then they might separate parts of the feasible set and the algorithm would not reach a minimum in one part if started in the other.

The same considerations apply to sampling.

7.3.3 Sampling with and without Constraints

If there are no constraints then sampling is the case $H_n = H$. The bounds Δ_j do not depend on j and all assumptions of Theorem 7.2.1(a) (besides (8.10)) are automatically fulfilled. The algorithm samples from $\Pi^H = \mu_n = \mu_\infty$. Similarly, part (b) of the theorem holds true under (8.10) alone and allows to approximate means w.r.t. Gibbs fields by means in time.

To sample from Π^H restricted to the feasible set $\mathbf{X}^{\mathrm{f}}$ choose $V \geq 0$ with $V \left| \mathbf{X}^f \right. \equiv 0$ and set

$$H_n = H + \lambda(n) \cdot V$$

Again, conditions (7.8) and (7.9) are met. Condition (7.14) holds if eventually

$$\lambda(k) \leq \frac{1}{\sigma\Gamma} \cdot \ln k + c$$

for some c and similarly (7.15) is implied by

$$\lambda(\tau(k)) \leq \frac{(1-\varepsilon)}{\sigma\Gamma} \cdot \ln k + c$$

eventually for some $\varepsilon > 0$.

Part III

More on Sampling and Annealing

8. Metropolis Algorithms

This chapter introduces Metropolis type algorithms which are popular alternatives to the Gibbsian versions considered previously. For low temperature and many states these methods usually are preferable. Metropolis methods are not restricted to product spaces and therefore lend themselves to many applications outside imaging, for example in combinatorial optimization. Related and more general samplers will be described as well.

We started our discussion with Gibbsian algorithms since their theory formally is more pleasant. It will serve us now as a guide line to the theory of other samplers.

8.1 The Metropolis Sampler

A popular alternative to the Gibbs sampler is the Metropolis algorithm (METROPOLIS, ROSENBLUTH, TELLER and TELLER (1953)). Let H denote the energy function of interest (possibly replaced by a parametrized energy βH) and let x be the configuration currently to be modified. Updating is then performed in two steps:

1. The proposal step.
   A new configuration y is proposed by sampling from a probability distribution $G(x, \cdot)$ on $\mathbf{X}$.
2. The acceptance step.
   a) If $H(y) \le H(x)$ then y is accepted as the new configuration.
   b) If $H(y) > H(x)$ then y is accepted with probability
   $$\exp(H(x) - H(y)).$$
   c) If y is not accepted then x is kept.

The matrix G is called the **proposal** or **exploration matrix** .

A new configuration y which is less favourable than x is not rejected automatically but accepted with a probability decreasing with the increment of energy $H(y) - H(x)$. This will - like annealing with the Gibbs sampler and unlike steepest descent - allow the annealing algorithm to climb hills in the energy landscape and thus to escape from local minima. Moreover, this allows the sampling algorithms to visit the states in a number of steps approximately proportional to their probability under the Gibbs field for H and thus to sample from this field.

Example 8.1.1. In image analysis a natural proposal procedure is to pick a site at random (i.e. sample fom the uniform distribution on the sites) and then to choose a new state at this site uniformly at random. More precisely,

$$G(x,y) = \begin{cases} \frac{1}{\sigma(N-1)} & \text{if } x_s \neq y_s \text{ for precisely one } s \in S \\ 0 & \text{otherwise} \end{cases} \tag{8.1}$$

where σ is the number of sites and N is the number of states in each site (we assume $|\mathbf{X}_s| = N$ for all s). Algorithms with such a proposal matrix are called **single flip algorithms.**

Note that the updating procedure introduced above is not restricted to product spaces $\mathbf{X}$; it may be adopted on arbitrary finite sets. Hence for the present it is sufficient to assume that $\mathbf{X}$ is a finite set and H is a real function on $\mathbf{X}$.

A further remark is in order here. Suppose that the number N of states in the last example is large. To update x one simply picks a y at random and then one either is done or has to toss a coin with probability $\exp(H(x)-H(y))$ of - say - head. If the energy only changes locally (which is the case in most of the examples) then this updating procedure may need less computing time than the evaluation of all exponentials in the partition function for the Gibbs sampler. In such cases the Metropolis sampler is preferable.

Before we are going to establish convergence of Metropolis algorithms let us note an explicit expression for the transition matrix π of the updating step:

$$\pi(x,y) = \begin{cases} G(x,y)\exp(-(H(y)-H(x))^+) & \text{if } x \neq y \\ 1 - \sum_{z \in \mathbf{X}\setminus\{x\}} \pi(x,z) & \text{if } x = y \end{cases} \tag{8.2}$$

If the energy function is of the form βH the transition matrix will be denoted by π^β.

8.2 Convergence Theorems

The basic limit theorems will be derived now. We follow the lines developed for the Gibbs sampler. In particular, the proofs will be based on Dobrushin's argument.

Let us first check invariance of the Gibbs fields.

Theorem 8.2.1. *Suppose that the proposal matrix G is symmetric and the energy function is of the form βH. Then Π^β and π^β fulfill the detailed balance equation*

$$\Pi^\beta(x)\pi^\beta(x,y) = \Pi^\beta(y)\pi^\beta(y,x)$$

for all $x, y \in \mathbf{X}$. *In particular, the Gibbs field* Π^β *is invariant w.r.t. the kernel* π^β.

Proof. It is sufficient to consider $x \neq y$. Since G is symmetric one only has to check the identity

$$\begin{aligned} & \exp(-\beta H(x)) \exp(-\beta(H(y) - H(x))^+) \\ = \; & \exp(-\beta H(y)) \exp(-\beta(H(x) - H(y))^+). \end{aligned}$$

If $H(y) \geq H(x)$ then the left-hand side equals

$$\begin{aligned} & \exp(-\beta H(x)) \exp(-\beta(H(y) - H(x))) \\ = \; & \exp(-\beta H(y)) \\ = \; & \exp(-\beta H(y)) \exp(-\beta(H(x) - H(y))^+). \end{aligned}$$

Interchanging x and y gives the detailed balance equation and thus invariance. □

Recall that it was important in Chapter 4 that every configuration y could be reached from each x after one sweep. The following condition yields a sufficient substitute for this requirement:

Definition 8.2.1. *A Markov kernel* G *on* $\mathbf{X}$ *is called* **irreducible** *if for all* $x, y \in \mathbf{X}$ *there is a chain* $x = u_0, u_1, \ldots, u_{\sigma(x,y)} = y$ *in* $\mathbf{X}$ *such that* $G(u_{j-1}, u_j) > 0$, $1 \leq j \leq \sigma(x, y) < \infty$.

The corresponding homogeneous Markov chain is called irreducible as well.

Extending the neighbourhood relation from Chapter 6 we shall call $y \in \mathbf{X}$ a **neighbour** of $x \in \mathbf{X}$ if $G(x, y) > 0$. In fact, if G is symmetric then

$$N(x) = \{y \in \mathbf{X} : x \neq y, G(x, y) > 0\} \tag{8.3}$$

defines a neighbourhood system in the sense of definition 3.1.1 (where symmetric neighbourhood relations were required). In terms of neighbourhoods the definition of irreducibility reads: There is a sequence $x = u_0, u_1, \ldots, u_{\sigma(x,y)} = y$ such that $x_{j+1} \in N(x_j)$ for all $j = 0, \ldots, \sigma(x, y) - 1$. In this case, we shall say that x and y **communicate**. This relation inherits symmetry from the neighbourhood relation.

Plainly, a primitive Markov kernel generates an irreducible Markov chain. We shall find that Metropolis algorithms with irreducible proposal are irreducible themselves (the samplers are even primitive and annealing has a similar property).

Example 8.2.1. Single-flip samplers are irreducible, i.e. for all x and y in $\mathbf{X}$ there is a chain $x = u_0, u_1, \ldots, u_{\sigma(x,y)} = y$ such that $\pi^\beta(u_{j-1}, u_j) > 0$ for all $j = 1, \ldots, \sigma(x, y)$ (this will be proved before long). On a product space $\mathbf{X} = \prod_s \mathbf{X}_s$, chains with an **exchange proposal** are not irreducible in general: A pair of sites is picked at random and their colours are exchanged. This way, proportions of colours are preserved and thus the Markov chain cannot be irreducible. On classes of images with the same proportions of colours the exchange proposal *is* irreducible. Such a class is not of product form and hence there is no Gibbsian counterpart to the exchange algorithm.

Conservation of proportions is one way to control the (colour) histograms. The exchange algorithm was used in CROSS and JAIN (1983) for texture synthesis (cf. Chapter 12). Fig. 8.1 shows samples from a Gibbs field on $\{0,1\}$ with a 64×64 square lattice. The energy is given by a pair potential with cliques $\langle s,t\rangle_h$ and $\langle s,t\rangle_v$ where s and t are nearest neighbours in the horizontal and vertical direction, respectively:

$$H(x) = -5.09\sum_s x_s + 2.16\sum_{\langle s,t\rangle_h} x_s x_t + 2.25\sum_{\langle s,t\rangle_v} x_s x_t.$$

The first term favours black (i.e. 'colour 1') pixels and the other terms are inhibitory, i.e. weight down neighbours which are both black. Irrespective of the initial configuration, the Gibbs sampler produces a typical configuration from $\{0,1\}^S$ (Fig. 8.1(b)). There are more white than black pixels since 'white-white' is not weighted down. The exchange algorithm started with a pepper and salt picture with about 50% black and white pixels ends up in a texture like Fig. (c) which has the same proportions of colours.

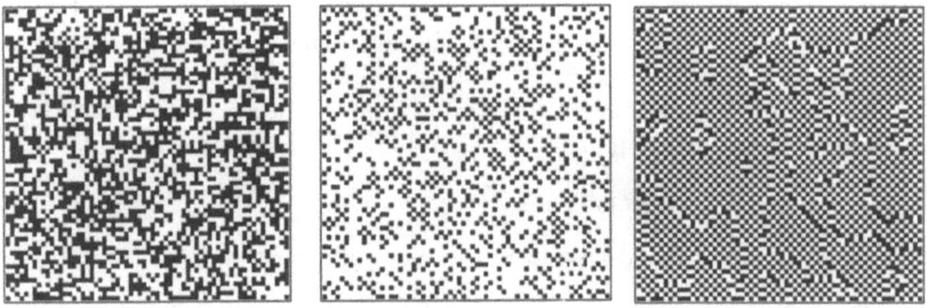

a b c

Fig. 8.1. Sampling. (**a**) initial configuration, (**b**) Metropolis sample, (**c**) sample from exchange algorithm

The crucial point in proving convergence of the algorithms was the estimation of the contraction coefficients and this will be crucial also for Metropolis methods. The role of maximal local oscillation will be played by maximal local increase

$$\Delta = \max\{H(y) - H(x) : x \in \mathbf{X}, y \in N(x)\}. \tag{8.4}$$

Two further constants will be used: Denote for $x, y \in \mathbf{X}$ the length of the shortest path along which x and y communicate by $\sigma(x,y)$ and set

$$\tau = \max\{\sigma(x,y) : x, y \in \mathbf{X}\}.$$

Finally, let

$$\vartheta = \min\{G(x,y) : x, y \in \mathbf{X}, G(x,y) > 0\}.$$

Lemma 8.2.1. *Suppose that H is not constant and that G is irreducible. Let $(\beta(n))_n$ be a sequence of positive numbers and set*

$$Q_k = \pi^{\beta((k-1)\tau+1)} \cdots \pi^{\beta(k\tau)}.$$

If $\beta(n) = \beta > 0$ for all n then Q_k is primitive. If $(\beta(n))_n$ increases to infinity then

$$c(Q_k) \le 1 - \vartheta^{\tau} \exp\left(-\beta(k\tau)\tau\Delta\right)$$

eventually.

Proof. For every x and $y \in N(x)$,

$$\pi^{\beta(n)}(x,y) \ge \vartheta \exp(-\beta(n)\Delta). \tag{8.5}$$

Since H is not constant and since G is irreducible, there is $\tilde{x} \in \mathbf{X}$ such that $H(\tilde{x})$ is minimal and $\tilde{x}$ has a neighbour z of higher energy. Let $\delta = H(z) - H(\tilde{x}) > 0$. Then

$$\begin{aligned}
&\sum_{y \in N(\tilde{x})} G(\tilde{x},y) \exp\left(-\beta(n)(H(y) - H(\tilde{x}))^+\right) \\
\le\ & G(\tilde{x},z) \exp\left(-\beta(n)\delta\right) + \sum_{y \in N(\tilde{x}), y \ne z} G(\tilde{x},y) \\
=\ & G(\tilde{x},z) \exp\left(-\beta(n)\delta\right) + 1 - \left(G(\tilde{x},\tilde{x}) + G(\tilde{x},z)\right) \\
=\ & 1 - G(\tilde{x},z)(1 - \exp(-\beta(n)\delta)) \\
\le\ & 1 - \delta\left(1 - \exp\left(-\beta(n)\delta\right)\right).
\end{aligned} \tag{8.6}$$

The minimizer $\tilde{x}$ communicates with every x along some path of length $\sigma(\tilde{x},x) \le \tau$ and by (8.5) x can be reached from $\tilde{x}$ with positive probability in $\sigma(\tilde{x},x)$ steps. The inequality (8.6) implies $\pi^{\beta(n)}(\tilde{x},\tilde{x}) > 0$ and hence the algorithm can rest in $\tilde{x}$ for $\tau - \sigma(\tilde{x},x)$ steps with positive probability. In summary, every x can be reached from $\tilde{x}$ in precisely τ steps with positive probability. This implies that the stochastic matrix Q_k has a (strictly) positive row and hence is primitive.

Let now $\beta(n)$ increase to infinity. Then (8.6) implies

$$\pi^{\beta(n)}(\tilde{x},\tilde{x}) \ge \vartheta(1 - \exp(-\beta(n)\delta) \ge \vartheta \exp(-\beta(n)\Delta)$$

for sufficiently large n. Together with (8.5) this yields

$$\begin{aligned}
c(Q_k) &\le 1 - \min_{x,y} \sum_z Q_k(x,z) \wedge Q_k(y,z) \le 1 - \min_x Q_k(x,\tilde{x}) \\
&\le 1 - \vartheta^{\tau} \exp\left(-\beta(k\tau)\tau\Delta\right).
\end{aligned}$$

which completes the proof. □

The limit theorems follow from the lemma in a straightforward way. We consider first the homogeneous case and prove convergence of one-dimensional marginals and the law of large numbers.

Theorem 8.2.2. *Let* $\mathbf{X}$ *be a finite set,* H *a nonconstant function on* $\mathbf{X}$ *and* Π *the Gibbs field for* H*. Assume further that the proposal matrix is symmetric and irreducible. Then:*

(a) For every $x \in \mathbf{X}$ *and every initial distribution* ν *on* $\mathbf{X}$*,*

$$\nu\pi^n(x) \longmapsto \Pi(x) \quad as \quad n \to \infty.$$

(b) For every initial distribution ν *and every function* f *on* $\mathbf{X}$*,*

$$\frac{1}{n}\sum_{i=1}^{n} f(\xi_i) \longrightarrow \mathsf{E}_\Pi(f) \quad as \quad n \to \infty$$

in L^2 *and in probability.*

Proof. Let Q denote the transition kernel for τ updates, i.e. $Q = Q_k$ in Lemma 8.2.1 for $\beta(n) \equiv 1$. By this lemma, Q is primitive. Moreover, Π is invariant w.r.t. π by Theorem 8.2.1. Hence the result follows from the theorems 4.3.1 and 4.3.2. □

A simple version of the limit theorem for simulated annealing reads:

Theorem 8.2.3. *Let* $\mathbf{X}$ *be a finite set and* H *a nonconstant function on* $\mathbf{X}$*. Let a symmetric irreducible proposal matrix* G *be given and assume that* $\beta(n)$ *is a cooling schedule increasing to infinity not faster than*

$$\frac{1}{\tau\Delta}\ln n.$$

Then for every initial distribution ν *on* $\mathbf{X}$ *the distributions*

$$\nu\pi^{\beta(1)}\ldots\pi^{\beta(n)}$$

converge to the uniform distribution on the set of minimizers of H*.*

Remark 8.2.1. We shall not care too much about good constants in the annealing schedules since HAJEK (1988) gives best constants (cf. Theorem 8.3.1).

Proof. We proceed like in the proof of Theorem 5.2.1 and reduce the theorem to Theorem 4.4.1. The distributions $\Pi^{\beta(n)}$ are invariant w.r.t. the kernels $\pi^{\beta(n)}$ by Theorem 8.2.1 and thus condition (4.3) in 4.4.1 holds by Lemma 4.4.2. Now we turn to the contraction coefficients.

Divide the time axis into epochs $((k-1)\tau, k\tau]$ of length τ and fix $i \geq 1$. For large n, the contraction coefficients of the transition probability Q_k over the k-th epoch (defined in Lemma 8.2.1) fulfill

$$
\begin{aligned}
& c(\pi^{\beta(i)} \dots \pi^{\beta(n)}) \\
\leq \; & c\left(\pi^{\beta(i)} \dots \pi^{\beta((p-1)\tau)}\right) c(Q_p \dots Q_q) c\left(\pi^{\beta(q\tau+1)} \dots \pi^{\beta(n)}\right) \\
\leq \; & \prod_{k=p}^{q} c(Q_k).
\end{aligned}
$$

By the estimate in Lemma 8.2.1 and the argument from Theorem 5.2.1 this tends to zero as q tends to infinity if

$$\sum_k \exp(-\beta(k\tau)\tau\Delta) = \infty.$$

Hence $\beta(k\tau) \leq (\tau\Delta)^{-1}\ln(k\tau)$ is sufficient. This proves the theorem. □

Remark 8.2.2. Requiring that H is not constant excludes such pathological (and not interesting) cases like the following one:

Let $\mathbf{X} = \{0,1\}$, H be constant and $G(0,1) = G(1,0) = 1$. Then irrespective of the values β and β',

$$\pi^\beta = \begin{pmatrix} 0 & 1 \\ 1 & 0 \end{pmatrix}, \pi^\beta \pi^{\beta'} = \begin{pmatrix} 1 & 0 \\ 0 & 1 \end{pmatrix}.$$

If the sampling or annealing algorithm is started at 0 then the one-dimensional marginals at even steps are (1,0) and those at odd steps are (0,1) and the respective limit theorem does not hold.

8.3 Best Constants

We did not care too much about good constants in the cooling schedule for two reasons: (i) we wanted to keep the theory as simple as possible, (ii) there are results even characterizing *best constants*. Two such theorems are reported now. The proofs are omitted since they are rather involved.

Before the theorems can be stated, some new notions and notations have to be introduced (the reader should not be discouraged by the long list – all notions are rather conspicuous). Let an irreducible and symmetric proposal matrix G be given. G induces a neighbourhood system or equivalently a graph structure on $\mathbf{X}$. A **path** linking two elements x and y in $\mathbf{X}$ is a chain $x = x_0, \dots, x_k = y$ such that $G(x_{j-1}, x_j) > 0$ for every $j = 1, \dots, k$. If there is a path linking x and y these two elements are said to **communicate**; they **communicate at level** h if either $x = y$ and $H(x) \leq h$ or if there is a path along which the energy never exceeds h, i.e. $H(x_i) \leq h$. A **proper local minimum** x does not communicate with any element y of lower energy at level $H(x)$, i.e. if $H(y) < H(x)$ then every path linking x and y visits an element z such that $H(z) > H(x)$. The elements x and y are **equivalent** if they are linked by a path of constant energy. This defines an equivalence

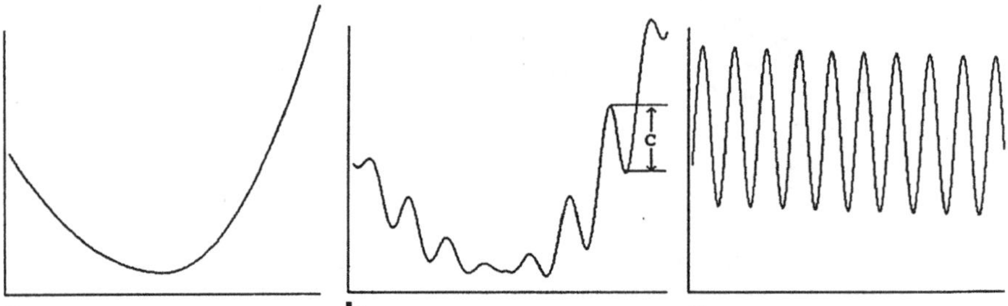

Fig. 8.2. Easy and hard problems

relation on the set of proper local minima; an equivalence class is called a **bottom**.

Let further $\mathbf{X}_{min}$ denote the set of minimizers of H and $\mathbf{X}_{loc}$ the set of proper local minima. A proper local minimum x is at the bottom of a 'cup' with a possibly irregular rim; if it is filled with water it will run over after the water has reached the lowest gap: the **depth** d_x of a proper local minimum x is the smallest number $d \geq 0$ such that x communicates with a y at height $H(x) + d$ and $H(y) < H(x)$ (if x is a global minimum then $d_x = \infty$).

Theorem 8.3.1 (HAJEK (1988)). *For every initial distribution* ν,

$$\mathsf{P}\left(\xi_n \in \mathbf{X}_{min}\right) = \nu\pi^{\beta(1)} \ldots \pi^{\beta(n)}(\mathbf{X}_{min}) \longrightarrow 1 \quad as \quad n \to \infty \tag{8.7}$$

if and only if

$$\sum_{n=1}^{\infty} \exp(-\beta(n)C) = \infty \tag{8.8}$$

where

$$C = \sup\left\{d_x : x \in \mathbf{X}_{loc} \backslash \mathbf{X}_{min}\right\}.$$

Usually we adopted logarithmic annealing schedules $\beta(n) = D^{-1} \ln n$. For them the sum becomes $\sum n^{-C/D}$ and HAJEK's result tells us that (8.7) holds if and only if $D \geq C$. In particular, if all proper local minima are global then $C = 0$ and we may cool as rapidly as we wish. On the other hand, we conclude that for $C > 0$ exponential cooling schedules $\beta(n) = A\rho^n$, $A > 0$, $\rho > 1$, cannot guarantee (8.7) since for them the sum in (8.8) is finite. Note that this result does not really cover the case of the Gibbs sampler; but the Gibbs sampler 'nearly' is a special case of the Metropolis algorithm and corresponding results should hold also there. Related results were obtained by GELFAND and MITTER (1985) and TSITSIKLIS (1989).

Fig. 8.2 symbolically displays hard and easy problems (JENNISON (1990)). Note that we met a situation similar to (c) in the Ising model.

The theorem states that the sets of minimizers of H have probability close to 1 as n gets large. The probability of some minimizers, however, might vanish in the limit. This effect does not occur for the annealing schedules fulfilling condition (7.18) (cf. Corollary 7.3.1). The following result gives the best constants for annealing schedules for which in the limit each minimum is visited with positive probability. Let for two elements $x, y \in \mathbf{X}$ the minimal height at which they communicate be denoted by $h(x, y)$.

Theorem 8.3.2 (CHIANG and CHOW (1988)). *The conditions*

$$\begin{aligned}\lim_{n\to\infty} \nu\pi^{\beta(1)}\ldots\pi^{\beta(n)}(x) &= 0 \quad \textit{if} \quad x \notin \mathbf{X}_{min},\\ \lim_{n\to\infty} \nu\pi^{\beta(1)}\ldots\pi^{\beta(n)}(x) &> 0 \quad \textit{if} \quad x \in \mathbf{X}_{min}\end{aligned}$$

hold if and only if

$$\sum_{n=1}^{\infty} \exp(-\beta(n)R) = \infty$$

where $R = CR'$ *with* $R' = \sup\{h(x,y) : x, y \in \mathbf{X}_{min}, x \neq y\}$.

8.4 About Visiting Schemes

In this section we comment on visiting schemes in an unsystematic way. First we ask if Metropolis algorithms can be run with deterministic visiting schemes and then we illustrate the influence of the proposal matrix on the performance of samplers.

8.4.1 Systematic Sweep Strategies

The Gibbs sampler is an irreducible Markov chain both for deterministic and random visiting schemes (with a symmetric and irreducible proposal matrix), i.e. each configuration can be reached from any other with positive probability. In the latter case (and for nonconstant energy) the Metropolis sampler is irreducible as well. On the other hand, H being nonconstant is not sufficient for irreducibility of the Metropolis sampler with *systematic* sweep strategy.

Consider the following modification of the one-dimensional Ising model: Let the σ sites be arranged on a circle and enumerated clockwise. Let in addition to the nearest neighbour pairs $\{i, i+1\}$, $1 \le i < \sigma$, the pixels $s = 1$ and $t = \sigma$ be neighbours of each other. This defines the one-dimensional **Ising model on the torus**. Given a configuration x, pick in the just visited site s a colour different from x_s uniformly at random (which amounts for the Ising model to propose a flip in s) and apply Metropolis' acceptance rule. If, for instance, $\sigma = 3$ and the sites are visited in order $1, \ldots, \sigma$ then the configuration $x = (1, -1, 1)$ is turned to $(-1, 1, -1)$ (and vice versa) after one sweep. In fact, starting with the first pixel, there is a neighbour with state 1 (site 3) and a neighbour with state -1 (site 2). Hence the energies for $x_s = 1$ and $x_s = -1$ are equal and the proposed flip is accepted. This

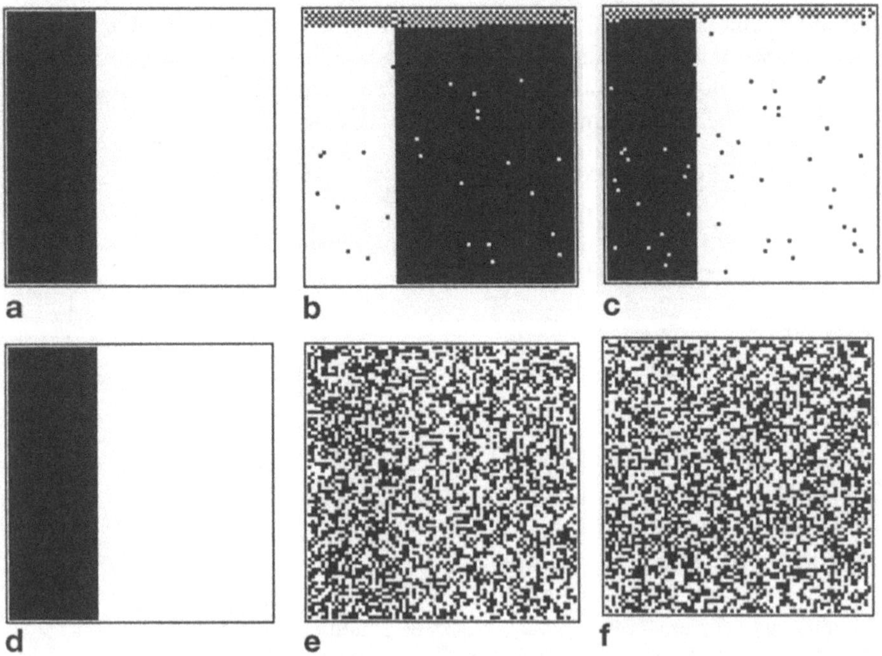

Fig. 8.3. High temperature sampling. (**a**)–(**c**) chequer board scheme, (**d**)–(**f**) random scheme

results in the configuration $(-1,-1,1)$. The situation for the second pixel is the same and consequently it is flipped as well. The third pixel is flipped for the same reason and the final configuration is $-x$. Hence x and $(1,1,1)$ do not communicate. The same construction works for every odd $\sigma \geq 3$. For even $\sigma = 2\tau$ one can distinguish between the cases (i) τ even and (ii)τ odd. Concerning (i) visit first the odd sites in increasing order and then the even ones. Starting with $x = (1,1,-1,-1,\ldots,1,1,-1,-1)$ all flips are accepted and one never reaches $(1,1,\ldots,1,1)$. For odd τ visit 1 and then $\tau+1$, then 2 and $\tau+2$, and so on. Then the configurations

$$(\underbrace{1,1,\ldots,1}_{\tau\ times},\underbrace{-1,-1,\ldots,-1}_{\tau\ times}),\quad (\underbrace{1,1,\ldots,1}_{2\tau\ times})$$

do not communicate (GIDAS (1991), 2.2.1).

You may construct the obvious generalizations to more dimensions (HWANG and SHEU (1991b)).

A similar phenomenon occurs also on finite lattices. For Figure 8.3, we adopted a chequer board scheme and a random proposal to the Ising model without external field. Figs. (b) and (c) show the outputs of the chequer board algorithm after the first and second sweep for inverse temperature 0.001 and initial configuration (a) (in the upper part one sees the beginning of the next

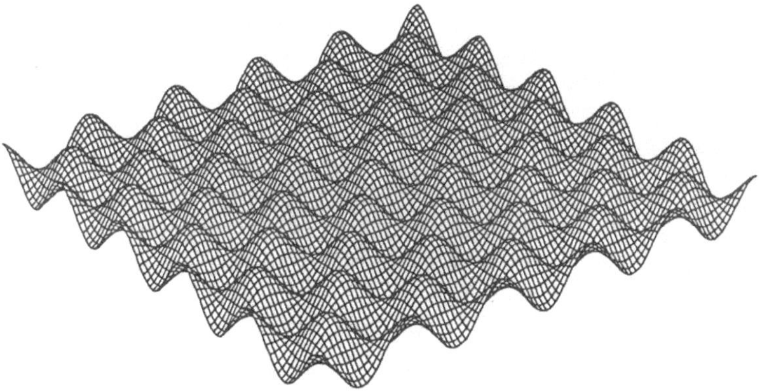

Fig. 8.4. The egg-box function with 25 minima. By courtesy of Ch. Jennison, Bath

half-sweep). For comparison, the outcomes for a random proposal at the same inverse temperature are displayed in the Figs. (e) and (f).

8.4.2 The Influence of Proposal Matrices

The performance of annealing considerably depends on the visiting scheme. For the Gibbs sampler the (systematic) chequer-board scheme is faster than (systematic) raster scanning. Similarly, for proposals with long range, annealing is more active than for short range proposals. This effect is illustrated by CH. JENNISON on a small-sample space. Let $\mathbf{X} = \{1, \ldots, 100\}^2$ and

$$H(x) = \cos\left(\frac{2\pi u_1}{20}\right)\cos\left(\frac{2\pi u_2}{20}\right).$$

The energy landscape of this function is plotted in Fig. 8.4. It resembles an egg box. There are 25 global minima of value -1. Annealing should converge to probability $1/25$ at each of these minima. The cooling schedule

$$\beta(n) = \frac{1}{3}\ln(1+n)$$

has a constant 3. A result by B. HAJEK shows that the best constant ensuring convergence is 1 for the above energy function (next chapter) and hence the limit theorem holds for this cooling schedule. Starting from the front corner, i.e. $\nu = \varepsilon_{(1,1)}$, the laws ν_n of annealing after n steps can be computed analytically. They are plotted below for two proposals and various step numbers n. The proposal G_1 suggests one of the four next neighbours of the current configuration x with probability $1/4$ each. The evolution of the marginals ν_n is plotted in Figs. 8.5(a)–(d) ($n = 100, 1000, 5000, 10000$). The proposal $G_{1,20}$ adds the four points with coordinates $u_1 \pm 20$, the probability being proposed $1/8$ for each of the eight near and far 'neighbours'. There is a considerable gain (Fig. 8.6). Marginals for the function

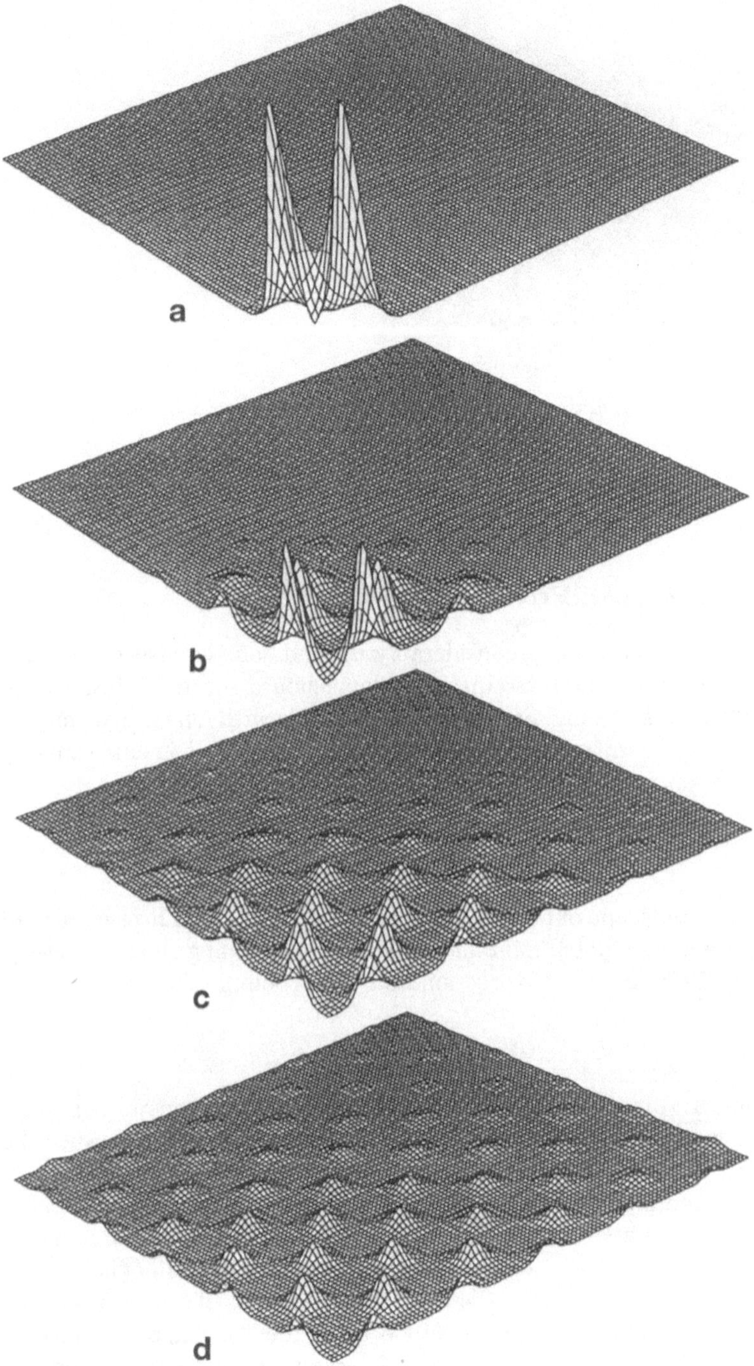

Fig. 8.5. (**a**) G_1, $n = 100$. (**b**) G_1, $n = 1000$. (**c**) G_1, $n = 5000$. (**d**) G_1, $n = 10000$. By courtesy of Ch. Jennison, Bath

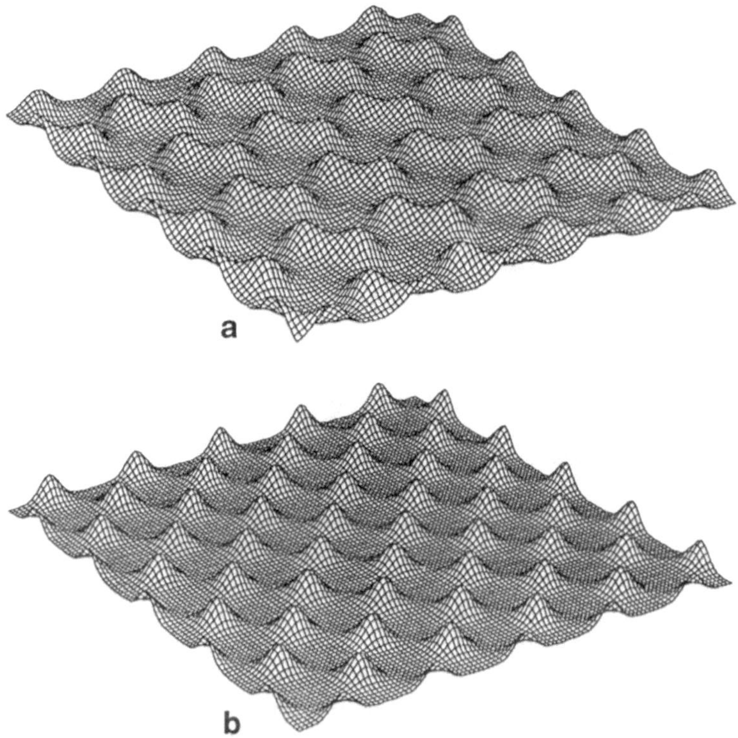

Fig. 8.6. (a) $G_{1,20}$, $n = 100$. (b) $G_{1,20}$, $n = 1000$. By courtesy of Ch. Jennison, Bath

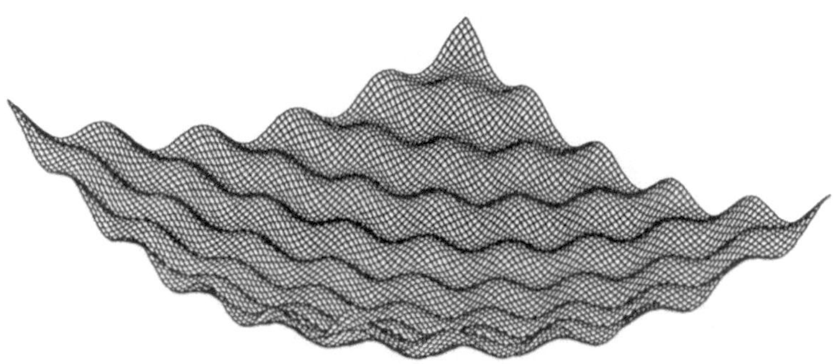

Fig. 8.7. A single minimum. By courtesy of Ch. Jennison, Bath

$$\tilde{H}(x) = H(x) + \frac{1}{500}\left((u_1 - 60)^2 + (u_2 - 50)^2\right)$$

(Fig. 8.7) which has a unique global minimum at $x = (60, 50)$ are displayed in the Figs. 8.8 and 8.9. Parameters are given in the captions. I thank Ch. Jennison for proofs.

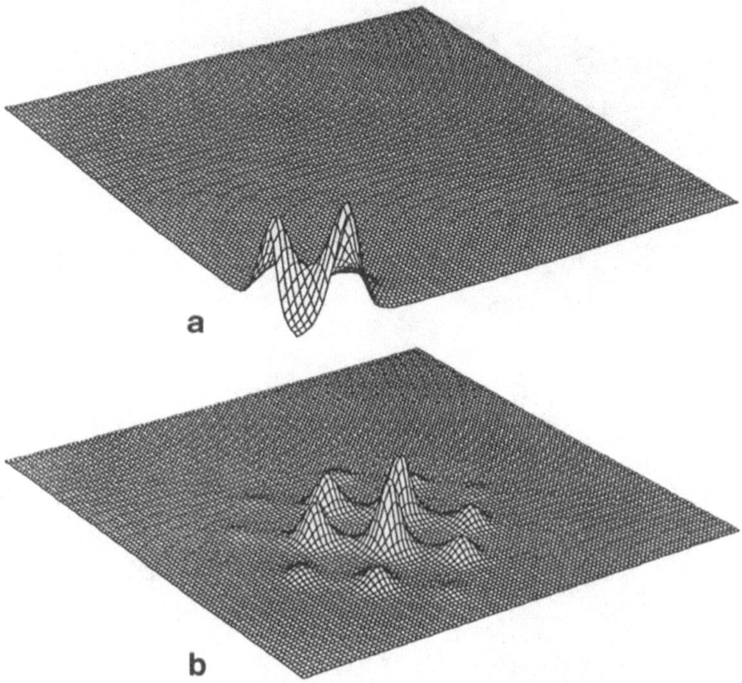

Fig. 8.8. (**a**) G_1, $n = 100$. By courtesy of Ch. Jennison, Bath; (**b**) G_1, $n = 1000$. By courtesy of Ch. Jennison, Bath

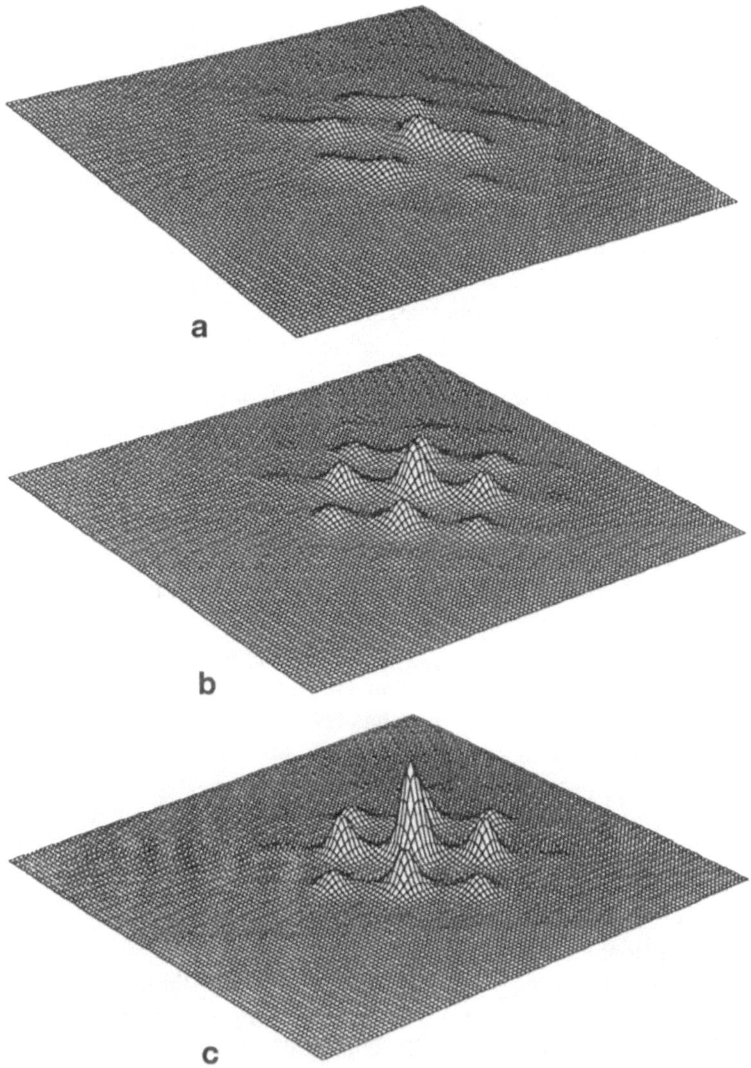

Fig. 8.9. (**a**) $G_{1,20}$, $n = 100$. (**b**) $G_{1,20}$, $n = 200$. (**c**) $G_{1,20}$, $n = 1000$. By courtesy of Ch. Jennison, Bath

8.5 The Metropolis Algorithm in Combinatorial Optimization

Annealing as an approach to combinatorial optimization was proposed in KIRKPATRICK, GELLATT and VECCHI (1982), BONOMI and LUTTON (1984) and ČERNY (1985). In combinatorial optimization, the sample space typically is not of the product form like in image analysis. The classical example, perhaps because it is so easy to state, is the travelling salesman problem. It is one of the best known NP-hard problems. It will serve as an illustration how dynamic Monte Carlo methods can be applied in combinatorial optimization.

Example 8.5.1 (Travelling salesman problem). A salesman has to visit each of N cities precisely once. He has to find a shortest route. Here is another formulation: A tiny 'soldering iron' has to solder a fixed number of joints on a microchip. The waste rate increases with the length of the path the iron runs through and thus the path should be as short as possible. Problems of this flavour arise in all areas of scheduling or design.

To state the problem in mathematical terms let the N cities be denoted by the numbers $1, \ldots, N$ and hence the set of cities is $\mathbf{C} = \{1, \ldots, N\}$. The distance between city i and j is $d(i,j) \geq 0$. A 'tour' is map $\varphi : \mathbf{C} \mapsto \mathbf{C}$ such that $\varphi^k(i) \neq i$ for all $k = 1, \ldots, N-1$ and $\varphi^N(i) = i$ for all i, i.e. a cyclic permutation of $\mathbf{C}$. The set $\mathbf{X}$ of all tours has $(N-1)!$ elements. The cost of a tour is given by its total length

$$H(\varphi) = \sum_{i \in \mathbf{C}} d(i, \varphi(i)).$$

We shall assume that $d(i,j) = d(j,i)$. This special case is known as the **symmetric travelling salesman problem.** For a reasonably small number of towns exact solutions have been computed but for large N exact solutions are known only in special cases (for a library cf. REINELT (1990), (1991)). To apply the Metropolis algorithm an initial tour and a proposal matrix have to be specified. An initial tour is easily constructed picking subsequently new cities until all are met. If the cooling schedule is close to the theoretical one it does not make sense to look for a good initial tour since it will be destroyed after few steps of annealing. For classical methods (and likewise for fast cooling), on the other hand, the initial tour should be as good as possible, since it will be improved iteratively. The simplest proposal exchanges two cities. The number Θ of neighbours will be the same for all tours and one will sample from the uniform distribution on the neighbours. A tour ψ is called a neighbour of the tour φ if it is obtained from φ in the following way: Think of φ as a directed graph like in Figure 8.10(a). Remove two nonadjacent arrows starting at p and $\varphi^{-1}(q)$, respectively, replace them by the arrows from p to $\varphi^{-1}(q)$ and from $\varphi(p)$ to q and finally reverse the arrows between $\varphi(p)$ and $\varphi^{-1}(q)$. This gives the graph in Fig. 8.10(b). A formal description of the procedure reads as follows:

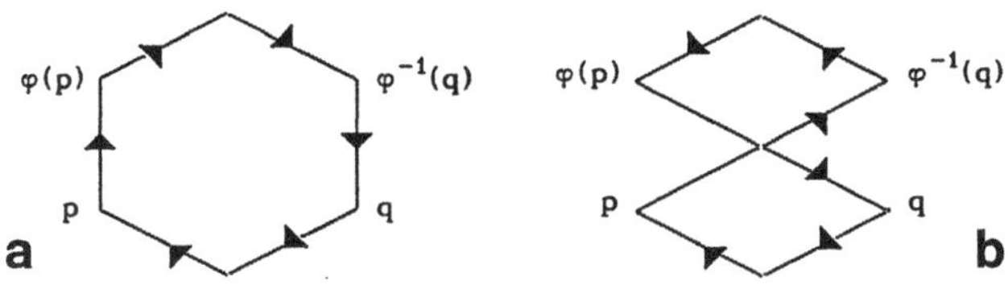

Fig. 8.10. A two-change

Let $q = \varphi^k(p)$ where by assumption $3 \leq k \leq N$. Set

$$\begin{aligned} \psi(p) &= \varphi^{-1}(q), \\ \psi(\varphi(p)) &= q, \\ \psi(\varphi^n(p)) &= \varphi^{n-1}(p) \quad \text{for} \quad n = 2, \dots, k-1, \\ \psi(r) &= \varphi(r) \quad \text{otherwise.} \end{aligned}$$

One says that ψ is obtained from φ by a **2-change**. We compute the number of neighbours of a given tour φ. The reader may verify by drawing some sketches the following arguments: Let $N \geq 4$. Given p, the above construction does not work if q is the next city. If q is the next but one, then nothing changes (hence we required $k \geq 3$). There remain $N-3$ possibilities to choose q. The city p may be choosen in N ways. Finally, choosing $p = q$ reverses the order of the arrows and thus gives the same tour for every p. In summary, we get $N(N-3)+1(=(N-1)(N-2)-1)$ neighbours of φ (recall that φ is not its own neighbour). The just constructed proposal procedure is irreducible. In fact, any tour ψ can be reached from a given tour φ by $N-2$ 2-changes; if γ_n, $n = 0, \dots, N-3$ is a member of this chain (except the last one) then for the next 2-change one can choose $p = \psi^n(1)$ and $q = \gamma_n(\psi^{n+1}(1))$.

In the symmetric travelling salesman problem the energy difference $H(\psi) - H(\varphi)$ is easily computed since only two terms in the sum are changed. For the asymmetric problem also the terms corresponding to reversed arrows must be taken into account. This takes time but still is computationally feasible.

More generally, one can use k-changes (LIN, KERNIGHAN (1973)).

Let us mention only some of the many authors who study annealing in special travelling salesman problems. In an early paper, ČERNY (1985) applies annealing to problems with known solution like N cities arranged uniformly on a circle and with Euclidean distance (an optimal tour goes round the circle; it was found by annealing). The choice of the annealing schedule in this paper is somewhat arbitrary. ROSSIER, TROYON and LIEBLING (1986) systematically compare the performance of annealing and the Lin-Kernighan (LK) algorithm. The latter proposes 2- (or k-) changes in a systematic way and accepts the change whenever it yields a shorter tour. Like many greedy algorithms, it terminates in a local minimum.

In the next examples, a quantity called **normalized length** will appear. For a tour φ it is defined by

$$l(\varphi) = H(\varphi)/\sqrt{AN}$$

for a measure A of an appropriate region containing the N cities.

- In the grid problem with $N = n^2$, n even, points (cities) on a square grid $\{1, \ldots, n\}^2 \subset Z^2$ and Euclidean distance the optimal solutions have tour length N. The cities are embedded into a $(n+1) \times (n+1)$-square, hence the optimal normalized tour length is $n/(n+1)$. For $N = 100$, the optimal normalized tour length is slightly larger than 0.909. All runs of annealing (with several cooling schedules) provided an optimal tour whereas the best normalized solution of 30 runs with different initial tours of the L-K algorithm was about 3.3% longer.
- For 'Grötschel's problem' with 442 cities nonuniformly distributed on a square and Euclidean distance, annealing found a tour better than that claimed to be the best known at that time. The best solution of L-K in 43 runs was about 8% larger and the average tour length was about 10% larger. (Grötschel's problem issued from a real world drilling problem of integrated circuit boards.)
- Finally, N points were independently and uniformly distributed over a square with area A. A theorem by BEARDWOOD, HALTON and HAMMERSLEY (1959) states that the shortest normalized tour length tends to some constant γ almost surely as $N \to \infty$. It is known that $0.625 \leq \gamma \leq 0.92$ and approximations suggest $\gamma \sim 0.749$. Annealing gave a tour of normalized length 0.7541 which is likely to be less than 1% from the optimum.

Detailed comparisons of annealing and established algorithms for the travelling salesman problem are also carried out in JOHNSON, ARAGON, MCGEOCH and SCHEVON (1989).

Another famous problem from combinatorial optimization, the **graph colouring problem** is of some interest for the limited or partially parallel implementation of relaxation techniques (cf. Section 10.1). The vertices of a graph have to be painted in such a fashion that no connected vertices get the same colour and this has to be done with a minimal number of colours.

We strongly recommend the thorough and detailed study by D.S. JOHNSON, C.R. ARAGON, L.A. MCGEOCH and C. SCHEVON (1989)–(1991) examining the competetiveness of simulated annealing in well-studied domains of combinatorial optimization: graph colouring, number partitioning and the travelling salesman problem. A similar study on matching problems is WEBER and LIEBLING (1986).

For applications in molecular biology cf. GOLDSTEIN and WATERMAN (1987) (mapping DNA) and DRESS and KRÜGER (1987).

8.6 Generalizations and Modifications

There is a whole zoo of Metropolis and Gibbs type samplers. They can be generalized in various ways. We shortly comment on the Metropolis-Hastings and the threshold acceptance method.

8.6.1 Metropolis-Hastings Algorithms

Frequently, the updating procedure is not formulated in terms of an energy function H but by means of the field Π from which one wants to sample. Given the proposal matrix G and a strictly positive probability distribution Π on $\mathbf{X}$ the Metropolis sampler can be defined by

$$\pi(x,y) = \begin{cases} G(x,y)\frac{\Pi(y)}{\Pi(x)} & \text{if} \quad \Pi(y) < \Pi(x) \\ G(x,y) & \text{if} \quad \Pi(y) \geq \Pi(x) \text{ and } x \neq y \\ 1 - \sum_{z \neq x} \pi(x,z) & \text{if} \quad x = y \end{cases}$$

If Π is a Gibbs field for an energy function H then this is equivalent to (8.2).

A more general and hence more flexible form of the Metropolis algorithm was proposed by HASTINGS (1970). For an arbitrary transition kernel G set

$$\pi(x,y) = \begin{cases} G(x,y)A(x,y) & \text{if} \quad x \neq y \\ 1 - \sum_{z \neq x} \pi(x,z) & \text{if} \quad x = y \end{cases}$$

where

$$A(x,y) = \frac{S(x,y)}{1 + \frac{G(x,y)\Pi(x)}{G(y,x)\Pi(y)}} \tag{8.9}$$

and S is a symmetric matrix such that $0 \leq A(x,y) \leq 1$ for all x and y. This makes sense if $G(x,y)$ and $G(y,x)$ are either both positive or both zero (since in the latter case $\pi(x,y) = 0 = \pi(y,x)$ regardless of the choice of $A(x,y)$). The detailed balance equation is readily verified and hence Π is stationary for π. Irreducibility must be checked in each specific application.

A special choice of S is

$$S(x,y) = \begin{cases} 1 + \frac{G(x,y)\Pi(x)}{G(y,x)\Pi(y)} & \text{if} \quad \frac{G(y,x)\Pi(y)}{G(x,y)\Pi(x)} \geq 1 \\ 1 + \frac{G(y,x)\Pi(y)}{G(x,y)\Pi(x)} & \text{if} \quad \frac{G(y,x)\Pi(y)}{G(x,y)\Pi(x)} \leq 1 \end{cases}. \tag{8.10}$$

The updating rule is similar as before: Given x draw y from the transition function $G(x,\cdot)$; accept y with probability

$$A(x,y) = \min\left\{1, \frac{\Pi(y)G(y,x)}{\Pi(x)G(x,y)}\right\}, \tag{8.11}$$

else reject y and stay at x. For symmetric G this boils down to the Metropolis sampler.

The Gibbs sampler fits into this framework too: $\mathbf{X}$ is a finite product space and the proposal matrix is defined as follows: a site s is chosen from S uniformly at random, and the proposed new colour is drawn from the local characteristic at s:

$$G(x,y) = \frac{1}{|S|} \sum_s \Pi\left(y_s | x_{S\setminus\{s\}}\right) \mathbf{1}_{\{y_{S\setminus\{s\}}=x_{S\setminus\{s\}}\}}.$$

For $x \neq y$ at most one term is positive. Hence for $x \neq y$, the proposal $G(x,y)$ is positive if and only if x and y differ in precisely one site and then $G(y,x)$ is positive too. In this case

$$\frac{G(x,y)}{G(y,x)} = \frac{\Pi(y)}{\Pi(x)}$$

and thus the acceptance probability $A(x,y)$ is identically 1 (and $S(x,y)$ is identically 2). From this point of view, the Gibbs sampler is an extreme form of the Hastings-Metropolis method where the proposed state is always accepted. The price is (i) a model-dependent choice of the proposal, (ii) normalization is required in $\Pi\left(\cdot|x_{S\setminus\{s\}}\right)$ which is expensive unless there are only few colours or the model is particularly adapted to the Gibbs sampler. There are other Metropolis methods giving zero rejection probability (cf. BARONE and FRIGESSI (1989)).

For $S(x,y) \equiv 1$ and symmetric G one gets

$$\pi(x,y) = G(x,y)\frac{\Pi(y)}{\Pi(x)+\Pi(y)}$$

which for random site visitation and binary systems again coincides with the Gibbs sampler. HASTINGS refers this to as BARKER'S method (BARKER (1965)). Like the Gibbs sampler, this is one of the 'heat-bath methods' (cf. BINDER (1978)); they are called 'heat-bath' methods since in statistical physics a Gibbs field corresponds to a 'canonical ensemble' which is a model for a system exchanging energy with a 'heat bath'.

Numerous modifications of Gibbs and Metropolis samplers were adopted (cf. GREEN (1991)). For instance P. GREEN (1986) suggests to modify the prior and use

$$\Pi^*(x) = \frac{\Pi(x)\exp(-\gamma D(x))}{\mathsf{E}_\Pi(\exp(-\gamma D(x))}$$

where $D(x)$ measures the extent to which x departs from some desired property. This shrinks the old prior Π towards the ideal property and may be regarded as kind of rejection method, since a sample x from Π is accepted with probability $\alpha\exp(-\gamma D(x))$. Formally, this simply amounts to a method to construct suitable priors. BARONE and FRIGESSI (1989) propose a modification which in the Gaussian case can give faster convergence. Following the lines sketched on the last pages, GREEN and HAN (1991) propose Gaussian approximations to the Gibbs sampler in the continuous case (they also give an outline of the arguments in BARONE and FRIGESSI (1990)) et cetera, et cetera.

The number of steps needed for a good approximation of the limit may be reduced by updating whole sets of sites simultaneously. The limit theorems hold if the single-site updating rules are replaced by such for subsets. For the Gibbs sampler and Gibbsian annealing this was proved in Chapter 7 and the reader may easily adapt the arguments to the Metropolis case. For large subsets the single steps become computationally expensive or even unfeasible. Applying the single-site rules on subsets simultaneously is cheap on parallel computers but there are theoretical limitations (which will be discussed later).

More literature about Metropolis algorithms can be found in the next chapter.

Let us finally compare the (standard version of the) Metropolis sampler with the Gibbs sampler by way of a simple example. On product spaces, both, the Gibbs and the Metropolis sampler can be adopted. Which one is preferable depends for example on the form of the energy function and on the computational load. For many colours, the Metropolis sampler usually is preferably in this respect. Performance of the algorithms also depends on the temperature. Roughly spoken, the Gibbs sampler is better at high temperature while for low temperature the Metropolis sampler is better. There are some recent results making this thumb rule precise. We shall shortly discuss this in the next chapter. Let us for the present just display the results of a simple experiment: For the Ising model without external field and inverse temperature $\beta = 9$ the Gibbs sampler (Figs. 8.11(a)–(c)) is opposed to the Metropolis sampler (Figs. 8.11(d)-(f)). A closer look at the illustrations shows that at this high inverse temperature the Metropolis sampler produces better configurations than the Gibbs sampler.

8.6.2 Threshold Random Search

Threshold search is a relaxation of the greedy (maximal descent) algorithm. Given a state x, a new state y is proposed by some deterministic or random strategy. The new state is not only accepted if it is better than x, i.e. $H(y) - H(x) \leq 0$, but also if $H(y) - H(x) \leq t$ for some positive threshold t. Such algorithms are not necessarily trapped in poor local minima.

In **threshold random search algorithms** a random sequence (ξ_k) of states (given an initial state ξ_0) are generated according to the following prescription:

Given $(\xi_0, \ldots, \xi_k)$ generate η_{k+1} by

$$\mathsf{P}(\eta_{k+1} = y | \xi_0 = x_0, \ldots, \xi_k = x_k) = G(x_k, y) \tag{8.12}$$

with a proposal matrix G. Then generate a random variable U_{k+1} uniformly distributed over $[0, 1]$ and set

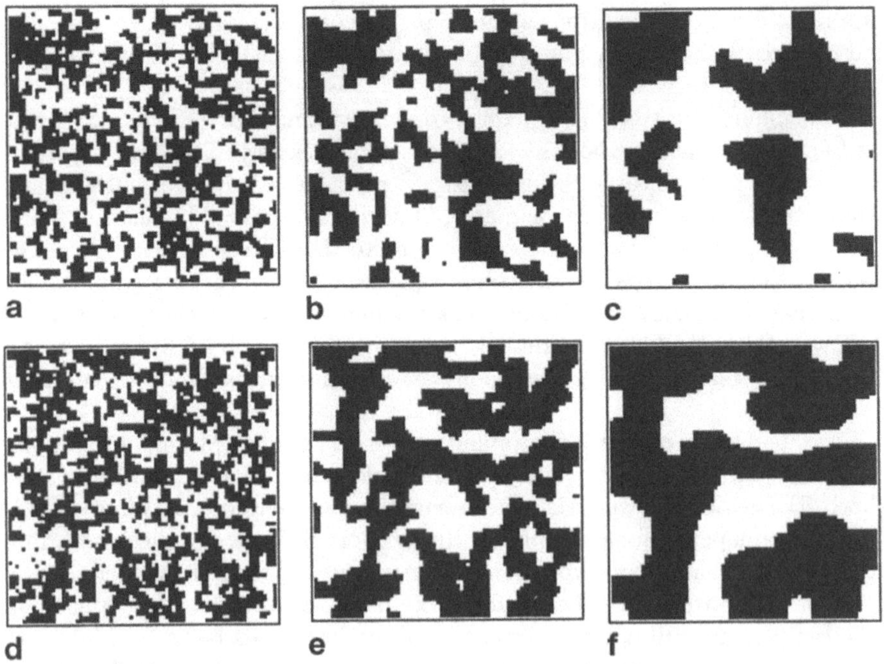

Fig. 8.11. Sampling at low temperature: the Gibbs samples (**a**)–(**c**) opposed to the Metropolis sampler (**d**)–(**f**)

$$\xi_{k+1} = \begin{cases} \eta_{k+1} & \text{if } H(\eta_{k+1}) - H(\xi_k) \le t_k, \\ \xi_k & \text{otherwise.} \end{cases} \tag{8.13}$$

If the thresholds t_k are real constants then this defines a 'deterministic-threshold, threshold random search'. More generally, the thresholds are random variables.

The proposal step in (Metropolis) simulated annealing is the same as (8.12). The acceptance step can be reformulated as follows:

$$\xi_{k+1} = \begin{cases} \eta_{k+1} & \text{if } U_k \le \exp(-\beta(k+1)(H(\eta_{k+1}) - H(\xi_k))) \\ \xi_k & \text{otherwise.} \end{cases} \tag{8.14}$$

Letting $t_k = -\beta(k+1)^{-1} \ln U_k$, we see that (8.14) and (8.13) are equivalent and Metropolis annealing is a special case of threshold random search.

The latter concept is a convenient framework to study generalizations of the Metropolis algorithm, for example with random, adaptive, cooling schedules. Such algorithms are not yet well understood. The paper HAJEK and SASAKI (1989) sheds some light on problems like this. These authors discuss also cooling and threshold schedules for finite time annealing. The reader may also consult LASSERRE, VARAIJA and WALRAND (1987).

9. Alternative Approaches

There are various approaches to stochastic relaxation methods. We started with the conceptually and technically simplest one adopting Dobrushin's contraction technique on finite spaces. Replacing the contraction coefficients by principal eigenvalues gives better estimates for convergence. This technique is adopted in most of the cited papers. Relaxation may also be introduced in continuous space and continuous time and then sampling and annealing is part of the theory of continuous-time Markov and diffusion processes. It would take quite a bit of space and time to present these and other important concepts in closed form. Therefore, we just sketch some ideas in the air. Neither of the topics is treated in detail. The chapter is intended as an incitement for further reading and work and we give a sample of recent papers at the end.

9.1 Second Largest Eigenvalues

We shall first reprove the convergence theorem for homogeneous Markov chains in terms of principal eigenvalues and then report some interesting recent results which were proved by this and similar methods.

9.1.1 Convergence Reproved

Let us first consider homogeneous algorithms. Let P be a Markov kernel on the finite space $\mathbf{X}$ with invariant distribution μ (for a while we shall not exploit the product structure). The general estimate

$$\|\nu P^n - \mu\| \leq 2c(P)^n$$

in (4.2) gives geometric convergence to equilibrium as soon as $c(P) < 1$. By inspection of P, in special cases upper bounds of the rate of convergence can be obtained (cf. Section 5.3). These estimates can be improved considerably. One way is to estimate the rate of convergence by means of the eigenvalues of P. We shall illustrate this technique reproving the convergence theorem for homogeneous Markov chains.

For the correct interpretation of the main Theorem 9.1.1 some facts about eigenvalues are useful. We shall also need some results concerning linear operators on the finite-dimensional Euclidean vector spaces $\mathbf{E} = \mathsf{R}^{\mathbf{X}}$ endowed with the inner product $\langle f, g\rangle_\mu = \sum_x f(x)g(x)\mu(x)$. Recall that P is reversible w.r.t. μ if and only if $\mu(x)P(x,y) = \mu(y)P(y,x)$ for all $x, y \in \mathbf{X}$ and selfadjoint if and only if $\langle Pf, g\rangle_\mu = \langle f, Pg\rangle_\mu$ for all $f, g \in \mathbf{E}$. For basic facts from linear algebra we refer to standard texts like HORN (1985). Recall also that P is primitive if it has a strictly positive power.

Lemma 9.1.1. *Let P be a Markov kernel on $\mathbf{X}$. Then:*

(a) If P is primitive then

$$|\lambda| \le c(P) \le 1$$

for every eigenvalue $\lambda \neq 1$ of P ('P primitive' can be dropped).

(b) P is reversible w.r.t. μ if and only if P is a selfadjoint operator on $(\mathsf{R}^{\mathbf{X}}, \langle\cdot,\cdot\rangle_\mu)$.

(c) If P is reversible then all eigenvalues are real and hence in $[-1, 1]$.

Proof. For the proof of (a) recall the elementary inequality (4.1), i.e.

$$|\rho(f) - \nu(f)| \le (1/2) \max_{x,y} |f(x) - f(y)| \|\rho - \nu\|$$

for distributions ρ and ν and real functions f on $\mathbf{X}$. Plugging in pairs of rows of P for ν and ρ yields

$$\max_{x,y} |Pf(x) - Pf(y)| \le c(P) \max_{x,y} |f(x) - f(y)|.$$

For every (possibly complex) eigenvalue λ with real right eigenvector f this implies

$$|\lambda| \max_{x,y} |f(x) - f(y)| \le c(P) \max_{x,y} |f(x) - f(y)|.$$

Every eigenvalue $\lambda \neq 1$ of P has a real nonconstant eigenvector (by the Perron-Frobenius theorem only $\lambda = 1$ has real constant eigenvectors and the real and imaginary parts of an eigenvector are eigenvectors for the same eigenvalue) and this implies $|\lambda| \le c(P)$. For a proof for general Markov kernels cf. SENETA (1981), thm. 2.10.

For equivalence of reversibility and selfadjointness cf. Remark 5.1.1. Given (b), assertion (c) is a well-known property of selfadjoint operators. □

We state now the main theorem for homogeneous Markov chains. As usual, $\mathsf{E}_\mu(f)$ will denote the expectation $\sum_x f(x)\mu(x)$ and $\mathsf{var}_\mu(f)$ the variance $\mathsf{E}_\mu((f - \mathsf{E}_\mu(f))^2)$ of a function f w.r.t. a distribution μ. For a reversible Markov kernel P let λ_s and λ_{sl} denote the smallest and the second largest eigenvalue, respectively, and set

$$\lambda_* = |\lambda_s| \vee \lambda_{sl}.$$

By the Perron-Frobenius theorem (Appendix B), $\lambda_* < 1$ if P is primitive.

Theorem 9.1.1. *Let P be a primitive Markov kernel reversible w.r.t. its invariant distribution μ. Then*

$$\|\nu P^n - \mu\| \leq c\lambda_*^n$$

for every initial distribution ν and each $n \geq 1$ where $c = \mathsf{var}_\mu(\rho_0)^{1/2}$ for $\rho_0(x) = \nu(x)/\mu(x)$. In particular,

$$\|P^n(x,\cdot) - \mu\| \leq \left(\frac{1-\mu(x)}{\mu(x)}\right)^{1/2} \lambda_*^n$$

for every $x \in \mathbf{X}$.

Remark 9.1.1. Physicists prefer another measure of convergence. Let the **relaxation time** τ be defined by

$$\lambda_* = \exp\left(-\frac{1}{\tau}\right).$$

Then

$$\|\nu P^n - \mu\| \leq c\exp\left(-\frac{n}{\tau}\right).$$

This shows that τ is a (arbitrarily chosen but generally accepted) time-unit for rates of convergence.

The theorem is propositon 3 in DIACONIS and STROOCK (1991). A proof can be based on the spectral radius formula $\lambda_* = \|P - Q\|_{op}$ where Q is the matrix with identical rows μ and $\|\cdot\|_{op}$ is the operator norm for $\langle\cdot,\cdot\rangle_\mu$ (cf. GIDAS (1991)). The more probabilistic proof below follows the lines in FILL (1991) (where it is extended to the nonreversible case). It uses the following characterization of eigenvalues.

Lemma 9.1.2. *Let L be a selfadjoint linear operator on $(\mathbf{E}, \langle\cdot,\cdot\rangle_\mu)$ for a strictly positive distribution μ. Then the smallest eigenvalue of L is given by*

$$\gamma_s = \min\left\{\frac{\langle Lf, f\rangle_\mu}{\langle f, f\rangle_\mu} : f \neq 0\right\}.$$

If, moreover, the eigenvectors of γ_s are the constant functions then the second smallest eigenvalue is given by

$$\gamma_{ss} = \min\left\{\frac{\langle Lf, f\rangle_\mu}{\mathsf{var}_\mu(f)} : f \text{ not constant}\right\}.$$

The minima are attained by the corresponding eigenvectors.

Proof. The first statement is an easy consequence of the minimax characterization of the eigenvalues of symmetric matrices (Rayleigh-Ritz theorem, HORN (1985), theorem 4.4.4) which states: The smallest eigenvalue of a symmetric matrix S is

$$\gamma_s^S = \inf\left\{\frac{\langle Sf, f\rangle}{\langle f, f\rangle} : f \neq 0\right\}$$

where $\langle f, g\rangle$ is the usual inner product $\sum_x f(x)g(x)$. The vectors $\mu(x)^{-1/2}\varepsilon_x$ form an orthonormal base in $(\mathbf{E}, \langle\cdot,\cdot\rangle_\mu)$ and w.r.t. *this base* L is represented by a symmetric matrix S and S has the same eigenvalues as L. Since μ is strictly positive,

$$\inf\left\{\frac{\langle Sf, f\rangle}{\langle f, f\rangle} : f \neq 0\right\} = \inf\left\{\frac{\langle Sg, g\rangle}{\langle g, g\rangle} : g = Df, f \neq 0\right\}$$

where D is the diagonal matrix with entries $\mu(x)^{1/2}$. Since $\langle g, g\rangle = \langle Df, Df\rangle = \langle f, f\rangle_\mu$ and similarly, $\langle Sg, g\rangle = \langle Pf, f\rangle_\mu$, the first equality is proved. Under the additional hypothesis, the orthocomplement of the eigenspace of γ_s consists of the functions $f - \mathsf{E}_\mu(f)$, $f \in \mathbf{E}$, the restriction $L^\perp$ of L to this space is selfadjoint and does *not* have eigenvalue γ_s and hence the smallest eigenvalue of $L^\perp$ is the second smallest of L. Since

$$\mathsf{var}_\mu(f) = \langle f - \mathsf{E}_\mu(f), f - \mathsf{E}_\mu(f)\rangle_\mu$$

the second equality follows from the first one.

If f is an eigenvector of γ_s then $\langle Lf, f\rangle_\mu = \gamma_s\langle f, f\rangle_\mu$ and hence the first minimum is attained by γ_s. The same holds for γ_{ss}. This completes the proof. □

Another simple identity will be useful (in FILL (1991) it is referred to as Mihail's identity, MIHAIL (1989)). Let I denote the identity operator.

Lemma 9.1.3. *If the Markov kernel P is reversible w.r.t. the distribution μ then*

$$\langle (I - P^2)f, f\rangle_\mu = \mathsf{var}_\mu(f) - \mathsf{var}_\mu(Pf).$$

Proof. Observe that $(I - P^2)$ is selfadjoint and use

$$\langle (I - P)f, f\rangle_\mu = \langle (I - P)(f - \mathsf{E}_\mu(f)), f - \mathsf{E}_\mu(f)\rangle_\mu$$

and

$$\langle P^2(f - \mathsf{E}_\mu(f)), f - \mathsf{E}_\mu(f)\rangle_\mu = \langle Pf - \mathsf{E}_\mu(Pf), Pf - \mathsf{E}_\mu(Pf)\rangle_\mu. \qquad \square$$

Proof (of Theorem 9.1.1). By the Perron-Frobenius theorem (Appendix B), P has a unique invariant distribution μ and μ is strictly positive. Let ν be any initial distribution and $\nu_n = \nu P^n$ the n-th marginal distribution of the chain. Set $\rho_n(x) = \nu_n(x)/\mu_n(x)$. Then

$$\begin{aligned}\|\nu_n - \mu\|^2 &= \left(\sum_x \frac{|\nu_n(x) - \mu(x)|}{\mu(x)}\mu(x)\right)^2 \\ &\le \sum_x \frac{|\nu_n(x) - \mu(x)|^2}{\mu(x)^2}\mu(x) \\ &= \mathsf{var}_\mu(\rho_n).\end{aligned}$$

The inequality follows from convexity of the square-function $a \mapsto a^2$ (cf. Appendix C). From reversibility follows

$$P\rho_n(x) = \sum_y P(x,y)\frac{\nu_n(y)}{\mu(y)} = \frac{1}{\mu(x)}\sum_y \nu_n(y)P(y,x) = \frac{\nu_{n+1}(x)}{\mu(x)} = \rho_{n+1}(x).$$

For $f = \rho_n$, Lemma 9.1.3 reads

$$\mathsf{var}_\mu(\rho_{n+1}) = \mathsf{var}_\mu(\rho_n) - \langle (I - P^2)\rho_n, \rho_n\rangle_\mu.$$

Since P is reversible it is selfadjoint (Lemma 9.1.1) and so is $L = I - P^2$. The eigenvalues γ of L and λ of P are related by $\gamma = 1 - \lambda^2$. In particular, the smallest eigenvalue of L is 0 with the constant functions as eigenvectors. Hence Lemma 9.1.2 yields

$$\langle L\rho_n, \rho_n\rangle_\mu \ge \gamma_{ss}\mathsf{var}_\mu(\rho)$$

and thus

$$\mathsf{var}_\mu(\rho_{n+1}) \le \mathsf{var}_\mu(\rho_n)(1 - \gamma_{ss}).$$

By induction,

$$\mathsf{var}_\mu(\rho_n) \le \mathsf{var}_\mu(\rho_0)(1 - \gamma_{ss})^n$$

and the result follows from the relation between the eigenvalues $\gamma = 1 - \lambda^2$ of L and λ of P. The rest is a straightforward calculation. □

Remark 9.1.2. The function $\rho_n = \nu_n/\mu$ is called the **likelihood ratio** and

$$\chi_n^2 = \sum \frac{(\nu_n(x) - \mu(x))^2}{\mu(x)} = \mathsf{var}_\mu(\rho_n)$$

is called the **chi-square distance** of ν and μ.

9.1.2 Sampling and Second Largest Eigenvalues

Let us now specialize to Gibbs fields. We indicate how second largest eigenvalues can be estimated and the applicaton of such estimates to the comparison of algorithms. Then we shortly comment on variance reduction.

Estimation of Second Largest Eigenvalues. To exploit the theorem, good estimates of λ_* have to be found for the various samplers. In general, this is a rather technical affair.

In the following statements about the Gibbs sampler we assume that $\mathbf{X}$ is a finite product space; some statements about the Metropolis sampler hold also for general $\mathbf{X}$. To simplify notation we assume without loss of generality that

$$\text{the minimal value of } H \text{ is } 0.$$

In addition to the notation introduced in Section 8.3 we need some more: The minimal elevation h at which x and y communicate will be denoted by $h_{x,y}$; plainly, $h_{x,y} = h_{y,x}$ and $h_{x,y} \leq h_{x,z} \wedge h_{z,y}$ for all $x, y, z \in \mathbf{X}$. Finally, we set

$$\eta = \max\{h(x,y) - H(x) - H(y) : x, y \in \mathbf{X}\}.$$

Note that $\eta > 0$ and $h(x_\eta, y_\eta) - H(x_\eta) - H(y_\eta) = \eta$ implies that either x_η or y_η is a global minimum. It is not difficult to show that

- $\eta = 0$ if and only if H has only one bottom (INGRASSIA (1991), Proposition 3.1 or (1990), proposizione 2.2.1).

For the next results, let $\mathbf{X}$ be of product form and for simplicity assume the same number of colours at every site. The Metropolis sampler in the single flip version, given x, will pick a neighbour of x (differing from x at precisely one site) uniformly at random and then choose or reject this neighbour by the Metropolis acceptance rule; the Gibbs sampler chooses a site uniformly at random and then picks a new (or the old) state there sampling from the one-site local characteristics. For the (general) Metropolis sampler at inverse temperature β (in continuous time) HOLLEY and STROOCK (1988) obtain estimates for $\lambda_* = \lambda_*(M, b))$ of the form

$$(1 - C\exp(-\beta\eta)) \leq \lambda_*(M, \beta) \leq (1 - c\exp(-\beta\eta)$$

where $0 < c \leq C > \infty$. Following ideas in HOLLEY and STROOCK (1988) and DIACONIS and STROOCK (1991), S. INGRASSIA (1990) and (1991) computes 'geometric' estimates of this form giving better constants. Similar bounds can be obtained adopting ideas by FREIDLIN and WENTZELL (1984); they are sketched in AZENCOTT (1988). For the Gibbs sampler with random visiting scheme INGRASSIA shows that for low temperature

$$\lambda_*(G, \beta) \leq (1 - c\exp(-\beta(\eta + \Delta))$$

where Δ is the maximal local oscillation of H. By the left inequality in the first expression, $\lambda_*(M, \beta)$ tends to 1 as β increases to infinity if $\eta > 0$. It can be shown that

- If H has at least two bottoms then $\lambda_*(\beta)$ converges to 1 as β tends to ∞ both for the Metropolis and the Gibbs sampler. This does not hold if H has only one bottom (FRIGESSI, HWANG, SHEU and DI STEFANO (1993), Theorem 5).

This indicates that the algorithms converge rather slow at high inverse temperature which is in accordance with the experiments. Moreover, at high inverse temperature the Metropolis sampler should converge faster than the Gibbs sampler since the Gibbs sampler is the local equilibrium distribution and the Metropolis sampler favours flips. At low inverse temperature the Gibbs sampler should be preferable: if, for instance, the Metropolis sampler for the Ising model is started with a completely white configuration it will practically always accept a flip since $\exp(\beta \Delta H)$ is close to 1 for all ΔH. Such phenomena (for single site updating dynamics) are studied in detail by FRIGESSI, HWANG, SHEU and DI STEFANO (1993) (and HWANG and SHEU (1991a)). They call a sampler better than another if the λ_* of the first one is smaller than that of the other. They find

- The Gibbs sampler is always better than the following version of the Metropolis sampler: after the proposal step the updating rule is applied twice,
- *for the Ising model* at low temperature the Metropolis sampler is better than the Gibbs sampler,
- *for the Ising model* at high temperature the Metropolis sampler is worse than the Gibbs sampler.

In the Ising case the authors compare a whole class of single site updating dynamics of which the Gibbs sampler is a member. It would be interesting to know more about the last items in the general case. An introduction to the circle of these ideas is contained in GIDAS (1991), 2.2.3.

Variance Reduction. Besides sampling from the invariant distribution, estimation of expectations is a main application of dynamic Monte Carlo methods. By the law of large numbers

$$\frac{1}{n}\sum_{i=1}^{n} f(\xi_i) \longrightarrow \mathsf{E}_\mu(f), \ n \to \infty,$$

and hence the empirical mean is a candidate for an estimator of the expectation. A distinction between accuracy, i.e. speed of convergence, and precision of the estimate has to be drawn. The latter can be measured by the variance of the estimator, i.e. the empirical mean. By the L^2-version of the law of large numbers,

$$\mathsf{var}\left(\frac{1}{n}\sum_{i=1}^{n} f(\xi_i)\right) \longrightarrow 0 \text{ as } n \to \infty,$$

independently of the initial distribution. Under the additional hypothesis of reversibility one can show (KEILSON (1979)) that even

$$n \operatorname{var}\left(\frac{1}{n}\sum_{i=1}^{n} f(\xi_i)\right)$$

converges to some limit $v(f, P, \mu)$. For good samplers this limit should be small for high precision. The asymptotic variance is linked to the eigenvalues and eigenvectors of P by the identities

$$\begin{aligned} v(f,P,\mu) &= \lim_{n\to\infty} n \operatorname{var}\left(\frac{1}{n}\sum_{i=1}^{n} f(\xi_i)\right) \\ &= \langle (I-P)^{-1}(I-P)(f-\mathsf{E}_\mu(f)), f-\mathsf{E}_\mu(f)\rangle_\mu \\ &= \sum_{k=2}^{N} \frac{1+\lambda_k}{1-\lambda_k}\langle f, e_k\rangle_\mu^2 \end{aligned}$$

where $1 = \lambda_1 > \lambda_2 \geq \ldots \geq \lambda_N$ are the $N = |\mathbf{X}|$ eigenvalues of P and the e_k are normalized eigenvectors (FRIGESSI, HWANG and YOUNES (1992); for a survey of related results cf. SOKAL (1989), GIDAS (1991)). This quantity is small if all eigenvalues are negative and small (except the largest one which equals 1) and explains the thumb rule 'negative eigenvalues help'. In contrast, rapid convergence of the marginals is supported by eigenvalues small in absolute value. Thus speeding up convergence of the marginals and reduction of the asymptotic variance are different goals: a chain with fast convergence may have large asymptotic variance and vice versa.

PESCUN (1973) compares Metropolis-Hastings algorithms (like (8.9). For a given proposal G, he proves that (8.11) gives best asymptotic variance (PESKUN (1973), thm. 2.2.1). Hence for symmetric G, the usual Metropolis sampler has least asymptotic variance. PESKUN also shows that Barker's method, a heat bath method closely related to the Gibbs sampler, performs worse. It is not difficult to show that the asymptotic variance $v(f, P, \mu)$ is always equal or greater than $1 - 2\min\{\mu(x) : x \in \mathbf{X}\}$. FRIGESSI et al. (1992) describe a sampler which attains this lower bound (see also GREEN and HAN (1991)).

Importance sampling is a trick to reduce the asymptotic variance. It is based on the simple observation that for any strictly positive distribution ρ,

$$\mathsf{E}_\mu(f) = \sum_x f(x)\frac{\mu(x)}{\rho(x)}\rho(x).$$

Hence estimation of the mean of $(f(x)\mu(x)/\rho(x)$ w.r.t. ρ is equivalent to the estimation of the mean of f w.r.t. μ. The variance of the fraction is minimized by

$$\rho(x) = \sum_y \frac{|f(x)|\mu(x)}{|f(y)|\mu(y)}.$$

There remains the problem to find computationally feasible approximations to ρ.

These ideas can be used to study annealing algorithms too. We shall not pursue this aspect.

9.1.3 Continuous Time and Space

Relaxation techniques can also be studied in continuous space and/or time. Most authors mentioned below base their proofs on the study of eigenvalues.

For a deeper understanding of their results, foreknowledge about continuous Markov and diffusion processes is required. The reader may wish to have a look at the subsequent remarks although he or she is perhaps not familiar with these concepts.

Besides discrete time and finite state space, there are the following combinations:

Discrete Time, Continuous State Space. The continuous state Metropolis chain, where usually $\mathbf{X} = \mathsf{R}^d$ and H is a real function on R^d, formally is similar to the discrete-space version. The Gibbs fields are given by densities $Z_\beta^{-1}\exp(-\beta H(x))$ w.r.t. some σ-finite measure on $\mathbf{X}$, in particular Lebesgue measure λ on R^d. The proposal $g(x,y)$ is a (conditional) density in the variable y. The densities for acceptance or rejection are formally given by the same expression as for finite state space (plainly, sums are replaced by integrals). Under suitable hypothesis one can procede along the same lines as in the finite case since Dobrushin's theorem holds for general spaces (even with the same proof). On the other hand, it does not lend itself to densities with unbounded support (in measure), in particular to the important Gaussian case (cf. Remark 5.1.2). A systematic study of Metropolis annealing for bounded measurable functions H on general probability spaces is started in HAARIO and SAKSMAN (1991).

Continuous Time, Discrete State Space. The discrete time-index set N_0 is replaced by R_+ and the paths are functions $x(\cdot) : \mathsf{R}_+ \to \mathbf{X}$, $t \mapsto x(t) \in \mathbf{X}$ instead of sequences $(x(0), x(1), \ldots)$. The Gibbs fields and the proposals are given like in the last chapter. If the process is at state x then it waits an exponential time with mean 1 and then updates x according to Metropolis' rule. To define the time-evolution precisely, introduce for inverse temperature β operators on $\mathsf{R}^{\mathbf{X}}$ by

$$L_\beta f(x) = \sum_y (f(y) - f(x))\pi^\beta(x,y).$$

Given a cooling schedule $\beta(t)$ the transition probabilities P_{st} between times $s < t$ are then determined by the **forward** or **Fokker-Planck** equation, i.e. for all f,

$$\begin{aligned}\frac{\partial}{\partial t} P_{st}f(x) &= \left(P_{st}L_{\beta(t)}f\right)(x),\ s<t,\\ P_{ss}(x,y) &= 1_{\{x=y\}},\end{aligned}$$

(where $Pf(x) = \sum_y P(x,y)f(y)$). For sampling, keep $\beta(t)$ constant. These Markov kernels fulfill the **Chapman-Kolmogorov equations**

$$P_{st}(x,y) = P_{sr}P_{rt}(x,y) = \sum_z P_{sr}(x,z)P_{rt}(z,y),\ 0 \le s < r < t,$$

which correspond to the continuous-time Markov property. They also satisfy the **backward equation**

$$\frac{\partial}{\partial s} P_{st}f(x) = -L_{\beta(s)}P_{st}f(x).$$

This constitutes a classical framework in which sampling ($\beta(t) = \beta$) and annealing can be studied. To be more specific, define

$$\mathcal{E}(f,f) = (1/2)Z_\beta^{-1}\sum_{x,y}(f(y)-f(x))^2\exp(-\beta H(x)\vee H(y))G(x,y).$$

Then

$$-\langle f, L_\beta f\rangle_{\Pi^\beta} = -\sum_{x,y} f(x)(f(y)-f(x))\pi^\beta(x,y)\Pi^\beta(x) = \mathcal{E}(f,f).$$

By Lemma 9.1.2, the second smallest eigenvalue of $-L_\beta$ is given by

$$\gamma_{ss} = \min\left\{\frac{\mathcal{E}(f,f)}{\mathsf{var}_{\Pi^\beta}} : f \text{ not constant}\right\} > 0$$

and $\gamma_* = \gamma_{ss}$ is the gap between 0 and the set of other eigenvalues of $-L_\beta$. This indicates that $-L_\beta$ plays the role of $I - P$ in the time-discrete case and that the analysis can be carried out along similar lines (HOLLEY and STROOCK (1988)).

Continuous Time, Continuous State Space. These ideas apply to continuous spaces as well. The difference operators L_β are replaced by differential operators and $\mathcal{E}$ is given by a (continuous) Dirichlet form. This way, relaxation processes are embedded into the theory of diffusion processes. Examination of the transition semi-groups via forward and backward equations is only one (KOLMOGOROV's analytical) approach to diffusion processes. It yields the easiest connection between diffusion theory and the theory of operator semigroups. ITÔ's approach via stochastic differential equations gives a better (probabilistic) understanding of the underlying processes and helps to avoid heavy calculations.

Let us start from continuous-time gradient descent in R^d , i.e. from the differential equation

$$dx(t) = -\nabla H(x(t))\,dt,\ x(0) = x_0.$$

To avoid getting trapped in local minima, a noise term is added and one arrives at the stochastic differential equation (SDE)

$$dx(t,\omega) = -\nabla H(x(t,\omega))\,dt + \sigma(t)dB(t,\omega),\ x(0,\omega) = x_0(\omega),$$

where $(B(t,\cdot))_{t\geq 0}$ is some standard R^d-valued Brownian motion. This equation does not make sense path by path (i.e. for every ω) in the framework of classical analysis since the functions $t \mapsto B(t,\omega)$ are highly irregular. Formally rewriting these equations as integral equations results in

$$x(t) = x(0) - \int_0^t \nabla H(x(s))\,ds + \int_0^t \sigma(t)\,dB(t).$$

The last integral does not make sense as a Lebesgue-Stieltjes integral since the generic path of Brownian motion is not of finite variation on compact intervals. It *does* make sense as a Wiener or Itô integral (see every introduction to stochastic analysis like v.WEIZSÄCKER and WINKLER (1990)). Under suitable hypothesis, a solution $x(\cdot)$ exists and the distributions ν_t of the variables $x(t)$ concentrate on the set of global minima of H if $\sigma(t) \to 0$ as $t \to \infty$ and

$$\sigma^2(t) \geq \frac{D}{\ln t}$$

for a suitable constant D (GIDAS (1985b), ALUFFI-PENTINI, PARISI and ZIRILLI (1985), GEMAN and HWANG (1986), BALDI (1986), CHIANG, HWANG and SHEU (1987) – improved in ROYER (1989), GOLDSTEIN (1988)).

In this framework connections between the various samplers (or versions of annealing) can be established (GELFAND and MITTER (1991)). Besides the comparisons sketched in the last section, this is another and most interesting way to compare the algorithms.

Let $(\xi_n)_{n\geq 0}$ be a Markov chain for the Metropolis sampler in R^d (the variables ξ_n live on some space Ω, for example on $(\mathsf{R}^d)^{\mathsf{N}_0}$). For each $\varepsilon > 0$ define a right-continuous process $x^\varepsilon(\cdot)$ by

$$x^\varepsilon(t,\omega) = \xi_n(\omega) \text{ if } \varepsilon n \leq t < \varepsilon(n+1).$$

If H is continuously differentiable and ∇H is bounded and Lipschitz continuous then there is a standard R^d-Brownian motion B and a process $x^M(\cdot)$ (adapted to the natural filtration of B) such that $x^\varepsilon \to x^M$ as $\varepsilon \to 0$ weakly in the space of R^d-valued right-continuous functions on R_+ endowed with the Skorohod topology (cf. KUSHNER (1974)) and

$$\begin{aligned} dx^M(t) &= -\frac{\beta}{2}\nabla H(x^M(t))dt + dB(t),\ t \geq 0, \\ x^M(0) &= x_0 \text{ in distribution.} \end{aligned}$$

The authors do not compare the Metropolis sampler with the Gibbs sampler but with Barker's method (last chapter). The SDE for Barker's method reads

$$dx^B(t) = -\frac{\beta}{4}\nabla H(x^B(t))\,dt + \frac{1}{\sqrt{2}}\,dB(t),\ t \geq 0.$$

We conclude that the interpolated Metropolis and Barker chains converge to diffusions running at different time scales:

If the diffusion $z(\cdot)$ solves the SDE

$$dz(t) = -\nabla H(z(t))\,dt + \sqrt{\frac{\beta}{2}}\,dB(t),\ t \geq 0,$$

with $z(0) = x_0$ in distribution, then for the time-change $\tau(t) = (\beta t)/2$ the process $z(\tau(\cdot))$ has the same distribution as x^M whereas for $\tau(t) = (\beta t)/4$ the process $z(\tau(\cdot))$ has the same distribution as x^B. Thus the limit diffusion for the Metropolis chain runs at twice the speed as the limit diffusion for Barker's chain.

Letting β depend on t gives analoguous results for annealing. The authors promise related results in the forthcoming monograph on simulated annealing-type algorithms for multivariate optimization (1992).

Further References. Research on sampling and annealing is still growing and we can only refer to a small fraction of recent papers on the subject. Besides the papers cited above let us mention the work of Taiwanese scientists, for instance CHIANG and CHOW (1988), (1989), (1990) and CHOW and HSIEH (1990) and also HWANG and SHEU (1987)–(1988c). A lot of research is presently done by a group around R. AZENCOTT, see for example CATONI (1991a,b) and (1992). Some of these authors use ideas from FREIDLIN and WENTZELL (1984), a monograph on random perturbations of dynamical systems (in continuous time; for a discrete time version of their theory cf. KIFER (1990)). In fact, augmentation of the differential equation $dx(t) = -\nabla H(x(t))$ by the noise term $\sigma(t)dB(t)$ reveals relaxation as a disturbed version of a classical dynamical system. AZENCOTT (1988) is a concise exposition of the circle of such ideas. More about the state of the art can be learned from AZENCOTT (1992). A survey of large time asymptotics is also TSITSIKLIS (1988). See also D. GEMAN (1990), AARTS and KORST (1989) and LAARHOVEN and AARTS (1987) for more information and references. Gibbs samplers are embedded into the framework of adaptive algorithms in BENVENISTE, MÉTIVIER and PRIOURET (1990).

10. Parallel Algorithms

In the previously considered relaxation algorithms, current configurations were updated sequentially: The Gibbs sampler (possibly) changed a given configuration x in a systematically or randomly chosen site s, replacing the old value x_s by a sample y_s from the local characteristic $\Pi(x_s|x_{S\backslash\{s\}})$. The next step started from the *new* configuration $y = y_s x_{S\backslash\{s\}}$. More generally, on a (random) set $A \subset S$ the subconfiguration x_A could be replaced by a sample from $\Pi(y_A|x_{S\backslash A})$ and the next step started from $y = y_A x_{S\backslash A}$. The latter reduces the number of steps needed for a good estimate but in general does not result in a substantial gain of computing time. The computational load in each step increases as the subsets get larger; for large A ($A = S$) the algorithms even become computationally infeasible.

It is tempting to let a large number of simple processing elements work simultaneously thus reducing computing time drastically. In the extreme case of synchroneous or 'massively parallel' algorithms, a processor is assigned to each site s. It has access to the data on $\partial(s)$ and serves as a random state generator on $\mathbf{X}_s$ with law $\Pi(\cdot|x_{s\backslash\{s\}})$. All these units work independently of each other and simultaneously pick new states y_s at random thus simulating a whole 'sweep' in a single step. This can be implemented on parallel computers, which are presently developed for a broad market (a well known parallel computer is the Connection Machine invented by W.D. Hillis (1985)). Unfortunately, a naive application of this technique can produce absolutely misleading results. Therefore, a careful analysis of the performance of parallel algorithms and of the envisaged applications is needed.

A large number of parallel or partially parallel algorithms have been proposed and experimentally simulated, but there are only few rigorous results. We give two examples for which convergence to the desired distributions can be proved and study massively parallel implementation in some detail.

Before, let us mention some basic parallelization techniques which will not be covered by this text.

- Simultaneous independent searches. Run annealing independently on p identical processors for N steps and select the best terminal state.
- Simultaneous periodically interacting search. Again, let p processors $\rho_1, \ldots, \rho_p$ anneal independently, but let periodically each ρ_j restart from the best state produced by $\rho_1, \ldots .\rho_p$ (Laarhoven and Aarts (1987)).

- Multiple trials. Let p processors execute one trial of annealing and pick an outcome different from the previous state (if such an outcome was produced).

At high inverse temperature this improves the rate of convergence considerably. Note that it can be implemented sequentially as well: repeat the same trial until something changed. This algorithm can be studied rigorously, cf. CATONI and TROUVÉ, Chapter 9 of the last reference.

Note that these algorithms lend themselves to arbitrary finite spaces. The next algorithm works on finite spaces $\mathbf{X} = \prod_{s \in S} \mathbf{X}$:

- τ-synchroneous search. There is a processing unit for each site $s \in S$, which in each step with probability τ independently of the others decides to be active. With probability $1 - \tau$ it is inactive. Afterwards the active units independently pick new states.

For $\tau = 1$ the algorithm works synchroneous, $\tau = 0$ corresponds to sequential annealing. The former will be studied below. In Chapter 10 of the last reference, TROUVÉ shows that for $0 < \tau < 1$ and $\tau = 1$ the asymptotic behaviour of the algorithms differs substantially.

For (partial) rigorous results and simulations with these and other techniques cf. AZENCOTT (1992a).

To keep the formalism simple, we now return to the setting of Chapter 5. In particular, the underlying space $\mathbf{X}$ will be a finite product of finite spaces $\mathbf{X}_s$, and the algorithms will be based on the Gibbs sampler.

10.1 Partially Parallel Algorithms

We give two examples where several (but not all) sites are updated simultaneously and for which limit theorems in the spirit of previous chapters can be proved. The examples are chosen to illustrate opposite approaches: The first one is a simple all-purpose technique while the second one is specially tailored for a special class of models.

10.1.1 Synchroneous Updating on Independent Sets

Systematic sequential sweep strategies visit sites one by one. There are no restrictions on the order in which the sites are visited. On a finite square lattice, for example, raster scanning can be adopted, but one can as well visit first the sites $s = (i, j)$ with even $i + j$ ('black' fields on a chequer board) and then those with odd $i + j$ (the 'white' fields). For a 4-neighbourhood with northern, eastern, southern and western neighbours, an update at a 'black' site needs no information about the states in other 'black' sites. Hence, given a configuration x, all 'black' processing units may do their job simultaneously and produce a new configuration y' on the basis of x and then the white processors may update y' in the same way and end up with a configuration y. Thus a sweep is finished after two time steps and the transition probability is the same as for sequential updating over a sweep in $|S|$ time steps.

Let us make this idea more precise. We continue with the previously introduced notations. In particular, S denotes the finite set of sites and $\mathbf{X}$ the product of $\sigma = |S|$ finite spaces $\mathbf{X}_s$. There is a function H on $\mathbf{X}$ inducing a Gibbs field Π. Either H is to be minimized or a sample from Π is desired. Let now T be a set of sites (e.g. the set of black sites in the above example) and let x be a given configuration. Then the parallel updating step on T is governed by the transition probability

$$R_T(x,y) = \prod_{s\in T} \Pi_s(x,y)$$

where $\Pi_s = \Pi_{\{s\}}$. More explicitely,

$$R_T(x,y) = \begin{cases} \prod_{s\in T} \Pi(X_s = y_s | X_t = x_t, t \neq s) & \text{if } y_{S\setminus T} = x_{S\setminus T} \\ 0 & \text{otherwise} \end{cases} . \quad (10.1)$$

Let now $\mathbf{T} = \{T_1, \ldots, T_K\}$ be a partition of S into sets T_i. Then the composition

$$Q(x,y) = R_{T_1} \ldots R_{T_K}(x,y)$$

gives the probability to get y from x in a single sweep. Such algorithms are called **limited** or **partially synchroneous** (some authors call them **partially** or **limited parallel**) (τ-synchroneous algorithms deserve this name as well).

Let now a neighbourhood system $\partial = \{\partial(s) : s \in S\}$ on S be given and call a subset T of S **independent** if it contains no pair of neighbours; independent sets are also called **stable**. If the Gibbs field Π enjoys the Markov property w.r.t. ∂ then

$$\Pi(X_s = y_s | X_t = x_t, s \neq t) = \Pi(X_s = y_s | X_t = x_t, t \in \partial(s)).$$

For an independent set T, the conditional probabilities in $s \in T$ depend only on the values off T and

$$\Pi_s(x,y) = \Pi(x',y) \text{ for } s \in T \text{ whenever } x_{S\setminus T} = x'_{S\setminus T}.$$

Hence

$$R_T(x,y) = \Pi_{s_1} \ldots \Pi_{s_{|T|}}(x,y) \quad (10.2)$$

for every enumeration $s_1, \ldots, s_{|T|}$ of T. We conclude that Q coincides with the transition probability for one sequential sweep.

The limit theorem for sampling reads:

Theorem 10.1.1. *If* $\mathbf{T}$ *is a partition of* S *into independent sets then for every initial distribution* ν*, the marginals* νQ^n *converge to the Gibbs field* Π *as* n *tends to infinity. The law of large numbers holds as well. Partitions can be replaced by coverings* $\mathbf{T}$ *of* S *with independent sets.*

Proof. In view of the above arguments, the result is a reformulation of the sequential version in 5.1 if $\mathbf{T}$ is a partition. If it is a covering, specialize from 7.3.3. □

For annealing, let a cooling schedule $(\beta(n))$ be given and denote by $R_{T,n}$ the Markov kernel for parallel updating on T and the Gibbs field $\Pi^{\beta(n)}$ with energy $\beta(n)H$. Given the partition $\mathbf{T}$ of S into independent sets, the n-th sweep has transition kernel

$$Q_n = R_{T_1,n} \dots R_{T_K,n}.$$

Let us formulate the corresponding limit theorem. Recall that Δ is the maximal local oscillation of H.

Theorem 10.1.2. *Assume that* $\mathbf{T}$ *is a partition of* S *into independent sets. If* $(\beta(n))$ *is a cooling schedule increasing to infinity and satisfying*

$$\beta(n) \leq \frac{1}{\sigma\Delta} \ln n$$

then for each initial distribution ν *the marginals* $\nu Q_1 \dots Q_n$ *converge to the uniform distribution on the minimizers of* H *as* n *tends to infinity.*

More generally, partitions $\mathbf{T}$ *of* S *can be replaced by coverings by independent sets.*

Proof. The result is a reformulation of Theorem 5.2.1 and of 7.3.1, respectively. □

For many applications, partitioning the sites into independent sets is straightforward (like for the Ising model). For other models, it can be hard to find such a partition.

The smallest cardinality of a partition of S into independent sets is called the **chromatic number** of the neighbourhood system. In fact, it is the smallest number of colours needed to paint the sites in such a fashion that neighbours never have the same colour. The chromatic number of the Ising model is two; if the states in the sites are independent, then there are no neighbouring pairs at all and the chromatic number is 1; in contrast, if all sites interact then the chromatic number is $|S|$ and partially synchroneous algorithms are purely sequential. Loosely spoken, if the neighbourhoods become large then the chromatic number becomes large. In the general case, partitioning the sites into few independent sets can be extremely difficult. In combinatorial optimization this problem is known as the graph colouring problem. It is NP-hard and its (approximate) solution may consume more time than the original optimization problem. Especially in such cases, it would be desirable to have a massively parallel implementation, i.e. to update all sites simultaneously and independently of each other.

10.1.2 The Swendson-Wang Algorithm

Besides general purpose algorithms there are techniques taylored for special problem classes. As an example, let us shortly discuss the Swendson-Wang algorithm (1987). For the Ising model – and more generally for the Potts model – these authors adopt ideas from percolation theory to improve the rate of convergence.

Consider a generalized Potts model: Let S be a finite set of sites and G a finite set of colours. Each $x \in \mathbf{X} = G^S$ has energy

$$H(x) = -\sum_{\{s,t\}} \alpha_{st} \left(\mathbf{1}_{\{x_s = x_t\}} - 1\right)$$

with individual coupling constants $\alpha_{st} = \alpha_{ts} \geq 0$ (the '-1' is inserted for convenience only). This model originates from physics but it is of interest in texture synthesis as well. Note that 'long-range' interactions are allowed. To describe the algorithm for sampling from the Potts field Π proposed by SWENDSON and WANG, some preparations are needed.

Define a neighbourhood system by $s \in \partial(t)$ if and only if $\alpha_{st} > 0$. This induces a graph structure with bonds $\langle s,t \rangle$ where $\alpha_{st} > 0$. Let S^B denote the set of bonds. Like in Chapter 2, introduce bond variables $b_{st} = b_{\langle s,t \rangle}$ taking values 0 or 1. If $b_{st} = 1$ we shall say that the bond is active or on and else it is off or inactive. The set of active bonds defines a new - more sparse - graph structure on S. Let us call $C \subset S$ a **cluster** if for all $s, t \in C$ there is a chain $s = u_0, \ldots, u_k = t$ in C with active bonds between subsequent sites. A configuration x is updated according to the following rule:

- Between neighbours s and t *with the same colour*, i.e. formally $t \in \partial(s)$ and $x_s = x_t$, activate independently bonds with probability $p_{st} = (1 - \exp(-\alpha_{st}))$. Afterwards, no active bonds are present between sites of different colour. Now assign a random colour to each of the clusters and erase the bonds.

What is left is a new configuration which can differ substantially from the old one.

We present an explanation of the idea behind following the lines in GIDAS (1991). First, we introduce the bond process b coupled to the colour process x. To this end, we specify the joint distribution μ of x and b on $\mathbf{X} \times \{0,1\}^{S^B}$. To simplify notation we shall use the Kronecker symbol δ ($\delta_{ij} = 1$ if $i = j$ and $\delta_{ij} = 0$ otherwise), and write $q_{st} = \exp(-\alpha_{st})$. Let

$$\mu(x, b) = Z^{-1} \prod_{b_{st}=0} q_{st} \prod_{b_{st}=1} (1 - q_{st}) \delta_{x_s x_t}.$$

To verify that μ is a probability distribution with first marginal Π we compute the sum over the bond configurations:

$$\begin{aligned}
& Z^{-1}\sum_b \prod_{b_{st}=0} q_{st} \prod_{b_{st}=1} (1-q_{st})\delta_{x_s x_t} \\
= \; & Z^{-1} \prod_{\{s,t\}} \sum_{b_{st}=0}^{1} \left(q_{st}\delta_{b_{st},0} + (1-q_{st})\delta_{x_s x_t}\delta_{b_{st},1}\right) \\
= \; & Z^{-1} \prod_{\{s,t\}} \left(\exp(-\alpha_{st}) + (1-\exp(-\alpha_{st}))\delta_{x_s x_t}\right) \\
= \; & Z^{-1}\exp(-H(x)) \\
= \; & \Pi(x).
\end{aligned}$$

To compute the second marginal Γ, i.e. the law of the bond process b, we observe that

$$\prod_{b_{st}=1} (1-q_{st})\delta_{x_s x_t} = \prod_{b_{st}=1} (1-q_{st})$$

if for all $\langle s,t\rangle$ with $b_{st}=1$ the colours in s and t are equal. Let A denote the set of all x with this property. Off A the term vanishes. Hence

$$\begin{aligned}
\Gamma(b) &= Z^{-1} \prod_{b_{st}=0} q_{st} \sum_A \prod_{b_{st}=1} (1-q_{st}) \\
&= Z^{-1}|G|^{c(b)} \prod_{b_{st}=0} q_{st} \prod_{b_{st}=1} (1-q_{st})
\end{aligned}$$

where $c(b)$ is the number of clusters in the bond configuration b. To understand the alternative generation of a bond configuration from a colour configuration and a new colour configuration from this bond configuration, consider the conditional probabilites

$$\mu(b|x) = \exp(H(x)) \prod_{b_{st}=0} q_{st} \prod_{b_{st}=1} (1-q_{st})\delta_{x_s x_t}$$

and

$$\mu(x|b) = |G|^{-c(b)} \prod_{b_{st}=1} \delta_{x_s x_t}.$$

Sampling from these distributions amounts to the following rules:

1. Given x, set $b_{st}=0$ if $x_s \neq x_t$. For the bonds $\langle s,t\rangle$ with $x_s = x_t$ set $b_{st}=1$ with probability $1-\exp(-\alpha_{st})$ and $b_{st}=0$ with probability $\exp(-\alpha_{st})$ (independently on all these bonds).
2. Given b, paint all the sites in a cluster in the same colour, where the cluster colours are picked independently from the uniform distribution.

Executing first step (1) and then step (2) amounts to the Swendson-Wang updating rule. The transition probability from the old x to the new y is given by

$$P(x,y) = \sum_b \mu(b|x)\mu(y|b).$$

Plainly, each configuration can be reached from any other in a single step with positive probability; in particular, P is primitive. A straightforward computation shows that Π is invariant for P and hence the sampling convergence theorem holds.

The Swendson-Wang algorithm is nonlocal and superior to local methods concerning speed. The study of bond processes is a matter of percolation theory (cf. SWENDSON and WANG (1987), KASTELEYN and FORTUIN (1969), 1972)). For generalizations and a detailed analysis of the algorithm, in particular quantitative results on speed of convergence, cf. GOODMAN and SOKAL (1989), EDWARDS and SOKAL (1988), (1989), SOKAL (1989), LI and SOKAL (1989), MARTINELLI, OLIVIERI and SCOPPOLA (1990).

10.2 Synchroneous Algorithms

Notwithstanding the advantages of partially parallel algorithms, their range of applications is limited, sometimes they are difficult to implement and in some cases they even are useless. Therefore (and not alone therefore) it is natural to ask why not to update all sites simultaneously and independently of each other.

Before we go into some detail let us as usual look at the Ising model on a finite square grid with 4-neighbourhood and energy $H(x) = -\beta \sum_{\langle s,t \rangle} x_s x_t$, $\beta > 0$. The local transition probability to state x_t at site t is proportional to $\exp(\beta \sum_{\langle s,t \rangle} x_s)$. For a chequerboard-like configuration all neighbours of a given site have the same colour and hence the pixel tends to attain this colour if β is large. Consequently, parallel updating can result in some kind of oscillation, the black sites tending to become white and the white ones to become black. Once the algorithm has produced a chequer-board-like configuration it possibly does not end up in a minimum of H but gets trapped in a cycle of period two at high energy level. Hence it is natural to suppose that massively parallel implementation of the Gibbs sampler might produce substantially different results than a sequential implementation and a more detailed study is necessary.

10.2.1 Introduction

Let us first fix the setting. Given a finite index set S and the finite product space $\mathbf{X} = \prod_{s \in S} \mathbf{X}_s$, a transition kernel Q on $\mathbf{X}$ will be called **synchroneous** if

$$Q(x,y) = \prod_{s \in S} q_s(x,y)$$

where $q_s(x,\cdot)$ is a probability distribution on $\mathbf{X}$.

The synchroneous kernels we have in mind are induced by Gibbs fields.

Example 10.2.1. Given a random field Π the kernel

$$Q(x,y) = R_S(x,y) = \prod_{s \in S} \Pi(X_s = y_s | X_t = x_t, s \neq t)$$

is synchroneous. It will be called the **synchroneous kernel induced by** Π.

10.2.2 Invariant Distributions and Convergence

For the study of synchroneous sampling and annealing the invariant distributions are essential.

Theorem 10.2.1. *A synchroneous kernel induced by a Gibbs field has one and only one invariant distribution. This distribution is strictly positive.*

Proof. Since the kernel is strictly positive, the Perron-Frobenius Theorem (Appendix (B)) applies. □

Since Q is strictly positive, the marginals νQ^n converge to the invariant distribution μ of Q irrespective of the initial distribution ν and hence the synchroneous Gibbs sampler produces samples from μ:

Corollary 10.2.1. *If Q is a synchroneous kernel induced by a Gibbs field then for every initial distribution ν,*

$$\nu Q^n \longrightarrow \mu$$

where μ is the unique invariant distribution of Q.

Unfortunately, the invariant distribution μ in general substantially differs from Π.

For annealing, we shall consider kernels

$$Q_n(x,y) = \prod_{s \in S} \Pi^{\beta(n)}(X_s = y_s | X_t = x_t, s \neq t), \tag{10.3}$$

look for invariant distributions μ_n and enforce

$$\nu Q_1 \ldots Q_n \longrightarrow \mu_\infty = \lim_{n \to \infty} \mu_n$$

by a suitable choice of the cooling schedule $\beta(n)$. So far this will be routine. On the other hand, for synchroneous updating, there is in general no explicit expression for μ_n and it is cumbersome to find μ_∞ and its support. In particular, it is no longer guaranteed that μ_∞ is concentrated on the minimizers of H. In fact, in some simple special cases the support contains configurations of fairly high energy (cf. Examples 10.2.3 and 10.2.4 below).

In summary, the main problem is to determine the invariant distributions of synchroneous kernels. It will be convenient to write the transition kernels in Gibbsian form.

Proposition 10.2.1. *Suppose that the synchroneous kernel Q is induced by a Gibbs field Π. Then there is a function $U : \mathbf{X} \times \mathbf{X} \to \mathsf{R}$ such that*

$$Q(x,y) = Z_Q(x)^{-1} \exp(-U(x,y)).$$

If $V = (V_A)_{A \subset S}$ is a potential for Π then an energy function U for Q is given by

$$U(x,y) = \sum_{s \in S} \sum_{A \ni s} V_A(y_s x_{S \setminus \{s\}}).$$

We shall say that Q is of Gibbsian form or a **Gibbsian kernel** with energy function U.

Proof. Let V be a potential for Π. By definition and by the form of local characteristics in Proposition 3.2.1 the synchroneous kernel Q induced by Π can be computed:

$$\begin{aligned} Q(x,y) &= \prod_s \frac{\exp\left(-\sum_{A \ni s} V_A(y_s x_{S \setminus \{s\}})\right)}{\sum_s \exp\left(-\sum_{A \ni s} V_A(z_s x_{S \setminus \{s\}})\right)} \\ &= \frac{\exp\left(-\sum_s \sum_{A \ni s} V_A(y_s x_{S \setminus \{s\}})\right)}{\sum_z \exp\left(-\sum_s \sum_{A \ni s} V_A(z_s x_{S \setminus \{s\}})\right)} \end{aligned}$$

Hence an energy function U for Q is given by

$$U(x,y) = \sum_{s} \sum_{A \ni s} V_A(y_s x_{S \setminus \{s\}}).$$ □

For symmetric U, the detailed balance equation yields the invariant distribution.

Lemma 10.2.1. *Suppose that the kernel Q is Gibbsian with symmetric energy, i.e. $U(x,y) = U(y,x)$ for all $x, y \in \mathbf{X}$. Then Q has a reversible distribution μ given by*

$$\mu(x) = \frac{\sum_z \exp(-U(x,z))}{\sum_y \sum_z \exp(-U(y,z))}.$$

Proof. The detailed balance equation reads:

$$\rho(x) Z_Q(x)^{-1} \exp(-U(x,y)) = \rho(y) Z_Q(y)^{-1} \exp(-U(y,x)).$$

By symmetry, this boils down to

$$\rho(x) Z_Q(x)^{-1} = \rho(y) Z_Q(y)^{-1}$$

and hence $\rho(x) = const \cdot Z_Q(x)$ is a solution. Since the invariant distribution μ of Q is unique we conclude that μ is obtained from ρ by proper normalization and hence has the desired form. □

If Π is given by a pair potential then a symmetric energy function for Q exists.

Example 10.2.2 (Pair Potentials). Let the Gibbs field Π be given by a pair potential V and let U denote the energy function of the induced synchroneous kernel Q from Proposition 10.2.1. Then there is a symmetrization $\tilde{U}$ of U:

$$\begin{aligned}
\tilde{U}(x,y) &= U(x,y)+\sum_s V_{\{s\}}(x) = \sum_{\{s,t\}} V_{\{s,t\}}(y_s x_t)) + \sum_s V_{\{s\}}(x) \\
&= \sum_{s\neq t}(V_{\{s,t\}}(y_s x_t)) + \sum_s V_{\{s\}}(y_s) + \sum_s V_{\{s\}}(x_s) \\
&= \sum_{s\neq t}(V_{\{s,t\}}(x_s y_t)) + \sum_s V_{\{s\}}(y_s) + \sum_s V_{\{s\}}(x_s) \\
&= \tilde{U}(y,x).
\end{aligned}$$

Since the difference $\tilde{U}(x,y) - U(x,y)$ does not depend on y, $\tilde{U}$ is an energy function for Q. By Lemma 10.2.1 the reversible distribution μ of Q has energy

$$\tilde{H}(x) = -\ln\left(\sum_z \exp(-\tilde{U}(x,z))\right).$$

There is a representation of $\tilde{H}$ by means of a potential $\tilde{V}$. Extracting the sum in $\tilde{U}$ which does not depend on z yields

$$\mu(x) = Z_\mu^{-1}\exp\left(-\sum_s V_s(x_s)\right)\cdot c(x) \tag{10.4}$$

where $c(x)$ equals

$$\begin{aligned}
&\sum_z \prod_s \exp\left(-\sum_t V_{\{s,t\}}(z_s x_t) - V_{\{s\}}(z_s)\right) \\
&= \prod_s \sum_{z_s} \exp\left(-\sum_t V_{\{s,t\}}(z_s x_t) - V_{\{s\}}(z_s)\right).
\end{aligned}$$

Hence a potential for μ is given by

$$\begin{aligned}
\tilde{V}_{\{s\}}(x) &= V_{\{s\}}(x_s), s\in S, \qquad (10.5)\\
\tilde{V}_{\{s\}\cup\partial(s)}(x) &= -\ln\left\{\sum_{z_s}\exp\left(-\sum_{t:\langle s,t\rangle} V_{\{s,t\}}(z_s x_t) - V_{\{s\}}(z_s)\right)\right\}, s\in S,
\end{aligned}$$

and $\tilde{V}_A = 0$ otherwise.

Remark 10.2.1. This crucially relies on reversibility. It will be shown before long that *it works only if Π is given by a pair potential.* In absence of reversibility, little can be said.

The following lemma will be used to prove a first convergence theorem for annealing.

Lemma 10.2.2. *Let the energy function H be given by the pair potential V and let $(\beta(n))$ increase. Let Q_n be given by (10.3). Then every kernel Q_n has a unique invariant distribution μ_n. The sequences $(\mu_n(x))_{n\geq 1}$, $x \in \mathbf{X}$, are eventually monotone. In particular, condition (4.3) holds.*

Proof. By Example 10.2.2 and Lemma 10.2.1 the invariant distributions μ_n exist and have the form

$$\mu_n(x) = \mu^{\beta(n)}(x) = \frac{\sum_z \exp(-\beta(n)\tilde{U}(x,z))}{\sum_y \sum_z \exp(-\beta(n)\tilde{U}(y,z))}$$

with $\tilde{U}$ specified in Example 10.2.2. The derivative w.r.t. β has the form

$$\frac{d}{d\beta}\mu^{\beta}(x) = const(\beta)^{-1} \sum_{k\in K} g_k \exp(\beta h_k)$$

where $const(\beta)$ is the square of the denominator and hence strictly positive for all β, and where K, g_k and h_k do not depend on β. We may assume that all coefficients in the sum do not vanish and that all exponents are different. For large β, the term with the largest exponent (in modulus) will dominate. This proves that $\mu_n(x)$ eventually is monotone in n. Condition (4.3) follows from Lemma 4.4.2. □

The special form of $\tilde{U}$ derived in Example 10.2.2 can be exploited to get a more explicit expression for μ_∞. We prefer to compute the limit in some examples and give a conspicuous description for a large class of pair potentials.

In the limit theorem for synchroneous annealing the **maximal oscillation**

$$\tilde{\Delta} = \max\{|U(x,y) - U(x,z)| : x, y, z \in \mathbf{X}\}$$

of U will be used. The theorem reads:

Theorem 10.2.2. *Let the function H on $\mathbf{X}$ be given by a pair potential. Let Π be the Gibbs field with energy H and Q_n the synchroneous kernel induced by $\beta(n)H$. Let, moreover, the cooling schedule $(\beta(n))$ increase to infinity not faster than $\tilde{\Delta}^{-1}\ln n$. Then for any initial distribution ν the sequence $(\nu Q_1 \dots Q_n)$ converges to some distribution μ_∞ as $n \to \infty$.*

Proof. The assumptions of Theorem 4.4.1 have to be verified. Condition (4.3) holds by the preceding lemma. By Lemma 4.2.3, the contraction coefficients fulfill the inequality

$$c(Q_n) \leq 1 - \exp(-\beta(n)\tilde{\Delta})$$

and the theorem follows like Theorem 5.2.1. □

10.2.3 Support of the Limit Distribution

For annealing the support

$$\operatorname{supp}\mu_\infty = \{x \in \mathbf{X} : \mu_\infty(x) > 0\}$$

of the limit distribution is of particular interest. It is crucial whether it contains minimizers of H only or also high-energy states. It is instructive to compute invariant distributions and their limit in some concrete examples.

Example 10.2.3. (a) Let us consider a binary model with states 0 or 1, i.e.

$$H(x) = -\sum_{\{s,t\}} w_{st}x_sx_t, \ \ x_s \in \{0,1\}$$

where S is any finite set of sites. Such functions are of interest in the description of textures. They also govern the behaviour of simple neural networks like Hopfield nets and Boltzmann machines (cf. Chapter 15). Let a neighbour potential be given by

$$V_{\{s,t\}}(z_sx_t) = w_{st}z_sx_t, V_{\{s\}}(x_s) = w_{ss}x_s.$$

For updating at inverse temperature β the terms V_A are replaced by βV_A. Spezializing from (10.4) and (10.5), the corresponding energy function H becomes

$$\sum_s \beta w_{ss}x_s - \ln\left\{\sum_{z_s}\exp\left(-\beta\sum_{t\neq s} w_{st}z_sx_t - w_{ss}z_s\right)\right\}.$$

With the short-hand notation

$$v_s(x) = \sum_{t\neq s} w_{st}x_t - w_{ss} \tag{10.6}$$

we can continue with

$$\begin{aligned}
&= \sum_s \beta w_{ss}x_s - \ln(1+\exp(-\beta v_s(x))) \\
&= \sum_s \beta w_{ss}x_s + \beta v_s(x)/2 - \ln(\exp(\beta v_s(x)/2)+\exp(-\beta v_s(x)/2)) \\
&= \beta\sum_s\{-\beta^{-1}\ln(\cosh(\beta v_s(x)/2) + (2w_{ss}x_s + v_s(x))/2 - \ln 2\}.
\end{aligned}$$

Hence the invariant distribution μ^β is given by

$$\begin{aligned}
\mu^\beta(x) &= Z_\beta^{-1}\exp\left(-\sum_s -\ln(\cosh(\beta v_s(x)/2) + \beta(2w_{ss}x_s + v_s(x))/2\right) \\
&= Z_\beta^{-1}\prod_s \cosh(\beta v_s(x)/2)\exp(-\beta(2w_{ss}x_s + v_s(x))/2)
\end{aligned}$$

with a suitable normalization constant Z_β. Let now β tend to infinity. Since

$$\ln\cosh(a) \sim |a| \text{ for large } |a|,$$

the first identity shows that μ^β, $\beta \to \infty$, tends to the uniform distribution on the set of minimizers of the function

$$x \longmapsto \sum_s 2w_{ss}x_s + v_s(x) - |v_s(x)|.$$

(b) For the generalized Ising model (or the Boltzmann machine with states $\pm$ 1), one has

$$H(x) = -\sum_{\{s,t\}} w_{st}x_s x_t, \;\; x_s \in \{-1,1\}$$

The arguments down to (10.6) apply *mutatis mutandis* and $\tilde{H}^\beta$ becomes

$$\begin{aligned} &\sum_s \beta w_{ss}x_s - \ln(\exp(\beta v_s(x)) + \exp(-\beta v_s(x))) \\ = \;\; &\sum_s \{\beta w_{ss}x_s - \ln(\cosh(\beta v_s(x))) - \ln 2\}. \end{aligned}$$

Again, cancelling out $\ln 2$ gives

$$\begin{aligned} \mu^\beta(x) &= Z_\beta^{-1} \exp\left\{\sum_s -\beta w_{ss}x_s + \ln\cosh(\beta v_s(x))\right\} \\ &= Z_\beta^{-1} \prod_s \cosh(\beta v_s(x)) \exp(-\beta w_{ss}x_s). \end{aligned}$$

The energy function

$$\sum_s \{\beta w_{ss}x_s - \ln\cosh(\beta v_s(x))\}$$

in the second expression is called the **Little Hamiltonian** (PERETTO (1984)).

Similarly as above, μ^β tends to the uniform distribution on the set of minimizers of the function

$$x \longmapsto \sum_s w_{ss}x_s - \left|\sum_{s \neq t} w_{st}x_t - w_{ss}\right|.$$

In particular, for the simple Ising model on a lattice with

$$H(x) = -\sum_{\langle s,t\rangle} x_s x_t,$$

annealing minimizes the function

$$x \longmapsto -\sum_s \left| \sum_{\langle s,t \rangle} x_t \right| .$$

This function becomes minimal if and only if for each s all the neighbours have the same colour. This can only happen for the two constant configurations and the two chequer-board configurations. The former are the minima whereas the latter are the maxima of H. Hence synchroneous annealing produces minima and maxima with probability $1/2$ each.

By arguments of A. TROUVÉ (1988) the last example can be generalized considerably.

Let S be endowed with a a neighbour hood system ∂. Denote the set of cliques by $\mathbf{C}$ and let a neighbour potential $V = (V_C)_{C \in \mathbf{C}}$ be given. Assume that there is a partition $\mathbf{T} = \{T\}$ of S into independent sets and choose $T \in \mathbf{T}$. Since a clique meets T in at most one site and since $V_C(x)$ does not depend on the values x_t for $t \notin C$,

$$\sum_{s \in T} \sum_{s \in C \in \mathbf{C}} V_C(y_s x_{S \backslash \{s\}}) = \sum_{C \in \mathbf{C}, C \cap T \neq \emptyset} V_C(y_T x_{S \backslash T}).$$

Hence

$$\begin{aligned}
&R_T(x,y) \\
&= \frac{\exp\left(-\sum_{s \in T} \sum_{s \in C \in \mathbf{C}} V_C(y_s x_{S \backslash \{s\}})\right)}{\sum_{z_T} \exp\left(-\sum_{s \in T} \sum_{s \in C \in \mathbf{C}} V_C(z_s x_{S \backslash \{s\}})\right)} \\
&= \frac{\exp\left(-\sum_{C \in \mathbf{C}, C \cap T \neq \emptyset} V_C(y_T x_{S \backslash T})\right)}{\sum_{z_T} \exp\left(-\sum_{C \in \mathbf{C}, C \cap T \neq \emptyset} V_C(z_T x_{S \backslash T})\right)} \\
&= \frac{\exp\left(-\sum_{C \in \mathbf{C}, C \cap T \neq \emptyset} V_C(y_T x_{S \backslash T}) - \sum_{C \in \mathbf{C}, C \cap T = \emptyset} V_C(y_T x_{S \backslash T})\right)}{\sum_{z_T} \exp\left(-\sum_{C \in \mathbf{C}, C \cap T \neq \emptyset} V_C(z_T x_{S \backslash T}) - \sum_{C \in \mathbf{C}, C \cap T = \emptyset} V_C(z_T x_{S \backslash T})\right)} \\
&= \frac{\exp(-H(y_T x_{S \backslash T}))}{\sum_{z_T} \exp(-H(z_T x_{S \backslash T}))}.
\end{aligned}$$

Since

$$Q(x,y) = R_S(x,y) = \prod_{T \in \mathbf{T}} R_T(x,y)$$

we find that

$$U(x,y) = \sum_{T \in \mathbf{T}} H(y_T x_T) \tag{10.7}$$

defines an energy function for $Q = R_S$.

Example 10.2.4 (TROUVÉ *(1988))*. Let the chromatic number be 2.

Note that this implies that H is given by a neighbour potential. The converse does not hold: For $S = \{1,2,3\}$ the Ising model $H(x) = x_1x_2 + x_2x_3 + x_3x_1$ is given by a neighbour potential for the neighbourhood system with neighbour pairs $\{1,2\},\{2,3\},\{3,1\}$. The set S is a clique and hence the chromatic number is 3.

For chromatic number 2, S is the disjoint union of two nonempty independent subsets R and T. Specializing from (10.7) yields

$$U(x,y) = H(x_Ry_T) + H(y_Rx_T). \tag{10.8}$$

The invariant distribution μ_n of Q is given by

$$\mu_n(x) = Z_n^{-1}\sum_z \exp(-\beta(n)U(x,z))$$

where

$$Z_n = \sum_{y,z} \exp(-\beta(n)U(y,z))$$

is the normalization constant. To find the limit μ_∞ as $\beta(n)$ tends to infinity, set

$$m = \min\{U(x,y) : x,y \in \mathbf{X}\}$$

and rewrite μ_n in the form

$$\mu_n(x) = \frac{\sum_z \exp(-\beta(n)(U(x,z)-m)}{\sum_{y,z}\exp(-\beta(n)(U(y,z)-m)}.$$

The denominator tends to

$$q = |\{(y,z) : U(y,z) = m\}|$$

and the numerator to

$$q(x) = |\{z : U(x,z) = m\}|.$$

Hence

$$\mu_\infty(x) = \frac{q(x)}{q}.$$

In particular, $\mu_\infty(x) > 0$ if and only if there is a z such that $U(x,z)$ is minimal. Since U is given in terms of H by (10.8), the latter holds if and only if both, $H(x_Rz_T)$ and $H(z_Rx_T)$, are minimal. In summary, $\mu_\infty(x) > 0$ if and only if x equals a minimizer of H on R and a (possibly different) minimizer on T. Hence the support of μ_∞ is

$$\operatorname{supp}\mu_\infty = \{x_Ry_T : x \text{ and } y \text{ minimize } H\}.$$

Plainly, the minimizers of H are contained in this set, but it can also contain configurations with high energy. In fact, $\operatorname{supp}\mu_\infty$ is strictly larger than the set of minimizers of H if and only if H has at least two (different) minimizers.

For the Ising model $H(x) = -\sum_{\langle s,t \rangle} x_s x_t$, the support of μ_∞ consists of the two constant configurations and the two chequer-board-like configurations which are the minima and maxima of H, respectively, and we have reproved the reproved the last result in Example 10.2.3.

If the chromatic number is larger than 2 then the situation is much more complicated. We shall pursue this aspect in the next section.

Remark 10.2.2. We discussed synchroneous algorithms from a special point of view: A fixed function H has to be minimized or samples from a fixed field Π are needed. A typical example is the travelling salesman problem. In applications like texture analysis, however, the situation is different. A parametrized model class is specified and some field in this class is chosen as an approximation to some unknown law. This amounts to the choice of suitable parameters by some estimation or 'learning' algorithm, based on a set of observations or samples from the unknown distribution. Standard parametrized families consist of binary fields like those in the last examples (cf. the Hopfield nets or Boltzmann machines). But why should we not take synchroneous invariant distributions as the model class, determine their parameters and then use synchroneous algorithms (which in this case work correctly)? Research on such approaches is quite recent. In fact, for synchroneous invariant distributions generally there is no explicit description and statisticians are not familiar with them. On the other hand, for most learning algorithms an explicit expression for the invariant distributions is not necessary. This promises to become an exciting field of future research. First results have been obtained for example in AZENCOTT (1990a)–(1992b).

10.3 Synchroneous Algorithms and Reversibility

In the last section, we were faced with several difficulties involved in the parallel implementation of sampling and annealing. A description of the invariant distribution was found for pair potentials only; in particular, the invariant distributions were reversible. In this chapter we shall prove kind of 'converse': reversible distributions exist only for pair potentials. This severely hampers the study of synchroneous algorithms.

We shall establish a framework in which existence of reversible distributions and their relation to the kernels can be studied systematically. We essentially follow the lines of H. KÜNSCH (1984), a paper which generalizes and develops main aspects in D.A. DAWSON (1975), N. VASILYEV (1978) and O. KOZLOW and N. VASILYEV (1980) (these authors assume countable index sets S).

10.3.1 Preliminaries

For the computations it will be convenient to have (Gibbsian) representations for kernels in terms of potentials. Let $\mathcal{S}$ denote the collection of nonempty subsets of S and $\mathcal{S}_0$ the collection of all subsets of S.

A collection $\Phi = \{\Phi_{AB} : A \in \mathcal{S}_0, B \in \mathcal{S}\}$ of functions

$$\Phi_{AB} : \mathbf{X} \times \mathbf{X} \longrightarrow \mathsf{R}$$

is called a **potential** (for a transition kernel) if $\Phi_{AB}(x, y)$ depends on x_A and y_B only. Given a reference element $o \in \mathbf{X}$ the potential is **normalized** if $\Phi_{AB}(x, y) = 0$ whenever $x_s = o_s$ for some $s \in A$ or $y_s = o_s$ for some $s \in B$. A kernel Q on $\mathbf{X}$ is called Gibbsian with potential Φ if it has the form

$$Q(x, y) = Z_Q(x)^{-1} \exp\left(- \sum_{A \in \mathcal{S}_0} \sum_{B \in \mathcal{S}} \Phi_{AB}(x, y) \right).$$

Remark 10.3.1. Random fields – i.e. strictly positive probability measures on $\mathbf{X}$ – are Gibbs fields (and conversely). Similarly, transition kernels are Gibbsian if and only if they are strictly positive. For Gibbsian kernels there also is a unique normalized potential. This can be proved along the lines of Section 3.3. We shall not carry out the details and take this on trust.

Example 10.3.1. If

$$\Phi_{AB} = 0 \quad \text{if} \quad |B| > 1 \tag{10.9}$$

then Q is synchroneous with

$$q_s(x, y_s) = Z_{s,x}^{-1} \exp\left(- \sum_{A \in \mathcal{S}_0} \Phi_{A\{s\}}(x, y) \right).$$

Conversely, if Q is synchroneous then (10.9) must hold for normalized Φ.

The synchroneous kernel Q induced by a Gibbs field Π with potential V (cf. Example 10.2.1) is of the form

$$Q(x, y) = Z_Q(x)^{-1} \exp\left(- \sum_{s \in S} \sum_{s \notin A \in \mathcal{S}} V_{A \cup \{s\}}(y_s x_{S \setminus \{s\}}) \right)$$

(Proposition 10.2.1). Hence Q is Gibbsian with potential

$$\Phi_{A\{s\}}(x, y) = V_{A \cup \{s\}}(y_s x_{S \setminus \{s\}})$$

if $s \notin A$ and $\Phi_{AB} = 0$ otherwise. Note that Φ is normalized if V is normalized.

We are mainly interested in synchroneous kernels Q. But we shall deal with 'reversed' kernels $\hat{Q}$ of Q and these will in general not be synchroneous (cf. Example refex synchroneous two examples). Hence we had to introduce the more general Gibbsian kernels.

Recall that a Markov kernel Q is reversible w.r.t. a distribution μ if it fulfills the detailed balance equation

$$\mu(x)Q(x,y) = \mu(y)Q(y,x),\ x,y \in \mathbf{X}.$$

Under reversibility the distribution

$$\bar{\mu}((x,y)) = \mu \otimes Q((x,y)) = \mu(x)Q(x,y)$$

on $\mathbf{X} \times \mathbf{X}$ is symmetric i.e. $\bar{\mu}(x,y) = \bar{\mu}(y,x)$ and vice versa (we skipped several brackets). If x is interpreted as the state of a homogeneous Markov chain $(\xi_n)_{n\geq 0}$ with transition probability Q and initial distribution μ at time 0 (or n) and y as the state at time 1 (or $n+1$) then the two-dimensional marginal distribution $\bar{\mu}$ is invariant under the exchange of the time indices 0 and 1 (or n and $n+1$) and hence 'reversible'. For a general homogeneous Markov chain (ξ_n) the **time-reversed kernel** $\hat{Q}$ is given by

$$\hat{Q}(x,y) = \mathsf{P}(\xi_0 = y | \xi_1 = x) = \bar{\mu}(\{y\} \times \mathbf{X} | \mathbf{X} \times \{x\}).$$

Reversibility implies $\hat{Q} = Q$ which again supports the above interpretation. Moreover, it implies invariance of μ w.r.t. Q and therefore the one-dimensional marginals of $\bar{\mu}$ are equal to μ.

Why did we introduce this concept? We want to discuss the relation of transition kernels and their invariant distributions. The reader may check that all invariant distributions we dealt with up to now fulfilled the detailed balance equation. This indicates that reversibility is an important special case of invariance. We shall derive conditions under which distributions are reversible for synchroneous kernels and thus gain some insight into synchroneous dynamics. The general problem of invariance is much more obscure.

Example 10.3.2. (a) Let $\mathbf{X} = \{0,1\}^2$ and $q_s((x_0,x_1),y_s) = p$, $0 < p < 1$, for $y_s = x_s$. Let Q denote the associated synchroneous kernel and $q = 1-p$. Then Q can be represented by the matrix

$$\begin{pmatrix} p^2 & pq & pq & q^2 \\ pq & p^2 & q^2 & pq \\ pq & q^2 & p^2 & pq \\ q^2 & pq & pq & p^2 \end{pmatrix}$$

where the rows from top to bottom and the coloumns from left to right belong to $(0,0),(0,1),(1,0),(1,1)$, respectively. Q has invariant distribution $\mu = (1/4,1/4,1/4,1/4)$ and by the symmetry of the matrix μ is reversible. The reversed kernel $\hat{Q}$ equals Q and hence $\hat{Q}$ is synchroneous.

(b) Let now $q_s((x_0, x_1), y_s) = p$ for $y_s = x_0$. Then the synchroneous kernel has the matrix representation

$$\begin{pmatrix} p^2 & pq & pq & q^2 \\ p^2 & pq & pq & q^2 \\ q^2 & pq & pq & p^2 \\ q^2 & pq & pq & p^2 \end{pmatrix}$$

and the invariant distribution is

$$\mu = \left((p^2 + q^2)/2, pq, pq, (p^2 + q^2)/2\right).$$

We read off from the first coloumn in the tableau that for instance

$$\hat{Q}((0,0)) = const \cdot \left((p^2 + q^2)p^2/2, p^2pq, q^2pq, (p^2 + q^2)q^2/2\right).$$

This is a product measure if and only if $p = 1/2$ and else μ is not reversible for Q and the reversed kernel is not synchroneous.

10.3.2 Invariance and Reversibility

We are going now to establish the relation between an initial distribution μ, the transition kernel Q and the reversed kernel $\hat{Q}$ and also the relation between the respective potentials. In advance, we fix a reference element $o \in \mathbf{X}$, and a site $a \in S$; like in Chapter 3 the symbol ${}^a x$ denotes the configuration which coincides with x off a and with ${}^a x_a = o_a$. We shall need some elementary computations. The following identity holds for every initial distribution μ and every transition kernel Q:

$$\frac{\mu(x)}{\mu({}^a x)} = \frac{Q({}^a x, y)}{Q(x, y)} \frac{\hat{Q}(y, x)}{\hat{Q}(y, {}^a x)}. \tag{10.10}$$

Proof.

$$\begin{aligned} & \mu(x)Q(x,y)\hat{Q}(y,{}^a x) \\ = \quad & \mu(x)\frac{\bar{\mu}(x,y)}{\mu(x)} \cdot \frac{\bar{\mu}({}^a x, y)}{\mu Q(y)} \\ = \quad & \mu({}^a x)\frac{\bar{\mu}({}^a x,y)}{\mu({}^a x)} \cdot \frac{\bar{\mu}(x, y)}{\mu Q(y)} \\ = \quad & \mu({}^a x)Q({}^a x,y)\hat{Q}(y,x). \end{aligned}$$

In particular, both sides of the identity are defined simultaneously or neither of them is defined. □

Assume now that Φ is a normalized potential for the kernel Q. Then

$$\begin{aligned} \frac{Q({}^a x, y)}{Q(x,y)} &= \frac{\sum_u g(x,u)Q({}^a x,u)}{g(x,y)}, \\ \text{where } g(x,y) &= \exp\left(-\sum_{a\in A}\sum_{B\in\mathcal{S}} \Phi_{AB}(x,y)\right), \qquad (10.11) \\ \sum_u g(x,u)Q({}^a x,u) &= \frac{Z_x}{Z_{a_x}}. \end{aligned}$$

We wrote Z_x for $Z_Q(x)$.

Proof. The first equality is verified by straightforward calculations:

$$\begin{aligned} &\frac{Q({}^a x,y)}{Q(x,y)} \\ &= \frac{Z_x}{Z_{^a x}} \cdot \frac{\exp\left(-\sum_{A\in\mathcal{S}_0}\sum_{B\in\mathcal{S}} \Phi_{AB}({}^a x,y)\right)}{\exp\left(-\sum_{A\in\mathcal{S}_0}\sum_{B\in\mathcal{S}} \Phi_{AB}(x,y)\right)} \\ &= \frac{1}{Z_{^a x}} \cdot \frac{\sum_z \exp\left(-\sum_{A\in\mathcal{S}_0}\sum_{B\in\mathcal{S}} \Phi_{AB}(x,z)\right)}{\exp\left(-\sum_{a\in A}\sum_{B\in\mathcal{S}} \Phi_{AB}(x,y)\right)} \\ &= \frac{1}{g(x,y)} \cdot \sum_z \exp\left(-\sum_{a\in A}\sum_{B\in\mathcal{S}} \Phi_{AB}(x,z)\right) \frac{\exp\left(\sum_{a\notin A}\sum_{B\in\mathcal{S}} \Phi_{AB}(x,z)\right)}{Z_{^a x}} \\ &= \frac{\sum_z g(x,z)Q({}^a x,z)}{g(x,y)}. \end{aligned}$$

The rest follows immediately from the last equation. □

Putting (10.10) and (10.11) together yields:

$$\frac{\mu(x)}{\mu({}^a x)} = \frac{\sum_z g(x,z)Q({}^a x,z)}{g(x,y)} \cdot \frac{\hat{Q}(y,x)}{\hat{Q}(y,{}^a x)}. \qquad (10.12)$$

Let us draw a first conclusion.

Theorem 10.3.1. *Suppose that the transition kernel Q has the normalized potential Φ. Then the invariant distribution μ of Q and the reversed kernel $\hat{Q}$ are Gibbsian. The normalized potential $\hat{\Phi}$ of $\hat{Q}$ fulfills*

$$\hat{\Phi}_{AB}(x,y) = \Phi_{BA}(y,x) \text{ for } A,B \in \mathcal{S}.$$

The normalized potential V of μ and the functions $\hat{\Phi}_{\emptyset A}$ determine each other by

$$\begin{aligned}\exp\left(-\sum_{a\in A} V_A(x)\right) &= \sum_u g(x,u)Q({}^ax,u)\cdot\exp\left(-\sum_{a\in A}\hat{\Phi}_{\emptyset A}(x)\right)\\ &= \frac{Z_x}{Z_{{}^ax}}\exp\left(-\sum_{a\in A}\hat{\Phi}_{\emptyset A}(x)\right).\end{aligned}$$

Proof. Q is Gibbsian and hence strictly positive. The invariant distribution of a strictly positive kernel is uniquely determined and itself strictly positive by the Perron-Frobenius Theorem (Appendix B). Hence the last fraction in (10.12) is (finite and) strictly positive and thus $\hat{Q}$ is Gibbsian since 'Gibbsian' is equivalent to strict positivity.

Assume now that μ and $\hat{Q}$ are Gibbsian with normalized potentials V and $\hat{\Phi}$. Then the left-hand side of (10.12) is

$$\frac{\mu(x)}{\mu({}^ax)} = \exp\left(-\sum_{a\in A} V_A(x)\right).$$

Setting

$$\gamma = \sum_u g(x,u)Q({}^ax,u)$$

the right-hand side becomes

$$\begin{aligned}&\frac{\sum_u g(x,u)Q({}^ax,u)}{g(x,y)}\cdot\frac{\hat{Q}(y,x)}{\hat{Q}(y,{}^ax)}\\ &= \gamma\cdot\exp\left(-\sum_{A\in\mathcal{S}_0}\sum_{a\in B}\hat{\Phi}_{AB}(x,y)+\sum_{a\in A}\sum_{B\in\mathcal{S}}\Phi_{AB}(x,y)\right)\\ &= \gamma\cdot\exp\left(-\sum_{a\in A}\hat{\Phi}_{\emptyset A}(x)-\sum_{a\in A}\sum_{B\in\mathcal{S}}(\hat{\Phi}_{BA}(x,y)-\Phi_{AB}(x,y)\right).\end{aligned}$$

Hence

$$\begin{aligned}&\exp\left(-\sum_{a\in A} V_A(x)\right)\\ &= \gamma\cdot\exp\left(-\sum_{a\in A}\hat{\Phi}_{\emptyset A}(x)-\sum_{a\in A}\sum_{B\in\mathcal{S}}(\hat{\Phi}_{BA}(y,x)-\Phi_{AB}(x,y))\right).\end{aligned}$$

For every x, the double sum on the right does not depend on y and vanishes for $y = o$. Thus it vanishes identically. This yields the representation of μ. By the uniqueness of normalized potentials even the single terms of the double sum must vanish and hence $\hat{\Phi}_{AB}(x,y) = \Phi_{BA}(y,x)$ for $A, B \in \mathcal{S}$. This completes the proof. □

The formulae show that the joint dependence of $\hat{Q}$ on x and y – expressed by the functions $\hat{\Phi}_{AB}$ – is determined by Q while the dependence on x alone – expressed by the functions $\hat{\Phi}_{\emptyset A}(x)$ – is influenced by μ. If μ is invariant for Q then because of the identity $\mu = \mu Q$ its potential depends on both, Q and $\hat{Q}$. If we are looking for a kernel leaving a given μ invariant we must take the reversed kernel into account which makes the examination cumbersome. For reversible (invariant) distributions we can say more.

Theorem 10.3.2. *Let Q be a Gibbsian kernel with unique invariant distribution μ. Let Φ denote a normalized potential for Q. Then μ is reversible if and only if*

$$\Phi_{AB}(x,y) = \Phi_{BA}(y,x) \text{ for all } A, B \in \mathcal{S}.$$

The normalized potentials V of μ and Φ of Q determine each other by

$$\begin{aligned}\exp\left(-\sum_{a\in A} V_A(x)\right) &= \sum_u g(x,u)Q(^a x, u)\cdot \exp\left(-\sum_{a\in A}\Phi_{\emptyset A}(x)\right)\\ &= \frac{Z_y}{Z_{^a x}}\exp\left(-\sum_{a\in A}\Phi_{\emptyset A}(x)\right).\end{aligned}$$

Proof. By the last theorem, μ and $\hat{Q}$ are Gibbsian. If μ is reversible then the reversed kernel coincides with Q and again by the last theorem

$$\Phi_{AB}(x,y) = \hat{\Phi}_B A(y,x) = \Phi_{BA}(y,x) \text{ for } A, B \in \mathcal{S}.$$

In addition, $\hat{\Phi}_{\emptyset B}(x) = \Phi_{\emptyset B}(x)$ and thus the representation of the potential V follows from the last theorem. That the symmetry condition implies reversibility will be proved in the next proposition. □

Proposition 10.3.1. *Let Q be a Gibbsian kernel with potential Φ satisfying the symmetry condition*

$$\Phi_{AB}(x,y) = \Phi_{BA}(y,x) \text{ for all } x, y \in \mathbf{X} \text{ and } A, B \in \mathcal{S}.$$

Then the invariant distribution of Q is reversible. It can be constructed in the following way: Consider the doubled index set $S \times \{0,1\}$ and define a potential

$$\begin{aligned}\Psi_{(A\times\{0\})\cup(B\times\{1\})}(x,y) &= \Phi_{AB}(x,y) \text{ for } A \in \mathcal{S}_0, B \in \mathcal{S},\\ \Psi_{A\times\{0\}}(x,y) &= \Phi_{\emptyset A}(x) \text{ for } A \in \mathcal{S}.\end{aligned}$$

(x denotes the coordinates $z_{s,0}$, $s \in S$, and y the coordinates $z_{s,1}$ of an element z of

$$\prod_{s\in S, i\in\{0,1\}} \mathbf{X}_{s,i},\ \mathbf{X}_{s,i} = \mathbf{X}_s).$$

Then the projection μ of the Gibbs field for Ψ onto the 0-th time coordinate is invariant and reversible for Q.

Proof. We are going to check the detailed balance equation. We denote the normalization constants of μ and $Q(x,\cdot)$ by Z_μ and $Z_Q(x)$, respectively, and write $\Phi_{A\emptyset}$ for $\Psi_{A\times\{0\}}$. Then

$$Z_\mu\mu(x) = \sum_z \exp\left(-\sum_{A,B\in\mathcal{S}_0} \Phi_{AB}(x,z)\right) = \exp\left(-\sum_{A\in\mathcal{S}} \Phi_{A\emptyset}(x)\right)\cdot Z_Q(x).$$

Hence

$$\begin{aligned} &Z_\mu\mu(x)Q(x,y) \\ &= \exp\left(-\sum_{A\in\mathcal{S}}\Phi_{A\emptyset}(x)\right)\exp\left(-\sum_{B\in\mathcal{S}}\Phi_{\emptyset B}(y)+\sum_{A,B\in\mathcal{S}}\Phi_{AB}(x,y)\right). \end{aligned}$$

By symmetry, this equals $Z_\mu\mu(y)Q(y,x)$ and detailed balance holds. □

Let us now spezialize to synchroneous kernels Q. The symmetry condition for the potential is rather restrictive.

Proposition 10.3.2. *A synchroneous Gibbsian kernel with normalized potential Π has a reversible distribution only if all terms of the potential vanish except those of the form*

$$\Phi_{AB}(x,y) = \Phi_{st}(x_s,y_t),\ \ \Phi_{\emptyset B}(y) = \Phi_s(y_s).$$

The kernel is induced by a Gibbs field with a pair potential given by

$$\begin{aligned} V_{\{s\}}(x) &= \Phi_s(x_s),\ \ s\in S, \\ V_{\{s,t\}}(x) &= 2\Phi_{\{s,t\}}(x_s x_t),\ \ s,t\in S, s\neq t, \\ V_A(x) &= 0,\ \ |A|>2. \end{aligned}$$

Proof. Let Q denote the synchroneous kernel. Then $\Phi_{AB}=0$ if $|B|>1$, and by symmetry, $\Phi_{AB}=0$ if $|B|>1$ or $|A|>1$. This proves the first assertion. That a Gibbs field with potential V induces Q was verified in Example 10.2.2. □

10.3.3 Final Remarks

Let us conclude our study of synchroneous algorithms with some remarks and examples.

Example 10.3.3. Let the synchroneous kernel Q be induced by a random field with potential V like in Example 10.2.1 and Proposition 10.2.1:

$$\Phi_{A\{s\}}(x,y) = V_{A\cup\{s\}}(y_s x_{S\setminus\{s\}}). \tag{10.13}$$

By the last result, V is a pair potential, i.e. only V_A of the form $V_{\{s,t\}}$ or $V_{\{s\}}$ do not vanish. This shows that the invariant distribution of Q satisfies the detailed balance equation if and only if Π is a Gibbs field for a pair potential.

By Proposition 10.3.2 and Example 10.2.2 (or by Proposition 10.3.1) the reversible distribution of a Gibbsian synchroneous kernel has a potential $\tilde{V}$ given by

$$\begin{aligned} \tilde{V}_{\{s\}}(x) &= \Phi_s(x_s),\ s \in S, \\ \tilde{V}_{\{s\}\cup\partial(s)}(x) &= -\ln\left\{\sum_{z_s}\exp\left(-\sum_{t\in\partial(s)}\Phi_{st}(z_s,x_t)-\Phi_s(z_s)\right)\right\},\quad s\in S, \\ \tilde{V}_A(x) &= 0 \text{ otherwise.} \end{aligned} \tag{10.14}$$

We conclude:

If the Gibbsian synchroneous kernel Q has a reversible distribution, then there is a neighbourhood system ∂, such that

$$q_s(x,y_s) = q_s(x_{\{s\}\cup\partial(s)}, y_s).$$

Define now a second order neighbourhood system by

$$\tilde{\partial}(s) = \partial(\partial(s)).$$

Then the singletons and the sets $\{s\}\cup\partial(s)$ are cliques of $\tilde{\partial}$ and μ is a 'second order' Markov field, i.e. a Markov field for $\tilde{\partial}$.

Let us summarize:

1. Each Markov field Π induces a synchroneous kernel Q. If Π is Gibbsian with potential V then Q is Gibbsian with the potential Φ given by (10.13). Q has an invariant Gibbsian distribution μ. In general, μ is different from Π and there is no explicit description of μ.
2. Only a Gibbs fields Π for a pair potential induces a reversible synchroneous kernel Q. If so, then the invariant distribution μ is Gibbsian with the potential in (10.14). This μ is Markov for a neighbourhood system with larger neighbourhoods than those of Π. Conversely, each synchroneous kernel is induced by a Gibbs field with pair potential.
3. Let $\Pi^{(n)}$ be the Gibbs field for pair potential $\beta(n)V$, let $Q^{(n)}$ be the induced synchroneous kernel $\beta(n) \nearrow \infty$. These kernels have reversible (invariant) distributions μ_n. In general, $\lim_{n\to\infty}\Pi^{(n)} \neq \lim_{n\to\infty} = \mu_\infty$. In particular, the support of μ_∞ can be considerably larger than the set of minima of the energy function $H = \sum_A V_A$.

Note that the potentials for generalized Ising models or Boltzmann machines are pair potentials and μ_∞ *can* be computed. The models for imaging we advocate rarely are based on pair potentials. On the other hand, for them limited parallelism is easy to implement. If there is long range dependence or if random interactions are introduced (like in partitioning) this can be hard. But even if synchroneous reversible dynamics exist one must be aware of (3).

Let us finally mention another naive idea. Given a function H to be minimized, one might look for a potential V which gives the desired minima and try to find corresponding synchroneous dynamics. Plainly, the detailed balance equation would help to compute the kernel. An example by DAWSON (1975) shows that even in simple cases no natural synchroneous dynamics exist.

Example 10.3.4. DAWSON's result applies to infinite volume Gibbs fields. It implies:

For the Ising field Π on $\mathbb{Z}^2$ there is no reversible synchroneous Markov kernel Q for which Π is invariant and for which the local kernels q_s are symmetric and translation invariant.

The result extends to homogeneous Markov fields (for the Ising neighbourhood system) the interactions of which are not essentially one-dimensional. The proof relies on explicit calculations of the local probabilites for all possible local configurations. For details we refer to the original paper.

Part IV

Texture Analysis

Having introduced the Bayesian framework and discussed algorithms for the computation of estimators we report now some concrete applications to the segmentation and classification of textures. The first approach once more illustrates the range of applicability of dynamic Monte Carlo methods. The second one gives us the opportunity to introduce a class of random field models, generalizing the Ising type and binary models. They will serve as examples for parameter estimation to be discussed in the next part of the text.

Parts of natural scenes often exhibit a repetitive structure similar to the texture of cloth, lawn, sand or wood, viewed from a certain distance. We shall freely use the word 'texture' for such phenomena. A commonly accepted definition of the term 'texture' does not exist and most methods in texture discrimination are *ad hoc* techniques. (For recent attempts to study textures systematically see GRENANDER (1976), (1978) and 1981)).

Notwithstanding these misgivings, something can be done. Even without a precise notion of textures, one may tell textures apart just comparing several features. Or, very restricted texture models can be formulated and parameters in these models fitted to samples of real textures. This way, one can mimic nature to a degree, which is sufficient or at least helpful for applications like quality control of textile or registration of damages done to forests (and many others).

Let us stress that the next two chapters are definitely not intended to serve as an introduction to texture segmentation. This is a field of its own. Even a survey of recent Markov field models is beyond the scope of this text. We confine ourselves to illustrate such methods by way of some representative examples.

11. Partitioning

11.1 Introduction

In the present chapter, we focus on partitioning or segmenting images into regions of similar texture. We shall not 'define' textures. We just want to tell different textures apart (in contrast to the classification methods in the next chapter).

A segmentor subdivides the image; a classifier recognizes or classifies individual segments as belonging to a given texture. Direct approaches to classification will be addressed in the next chapter. However, partitioning can also be useful in classification. A 'region classifier' which decides to which texture a region belongs can be put to work after partitioning. This is helpful in situations where there are no *a priori* well-defined classes; perhaps, these can be defined after partitioning.

Basically, there are two ways to partition an area into regions of different textures: either different textures are painted in different colours or boundaries are drawn between regions of different textures. We shall give examples for both approaches. They are constructed along the lines developed in Chapter 2 for the segmentation of images into smooth regions.

Irrespective of the approach, we need criteria for similarity or disparity of textures.

11.2 How to Tell Textures Apart

To tell a white from a black horse it is sufficient to note the different colours. To discriminate between horses of the same colour, another feature like their height or weight is needed. Anyway, a relatively small amount of data should suffice for discrimination and a full biological characterization is not necessary. In the present context, one has to decide whether the textures in two blocks of pixels are similar or not. The decision is made on the basis of texture features, for example primitive characteristics of grey-value configurations, hopefully distinguishing between the textures. The more textures one has and the more similar they are, the more features are necessary for reliable partitioning. Once a set of features is chosen, a deterministic decision rule can be formulated: Decide that the textures in two blocks are different if they differ noticeable in at least one feature and otherwise treat them as equal. Let us make this precise. Let $(y_s)_{s\in S^P}$ be a grey value configuration on a finite square lattice S^P and let B and D denote two blocks of pixels. The blocks will get the same label if they contain similar textures and for different textures there will be different labels. For simplicity, labeling will be based on the grey-value configurations y_B and y_D on the blocks. Let L be a supply of labels or symbols large enough to discriminate between all possible pairs of textures. Next, a set $(\phi^{(i)})$ of features is chosen. For the present, features may be defined as mappings $y_B \mapsto \phi^{(i)}(y_B) \in \Phi^{(i)}$ to a suitable space $\Phi^{(i)}$, typically a Euclidean space R^d. Each space $\Phi^{(i)}$ is equipped with some measure $d^{(i)}$ of distance. A rigid condition for equality of textures (and assigning equal labels to B and D) is $d^{(i)}(\phi^{(i)}(y_B), \phi^{(i)}(y_D)) < c^{(i)}$ for all i and thresholds $c^{(i)}$. If one of these constraint is violated the labels will be different. This way a family $(l_B)_{B\text{ a block}}$ of labels – called a labeling – is defined. The set of constraints may then be augmented by requirements on organization of label configurations. Then the Bayesian machinery is set to work: the rigid constraints are relaxed to a prior distribution, and, given the observation, the posterior serves as a basis for Bayes estimators.

11.3 Features

Statistics provides a whole tool-kit of features, usually corresponding to estimators of relevant statistical entities. The most primitive features are based on first-order grey value histograms. If $G \in \mathsf{R}$ is the set of grey-values the **histogram** of a configuration on a pixel block B is defined by

$$h(g) = \frac{|\{s \in B : y_s = g\}|}{|B|}, \quad g \in G.$$

The shape of histograms provides many clues as to characterizes textures. There are the empirical mean

$$\mu = \sum_{g\in G} g h(g)$$

or the (empirical) variance or second centered moment

$$\sigma^2 = \sum_{g\in G} (g-\mu)^2 h(g).$$

The latter can be used to establish descriptors of relative smoothness like

$$1 - \frac{1}{1+\sigma^2}$$

which vanishes for blocks of constant intensity and is close to 1 for rough textures. The third centered moment

$$\sum_{g\in G}(g-\mu)^3 h(g)$$

is a measure of skewness. For example, most natural images possess more dark than bright pixels and their histograms tend to fall off exponentially at higher luminance levels. Still other measures are the energy and entropy, given by

$$\sum_{g\in G} h(g)^2, \quad -\sum_{g\in G} h(g)\log_2(h(g)).$$

Such functions of the first-order histogram do not carry any information regarding the relative position of pixels with respect to each other. **Second-order histograms** do: Let S be a subset of Z^2, y a grey-value configuration and $\tau \in \mathsf{Z}^2$. Let A_τ be the $|G| \times |G|$-matrix with entries $A_\tau(g,g')$, $g,g' \in G$. $A_\tau(g,g')$ is the number of pairs $(s, s+\tau)$ in $S \times S$ with $y_s = g$ and $y_{s+\tau} = g'$. Normalization, i.e. division of $A_\tau(g,g')$ by the number of pairs $(s, s+\tau) \in S \times S$ gives the second-order histogram or **cooccurence matrix** C_τ. For suitable τ, the entries will cluster around the diagonal in $S \times S$ for coarse texture, and will be more uniformly dispersed for fine texture. This is illustrated by two binary patterns and their matrices A_τ for $\tau = (0,1)$ in Fig. 11.1.

1	1	1	1	1
1	1	1	1	0
1	1	1	0	0
1	1	0	0	0
1	0	0	0	0

	0	1
0	6	0
1	4	10

1	0	1	0	1
0	1	0	1	0
1	0	1	0	1
0	1	0	1	0
1	0	1	0	1

	0	1
0	0	10
1	10	0

Figure 11.1

Various descriptors for the shape were suggested by Haralick and others (1979), cf. also Haralick and Shapiro (1992), Chapter 9. For instance, element-difference moments

$$\sum_{g,g'}(g-g')^k C_\tau(g,g')$$

are small for even and positive k if the high values of C_τ are near the diagonal. Negative k have the opposite effect. The entropy

$$-\sum_{g,g'} C_\tau(g,g')\ln C_\tau(g,g')$$

is maximal for the uniform and small for less 'random' distributions. A variety of other descriptors may be derived from such basic ones (cf. PRATT (1978), 17.8) or HARALICK and SHAPIRO (1992).

The use of such descriptors is supported by a conjecture by B. JULESZ et al. (1973) (see also JULESZ (1975)), who argue that, in general, it is hard for viewers to tell a texture from another with the same first- and second-order statistics. This will be discussed in Section 11.5.

11.4 Bayesian Texture Segmentation

We are going now to describe a Bayesian approach to texture segmentation. We sketch the circle of ideas behind the comprehensive paper by D. and S. GEMAN, CHR. GRAFFIGNE and PING DONG (1990), cf. also D. GEMAN (1990).

11.4.1 The Features

These authors use statistics of higher order, derived from a set of transformations of the raw data. Thus the features are now grey-value histograms.

The simplest transformation is the identity

$$y^{(1)} = y$$

where y is the configuration of grey values. Let now s be a label site (labeling is usually performed on a subset of pixel sites) and let B_s be a block of pixel sites centering around s. Then

$$y_s^{(2)} = \max\{y_t : t \in B_s\} - \min\{y_t : t \in B_s\},$$

is the intensity range in B_s. If ∂B_s denotes the perimeter of B_s then the 'residual' is given by

$$y_s^{(3)} = \left| y_s - \frac{1}{|\partial B_s|} \sum_{t \in \partial B_s} y_t \right|.$$

Similarly,

$$\begin{aligned} y_s^{(4)} &= \left| y_s - (y_{s+(1,0)} + y_{s-(1,0)})/2 \right|, \\ y_s^{(5)} &= \left| y_s - (y_{s+(0,1)} + y_{s-(0,1)})/2 \right|, \end{aligned}$$

are the directional residuals (we have tacitly assumed that the pixels are arranged on a finite lattice; there are modifications near its boundary). The residuals gauge the distance of the actual value in s to the linear prediction based on values nearby. One may try other transformations like mean or variance, but not all add sufficient information. The block size may vary from transformation to transformation and from pixel to pixel.

11.4.2 The Kolmogorov-Smirnov Distance

The basis of further investigation are the histograms of arrays $y^{(i)}$ in pixel blocks around label sites. For label sites s and t, blocks D_s and D_t of pixels around s and t are chosen and the histograms of $(y_r^{(i)} : r \in D_s)$ and $(y_r^{(i)} : r \in D_t)$ are compared. The distance between the two histograms will be measured in terms of the Kolmogorov-Smirnov distance. This is simply the max-norm of the difference of the sample distribution functions corresponding to the histograms (cf. any book on statistics above the elementary level). It plays an important role in Kolmogorov-Smirnov tests, whence the name. To be more precise, let the transformed data in a block be denoted by $\{v\}$. Then the sample or empirical distribution function $F : \mathsf{R} \mapsto [0,1]$ is given by

$$F(\tau) = |\{v\}|^{-1}\,|\{v : v \le \tau\}|$$

and the **Kolmogorov-Smirnov distance** of data $\{v\}$ and $\{w\}$ in two blocks is

$$d(\{v\},\{w\}) = \max\{|F_{\{v\}}(\tau) - F_{\{w\}}(\tau)| : \tau \in \mathsf{R}\}.$$

This distance is invariant under strictly monotone transformations ρ of the data since

$$|\{\rho v : \rho v \le \rho\tau\}| = |\{v : v \le \tau\}|.$$

In particular, the distance does not change for the residuals, if the raw data are linearly transformed. In fact, setting

$$y'_s = \left|y_s - \sum \vartheta_t y_t\right|, \sum \vartheta_t = 1;$$

one gets

$$(ay+b)'_s = \left|ay_s + b - \sum \vartheta_t(ay_t + b)\right| = |a|y'_s$$

and for $a \ne 0$ this transformation is strictly monotone and does not affect the distance.

Invariance properties of features are desirable, since they contribute to robustness against shading etc.. Let us now turn to partioning.

11.4.3 A Partition Model

There are a pixel and a label process y and x. The array $y = (y_s)_{s\in S^P}$ describes a pattern of grey values on a finite lattice $S^P = \{(i,j) : 1 \le i,j \le N\}$. The array $x = (x_s)_{s\in S^L_\rho}$ represents labels from set L on a sublattice

$$S^L_\rho = \{(i\rho+1, j\rho+1) : 0 \le i,j \le (N-1)/\rho\}.$$

The number ρ corresponds to resolution: low resolution – i.e. large ρ – suppresses boundary effects and gives more reliability but looses details. There is some neighbourhood system on S^L_ρ and - as usual - the symbol $\langle s,t\rangle$ will indicate that $s,t \in S^L_\rho$ are neighbours. The pixel-label interaction is given by

$$K(y,x) = \sum_{\langle s,t\rangle} \Psi_{s,t}(y)\Phi_{s,t}(x)$$

where usually $\Phi_{s,t}(x) = 1_{\{x_s=x_t\}}$. Ψ measures disparity of the textures around s and t – hence Ψ must be small for similar textures and large for dissimilar ones. Later on, a term will be added to K, weighting down undesired label configurations.

Basically, the textures around label sites $s,t \in S^L_\rho$ are counted as different, if for some i the Kolmogorov-Smirnov distance of the transformed data $y^{(i)}_{D_s}$ in a block D_s around s and $y^{(i)}_{D_t}$ in a block D_t around t exceeds a certain threshold $c^{(i)}$. This leads to the choice

$$\Psi_{s,t}(y) = \max\left\{2\cdot 1_{\left\{d\left(y^{(i)}_{D_s},y^{(i)}_{D_t}\right)>c^{(i)}\right\}}(y) - 1 : i\right\}.$$

In fact, $\Psi_{s,t}(y) = +1$ or -1 depending on whether $d^{(i)} > c^{(i)}$ for some index i or $d^{(i)} \le c^{(i)}$ for all i. Thus $\Psi_{s,t}(y) = 1$ corresponds to dissimilar blocks and is coupled with distinct labels; similarly, identical labels are coupled with $\Psi_{s,t}(y) = -1$.

Note the similarity to the prior in Example 2.3.1. The function Ψ there was a disparity measure for grey values.

Remark 11.4.1. Let us stress that the disparity measure might be based on any combination of features and suitable distances. One advantage of the features used here is the invariance property. On the other hand, their computation requires more CPU-time.

In their experiments, GEMAN, GEMAN et al. (1990) use one (i.e. the raw grey values) to five transformations. In the first case, the model seems to be relatively robust to the choice of the threshold parameter c and it was simply guessed. For more transformations, parameters were adjusted to limit the percentage of false alarms: Samples from homogeneous regions of the textures were chosen; then the histograms for the Kolmogorov-Smirnov distance for pairs of blocks inside these homogeneous regions were computed and thresholds were set such that no more than three or four percent of the intra region distances were above the thresholds. 'Learning the parameters' $c^{(i)}$ is 'supervised' since texture samples are used.

To complete the model, undesired label configurations are penalized, in particular small and narrow regions. A region is 'small' at label site s if less than 9 labels in a 5×5-block E_s in S^L_ρ around s agree with x_s . 'Thin' regions are only one label-site wide (at resolution ρ) in the horizontal or vertical direction. Hence the number of penalties for small regions is

$$\sum_s \mathbf{1}_{\{\sum_{t \in E_s} \mathbf{1}_{\{x_t = x_s\}} < 9\}}(x)$$

and the number of thin regions is

$$\sum_s \mathbf{1}_{\{x_{s-(1,0)} \neq x_s, x_s \neq x_{s+(1,0)}\}} + \mathbf{1}_{\{x_{s-(0,1)} \neq x_s, x_s \neq x_{s+(0,1)}\}}.$$

The total number $V(x)$ of penalties is the sum of these two terms. In summary, the complete energy function takes the form

$$H(y,x) = K(y,x) + V(x).$$

11.4.4 Optimization

Some final remarks concern optimization of H. The authors experiment with sampling and annealing methods or with combinations of these. They adopt sequential visiting schedules as well as setwise updating.

Recall that y is fixed. Given a site s, either the label in site s is updated or a small set of labels around s is updated simultaneously. The latter is feasible by the results in Chapter 7. The authors frequently use a cross of 5 sites in S_ρ^L with center s. Following the lines of early chapters, one would minimize the overall energy function $K(x) + V(x)$ by annealing or sample from $\beta(K(x) + V(x))$ at sufficiently high temperature. The authors argue, that the expectations about certain types of labels are quite precise and rigid. Hence they introduce hard constraints for the forbidden configurations counted by V. The set of feasible solutions is $\{V(x) = 0\}$ and H is minimized on this set only. By the theory in Chapter 7 this can be done introducing $\beta(K(x) + \lambda V(x))$ and then run annealing with $\beta, \lambda \nearrow \infty$. In practice, the authors fix some high inverse temperature β_0 and let λ tend to infinity in order to gradually introduce the hard constraints.

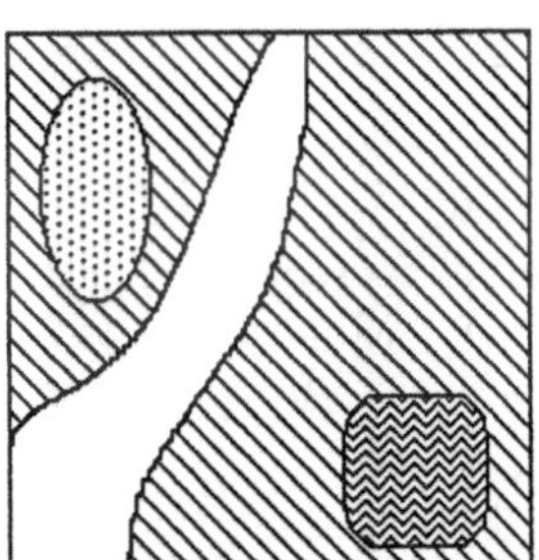

Fig. 11.2.

There are two main drawbacks in these algorithms. The energy landscape of H contains wide local minima like the Ising model. Thus convergence is extremely slow. Secondly, regions of the same texture but with nonoverlapping boundaries like the striped ones in Fig. 11.2 may get different labels and such of different texture like the smaller patches in the Figure may be labeled identically. This undesired effect is illustrated by a simple example below. As a remedy, the authors introduce random neighbourhoods. From time to time, given a label site s, they randomly choose 'neighbours' t which possibly are far away. The labels are then updated as usual using these random neighbours. Introduction of such long range interactions suppresses spurious labelings. There is some evidence that the problem of wide local minima is also overcome. On the other hand, there is little theoretical support for such a conjecture.

Let us conclude this section with the announced example.

Example 11.4.1. Consider the following problem: Given a grey-value pattern find a labeling such that patches of the same grey values are uniformly labeled.

Let y denote a pattern of p grey values and x a pattern of $q \geq p$ labels. (Plainly, y itself *is* a labeling and thus the example is not of practical interest.) In view of the Ising or Potts model, an energy function appropriate for the above task is given by

$$H(y,x) = \sum_{\langle s,t \rangle} 1_{\{x_s = x_t\}} \Psi_{s,t}(y)$$

where $\Psi_{s,t}(y)$ weights the disparity of y_s and y_s. A reasonable choice is $\Psi_{s,t}(y) = -1$ if $y_s = y_t$ and $\Psi_{s,t}(y) = 1$ otherwise. If undegraded data are observed the posterior distribution is

$$\Pi(x|y) = Z(y)^{-1} \exp(-H(y,x)).$$

Let now S be a 3×3-lattice, $\partial(s)$ the usual 4-neighbourhood and $p = 2$. Consider two observations y:

1	1	0
1	0	0
0	0	0

1	0	0
0	0	0
0	0	1

For the left observation all labelings assigning one label to regions of grey-value 1 and another to regions of grey-value 0 is an MAP estimate. For $q = 3$ such labelings may look like

1	1	0
1	0	0
0	0	0

2	2	1
2	1	1
1	1	1

The right observation has MAP estimates like

0	1	1
1	1	1
1	1	0

2	1	1
1	1	1
1	1	0

Regions of the same grey value can break into regions of different labels if their neighbourhoods do not intersect. The model solves the problem of assigning the same label to *connected* patches of the same grey value but it does not necessarily label disconnected regions of the same grey value uniformly. To solve the latter problem long range interactions have to be introduced as indicated above.

11.4.5 A Boundary Model

Various types of boundaries correspond to sudden changes of image attributes in two-dimensional scenes. There may be sudden changes in shape (surface creases), depth (occluding boundaries) or surface composition. We focus on the latter now. Whereas in the models of Chapter 2 a boundary element was encouraged by disparity of intensity, disparity of textures will be the criterion now. The pixel lattice S^P is the same as above and the boundary lattice S^B is the $(N-1)\times(N-1)$-lattice interspersed among the pixels like in Example 2.4.1. S^B_ρ is the sublattice of S^B for resolution ρ. The boundary process is $b=(b_s)_{s\in S^B_\rho}$ with $b_s\in\{0,1\}$ and neighbourhoods consisting of the northern, southern, eastern and western nearest neighbours in S^B_ρ. Thus $\langle s,t\rangle$ in S^B_ρ corresponds to a horizontal or vertical string of $\rho+1$ sites in S^P including s,t and the sites inbetween. In Fig. 11.3, the pixel locations are indicated by $\circ$, the bars are the micro edges and the stars are the vertices of S^B (i.e. S^B_ρ for $\rho=1$). Vertices of S^B_ρ of boundary elements for resolution $\rho=3$ are marked by a diamond.

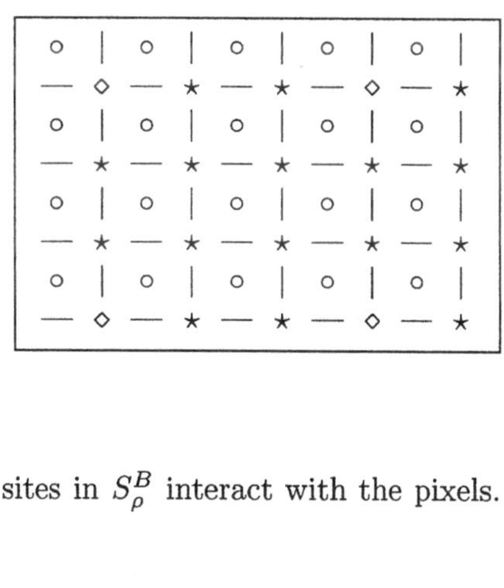

Figure 11.3

Only boundary sites in S^B_ρ interact with the pixels. The interaction has the general form

$$K(y,b) = \sum_{\langle s,t \rangle} \Psi(\Delta_{s,t}(y))(1 - b_s b_t).$$

$\Delta_{s,t}(y)$ will gauge the 'disparity flux' across the string $\langle s,t \rangle$. To make this precise, let $B(s,t)$ and $D(s,t)$ be adjacent blocks of pixels separated by $\langle s,t \rangle$ as displayed in Fig. 11.4.

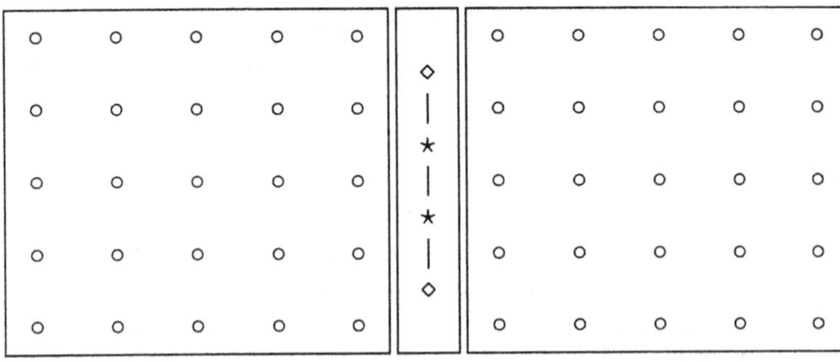

Figure 11.4

Let $y^{(i)}$ be the data under the i-th transformation, $y^{(i)}_{B(s,t)}$ and $y^{(i)}_{D(s,t)}$ the transformed data in the blocks and set

$$\Delta_{s,t}(y) = \max\left\{ \left(c^{(i)}\right)^{-1} d\left(y^{(i)}_{B(s,t)}, y^{(i)}_{D(s,t)} \right) : i \right\}$$

Similar to the partition model, the thresholds $c^{(i)}$ are chosen to limit false alarms. Plainly, a boundary string $\langle s,t \rangle = [\diamond - \star - \star - \diamond]$ should be switched on, i.e $(1 - b_s b_t) = 1$, if the adjacent textures are dissimilar. The function Ψ should be low for similar textures i.e. around the minimum of Δ which is 0. Furthermore, Ψ should be increasing with $\Psi(0) < 0$ (if Ψ were never negative then $b \equiv 1$ would minimize the interaction energy). The authors employ

$$\Psi(\Delta) = \left(\frac{\Delta - \gamma}{1 - \gamma} \right)^2, \ \Delta \geq \gamma, \quad \Psi(\Delta) = -\left(\frac{\Delta - \gamma}{\gamma} \right)^2, \ 0 \leq \Delta \leq \gamma.$$

Finally, forbidden configurations are penalized. There are selected undesidered local configurations in S^B_ρ, for instance

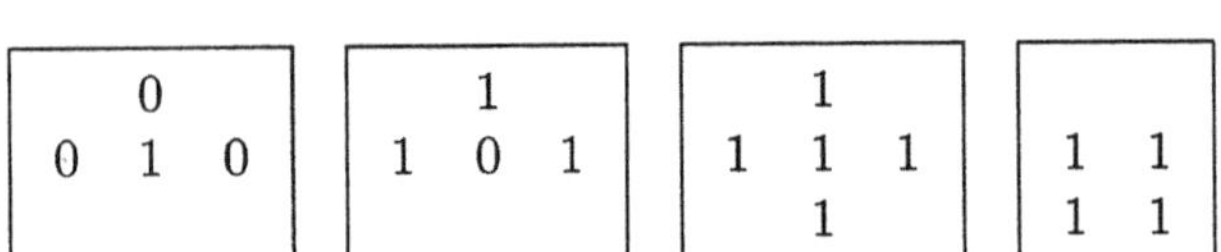

Figure 11.5

correspond to an isolated or abandoned segment, sharp turn, quadrupel junction and small structure, respectively. $V(b)$ denotes the number of these local configurations and defines the forbidden set. Then H is minimized under the constraint $V = 0$ like in partitioning.

For more information the reader is referred to the original paper and to D. GEMAN (1990). The authors perform a series of experiments with partioning and boundary maps and comment on details of modelling and computation.

11.5 Julesz's Conjecture

11.5.1 Introduction

In Section 11.3, a conjecture of Julesz and others was mentioned, concerning the ability of the human visual system to discriminate textures. We shall comment on its mathematical background and give a 'counterexample'. This gives the opportunity for an excursion to the theory of point processes.

The objective of the last pages was the design of systems which automatically discriminate different textures. Basically, one should be able to tell them apart by statistical means like suitable features. In practice, features often are chosen or discarded interactively, i.e. by visual inspection of the corresponding labelings. This brings up the question about human ability to discriminate textures. B. JULESZ (1975) and others (1973) systematically searched for a 'mathematical' or quantitative conjecture about the limits of human texture perception and carried out a series of experiments. They conclude that

> [] texture discrimination ceases rather abruptly when the order of complexity exceeds a surprisingly low value. Whereas textures that differ in the first- and second-order statistics can be discriminated from each other, those that differ in their third or higher order statistics usually cannot.
> (JULESZ (1975), p. 35).

Fig. 11.6 shows a simple example (for more complicated ones cf. the cited literature). Two textures are displayed. There is a large square with white $\sqcap$s on black background and a smaller one in which the $\sqcap$s are rotated. Rotation by 90° results in a texture with different second-order statistics and the difference is readily visible. If the $\sqcap$s are turned around (right figure) the second-order statistics do not change and discrimination requires deliberate effort.

11.5.2 Point Processes

Point processes are models for sparse random point patterns on the Euclidean plane (or, more generally, on R^d). One might be reminded of cities distributed over the country or stars scattered over the sky. Such a point pattern is a

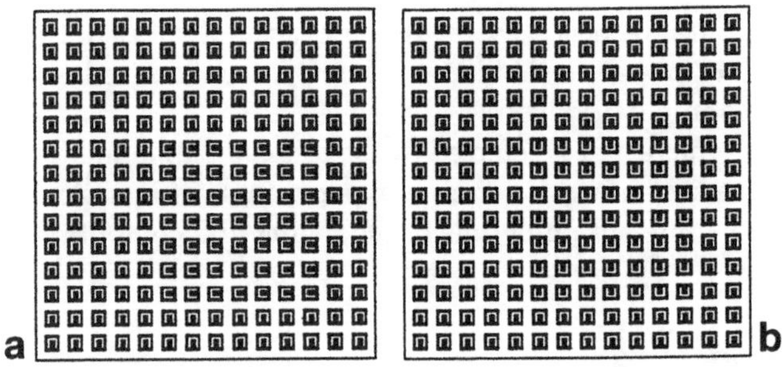

Fig. 11.6. Patterns with (**a**) different, (**b**) identical second-order statistics

countable subset $\omega \subset \mathsf{R}^2$ and the point process is a probability distribution P on the space Ω of all point clouds ω. Here we leave discrete probability, but the arguments should be plausible. The space Ω is a continuous analogue of the discrete space $\mathbf{X}$ and P corresponds to the former Π. One is particularly interested in the number of points falling into test sets; for every (measurable and) bounded subset A of the plane this number is a random variable given by

$$N(A) : \Omega \longrightarrow \mathsf{N}_0, \omega \longmapsto N(A)(\omega) = |A \cap \omega|.$$

The **homogeneous Poisson process** is characterized by two properties

(i) For each measurable bounded nonempty subset A of the plane the number $N(A)$ of counts in A has a Poisson distribution with parameter $\lambda \cdot \mathsf{area}(A)$.

(ii) The counts $N(A)$ and $N(B)$ for disjoint subsets A and B of R^2 are independent.

The constant $\lambda > 0$ is called **intensity**. A homogeneous Poisson process is automatically isotropic. To realize a pattern ω, say on a unit square, draw a number N from a Poisson distribution of mean λ, and distribute N points uniformly and independently of each other over the square. Hence Poisson processes may be regarded as continuous parameter analogues of independent observations.

Second-order methods are concerned with the covariances of a process. In the independent case, only the variances of the single variables have to be known and this property is shared by the Poisson process. In fact, let A and B be bounded, set $A' = A \backslash B$, $B' = B \backslash A$ and $C = A \cap B$. Then by (ii),

$$\begin{aligned} & \mathsf{cov}(N(A), N(B)) \\ = \; & \mathsf{cov}(N(A') + N(C), N(B') + N(C)) \\ = \; & \mathsf{var}(N(C)) = \mathsf{var}(N(A \cap B)). \end{aligned}$$

A.J. BADDELEY and B. W. SILVERMAN (1984) construct a point process with the same second-order properties as the Poisson process which easily can be discriminated by an observer. The design principle is as follows: Divide the plane into unit squares, by randomly throwing down a square grid. For each cell C, choose a random occupation number $N(C)$ independently of the others, and with distribution

$$\mathsf{P}(N(C)=0)=\frac{1}{10},\mathsf{P}(N(C)=1)=\frac{8}{9},\mathsf{P}(N(C)=10)=\frac{1}{90}.$$

Then distribute N(C) points uniformly over the cell C. The key feature of this distribution is

$$\mathsf{E}(N(C))=\mathsf{var}(N(C))(=1). \tag{11.1}$$

This is used to show

Proposition 11.5.1. *For both, the cell process and the Poisson process with intensity 1,*

$$\mathsf{E}(N(A))=\mathsf{var}(N(A))=\mathsf{area}(A)$$

for every Borel set A in R^2.

Proof. For the Poisson process, $N(A)$ is Poissonian with mean – and therefore variance – $a=\mathsf{area}(A)$. Let E_G and var_G denote expectation and variance conditional on the position and orientation of the grid. Let C_i denote the cells and a_i the area of $A\cap C_i$ (recall $\mathsf{area}(C_i)=1$). *Conditional* on the grid *and* on the chosen number of points in C_i, $N(A\cap C_i)$ has a binomial distribution with parameters $N(C_i)$ and a_i. By (11.1),

$$\mathsf{E}_G(N(A\cap C_i))=\mathsf{E}_G(\mathsf{E}(N(A\cap C_i)|N(C_i)))=\mathsf{E}(a_iN(C_i))=a_i.$$

Similarly,

$$\begin{aligned} &\mathsf{var}(N(A\cap C_i))\\ =\;&\mathsf{E}_G(\mathsf{var}_G(N(A\cap C_i)|N(C_i)))+\mathsf{var}_G(\mathsf{E}(N(A\cap C_i)|N(C_i)))\\ =\;&\mathsf{E}_G(N(C_i)a_i(1-a_i))+\mathsf{var}_g(a_iN(C_i)))\\ =\;&a_i(1-a_i)+a_i^2=a_i.\end{aligned}$$

Plainly,

$$\mathsf{E}_G(N(A))=\sum\mathsf{E}_G(N(A\cap C_i))=a.$$

Conditional on the grid, the random variables $N(A\cap C_i)$ are independent and hence

$$\mathsf{var}_G(N(A))=\sum\mathsf{var}_G(N(A\cap C_i))=a.$$

We conclude

$$\mathsf{E}(N(A))=\mathsf{E}(\mathsf{E}_G(N(A)))=a$$

and

$$\mathsf{var}(N(A))=\mathsf{var}_G(N(A))+\mathsf{var}(\mathsf{E}_G(N(A)))=a+0=a.$$

This completes the proof. □

The relation between the two processes, revealed by this result, is much closer than might be expected. B. RIPLEY (1976) shows that for a homogeneous and isotropic processes the noncentered covariances can be reduced to a nonnegative increasing function K on $(0, \infty)$. By homogeneity, $\mathsf{E}(N(A)) = \lambda \cdot \mathsf{area}(A)$. K is given by (don't worry about details)

$$E(N(A)N(B)) = \lambda(A \cap B) + \lambda^2 \int_0^\infty \nu_t(A \times B) dK(t)$$

where

$$\nu_t(A \times B) = \int_A \sigma_t(\{v - u | v \in B, \|v - u\| = t\}) du$$

and σ_t is the uniform distribution on the surface of the sphere of radius t centered at the origin. For a Poisson process, $K(t)$ is the volume of a ball of radius t (hence $K(t) = \pi t$ in the plane). Two special cases give intuitive interpretations (RIPLEY (1977)):

(i) $\lambda^2 K(t)$ is the expected number of (ordered) pairs of distinct points not more than distance t apart and with the first point in a set of unit area.

(ii) $\lambda K(t)$ is the expected number of further points within radius t of an arbitrary point of the process.

By the above proposition,

Corollary 11.5.1. *The cell and the Poisson process have the same K-function.*

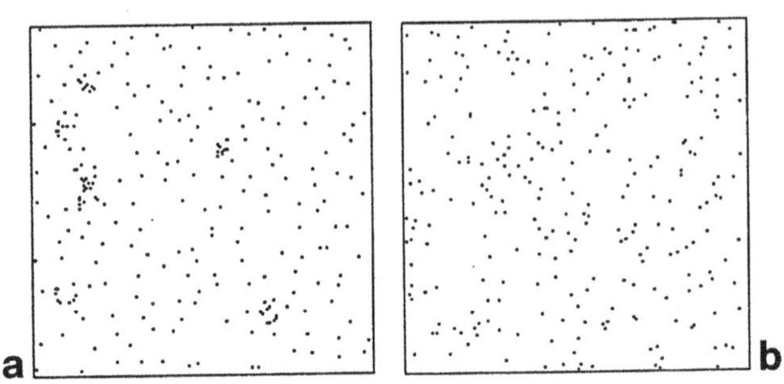

Fig. 11.7. (a) A sample from the cell process, (b) a sample from the Poisson process

Hence these processes share a lot of geometric properties based on distances of pairs of points. Nevertheless, realizations from these processes can easily be discriminated by the human visual system as Fig. 11.7 shows.

12. Texture Models and Classification

12.1 Introduction

In contrast to the last chapter, regions of pixels will now be classified as belonging to particular types or classes of texture. There are numerous deterministic or probabilistic approaches to classification, and in particular, to texture classification. We restrict our attention to some model-based methods.

For a type or class of textures there is a Markov random field on the full space $\mathbf{X}$ of grey value configurations and a concrete instance of this type is interpreted as a sample from this field. This way, texture classes correspond to random fields. Given a random field, Gibbs- or Metropolis samplers may be adopted to produce samples and thus to synthesize textures. By the way, well-known autoregressive techniques for synthesis will turn out to be special Gibbs samplers.

The inverse – and more difficult – problem is to fit Gibbs fields to given data. In other words, Gibbs fields have to be determined, samples of which are likely to resemble an initially given portion of pure texture. This is an own and difficult topic and will be addressed in the next part of the text.

Given the random fields corresponding to several texture classes, a new texture can be classified as belonging to that random field from which it is most likely to be a sample.

Pictures of natural scenes are composed of several types of texture, usually represented by certain labels. The picture is covered with blocks of pixels, and the configuration in each block is classified. This results in a pattern of labels – one for each texture class – and hence a segmentation of the picture. In contrast to the methods in the last chapter, those to be introduced provide information about the texture type in each segment. Such information is necessary for many applications. The labelling is a pattern itself, possibly supposed to be structured and organized. Such requirements can be integrated into a suitable prior distribution.

Remark 12.1.1. Intuitively, one would guess that such random field models are more appropriate for pieces of lawn than for pictures of a brick wall. In fact, for regular 'textures' it is reasonable to assume, for example, that they are composed of texture elements or primitives – such as circles, hexagons or dot patterns – which are distributed over the picture by some (deterministic) placement rule. Natural microtextures are not appropriately described by such a model since possible primitives are very random in shape. CROSS and JAIN (1983) (see below) carried out experiments with random field models of maximum fourth-order dependence i.e. about 20 neighbours mostly on 64×64 lattices (for higher order one needs larger portions of texture to estimate the parameters). The authors find that synthetic microtextures closely resemble their real counterparts while regular and inhomogeneous textures (like the brick wall) do not. Other models used to generate and represent textures include (CROSS and JAIN (1987)): (1) time series models, (2) fractals, (3) random mosaic methods, (4) mathematical morphology, (5) syntactic methods, (6) linear models.

12.2 Texture Models

We are going now to describe some representative Markov random field models for pure texture. The pixels are arranged on a finite subset S of $\mathbb{Z}^2$, say a large rectangle (generalization to higher dimension is straightforward). There is a common finite supply G of grey values. A pure texture is assumed to be a sample from a Gibbs field Π on the grey value configurations $y \in \mathbf{X} = G^S$. All these Gibbs fields have the following invariance property: The neighbourhoods are of the form $(\partial(0)+s)\cap S$ for a fixed 'neighbourhood' $\partial(0)$ of $0 \in \mathbb{Z}^2$, and, whenever $(\partial(0)+s),(\partial(0)+t) \subset S$ then

$$\Pi\left(X_s = x_s | X_{\partial(s)} = x_{\partial(s)}\right) = \Pi(X_t = (\theta_{t-s}x)_t | X_{\partial(t)} = (\theta_{t-s}x)_{\partial(t)}\right)$$

where $(\theta_u x)_t = x_{t-u}$. The energy functions depend on multidimensional parameters ϑ corresponding to various types of texture.

12.2.1 The Φ-Model

We start with this model because it is constructed like those previously discussed. It is due to CHR. GRAFFIGNE (1987) (cf. also D. GEMAN and CHR. GRAFFIGNE (1987)). The energy function is of the form

$$K(y) = \sum_{i=1}^{6} \sum_{\langle s,t\rangle_i} \vartheta_i \Psi(y_s - y_t).$$

The symbol $\langle s,t\rangle_i$ indicates that s and t form one of six types of pair cliques like in Fig. 12.1.

The disparity function Ψ is for example

$$\Psi(\Delta) = \frac{-1}{1+|\Delta/\delta|^2}$$

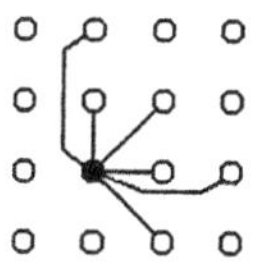

Fig. 12.1. Six types of pair cliques

with a positive scaling parameter δ. Any other disparity function increasing in $|\Delta|$ may be plugged in. On the other hand, functions like the square penalize large grey value differences too hard and the above form of Ψ worked reasonably. DERIN and ELLIOTT (1987) adopt the degenerate version $\Psi(\Delta) = -\gamma$ if $\Delta = 0$, i.e. $y_s = y_t$, and $\Psi(\Delta) = \gamma$ otherwise, for some $\gamma > 0$. The latter amounts to a generalized Potts model. Note that for positive ϑ_i, similar grey values of i-neighbours are favourable while dissimilar ones are favourable for negative ϑ_i. Small values $|\vartheta_i|$ correspond to weak and large values $|\vartheta_i|$ correspond to strong coupling. By a suitable choice of the parameters clustering effects (cf. the Ising model at different temperatures), anisotropic effects, more or less ordered patterns and attraction-repulsion effects can be incorporated into the model.

GRAFFIGNE calls the model Φ-model since she denotes the disparity function by Φ.

12.2.2 The Autobinomial Model

The energy function in the autobinomial model for a pure texture is given by

$$K(y) = -\sum_{i=1}^{T} \vartheta_i \sum_{\langle s,t\rangle_i} y_s y_t - \vartheta_0 \sum_s y_s - \sum_s \ln \binom{N}{y_s}$$

where the grey levels are denoted by $0, \ldots, N$ and $\binom{n}{m}$ are the binomial coefficients. This model was used for instance in CROSS and JAIN (1983) for texture synthesis and modeling of real textures. Like in the Φ-model, the symbol $\langle s, t\rangle_i$ indicates that s and t belong to a certain type of pair cliques. The single-site local characteristics are

$$\frac{\binom{N}{y_s}\left(\exp\left(\vartheta_0 + \sum_{i=1}^{T} \vartheta_i \sum_{\langle s,t\rangle_i} y_t\right)\right)^{y_s}}{\sum_{z_s} \binom{N}{z_s}\left(\exp\left(\vartheta_0 + \sum_{i=1}^{T} \vartheta_i \sum_{\langle s,t\rangle_i} y_t\right)\right)^{z_s}}.$$

Setting

$$a = \exp\left(\vartheta_0 + \sum_{i=1}^{T} \vartheta_i \sum_{\langle s,t\rangle_i} y_t\right), \tag{12.1}$$

the binomial formula gives $(1 + a)^N$ for the denominator and the fraction becomes

$$\binom{N}{y_s} a^{y_s}(1+a)^{-N} = \binom{N}{y_s} \left(\frac{a}{1+a}\right)^{y_s} \left(1 - \frac{a}{1+a}\right)^{N-y_s}.$$

Thus the grey level in each pixel has a binomial distribution with parameter $a/(1+a)$ controlled by its neighbours. In the binary case $N = 1$, where $y_s \in \{0,1\}$, the expression boils down to

$$\frac{\exp\left(y_s\left(\vartheta_0 + \sum_{i=1}^T \vartheta_i \sum_{\langle s,t\rangle_i} y_t\right)\right)}{1 + \exp\left(\vartheta_0 + \sum_{i=1}^T \vartheta_i \sum_{\langle s,t\rangle_i} y_t\right)}. \tag{12.2}$$

CROSS and JAIN use different kinds of neighbours. Given a pixel $s \in S$, the neighbours of first order are those next to s in the eastern, western, northern and southern direction, i.e. those with Euclidean distance 1 from s. Neighbours of order two are those with distance $\sqrt{2}$, i.e. the next pixels on the diagonals. Similarly, order three neighbours have distance 2 from s and order 4 neighbours have distance $\sqrt{5}$. The symbols for the various neighbours of a pixel s can be read off from Table 12.1.

Table 12.1

	$o1$	m	$q1$	
$o2$	v	u	z	$q2$
l	t	s	t'	l'
$q1'$	z'	u'	v'	$o1'$
	$q2'$	m'	$o2'$	

Because of translation invariance the parameters say for the pair $\langle s,t\rangle$ and $\langle s,t'\rangle$ must coincide. They are denoted by $\vartheta(1,1)$. Similarly, the parameter for $\langle s,u\rangle$ and $\langle s,u'\rangle$ is $\vartheta(1,2)$. These are the parameters for the first-order neighbours. The parameters for the third-order neighbours m, m' and l, l' are $\vartheta(3,1)$ and $\vartheta(3,2)$, respectively. Hence for a fourth-order model the exponent $(\ln a)$ takes the values

$$\begin{aligned}
&\vartheta(0) + \vartheta(1,1)(t+t') + \vartheta(1,2)(u+u') \\
+\;& \vartheta(2,1)(v+v') + \vartheta(2,2)(z+z') \\
+\;& \vartheta(3,1)(m+m') + \vartheta(3,2)(l+l') \\
+\;& \vartheta(4,1)(o1+o1'+o2+o2') + \vartheta(4,2)(q1+q1'+q2+q2').
\end{aligned}$$

(we wrote t for $y_t, \ldots$). For lower order, just cancel the lines with higher indices k in $\vartheta(k,\cdot)$.

Samples from GRAFFIGNE's model tend to be smoother than those from the binomial model.

12.2.3 Automodels

Gibbs fields with energy function

$$H(x) = -\sum_s G(y_s)y_s - \frac{1}{2}\sum_{\langle s,t\rangle} a_{st}y_sy_t$$

are called **automodels**. They are classified according to the special form of the single-site local characteristics. We already met the autobinomial model, where the conditional probabilities are binomial, and the autologistic model. If grey values are countable and the projections X_s conditioned on the neighbours obey a Poisson law with mean $\mu_s = \exp(a_s + \sum a_{st}y_t)$ then the field is **autopoisson**. For real-valued colours autoexponential and autogamma models may be introduced – corresponding to the exponential and gamma-distribution, respectively. Of main interest are **autonormal models**. The grey values are real with conditional densities

$$f_s(x_s|rest) = (2\pi\sigma^2)^{-1}\exp\left(-\frac{1}{2\sigma^2}\left(x_s - \left(\mu_s + \sum_{\langle s,t\rangle} a_{st}(x_t-\mu_t)\right)\right)^2\right)$$

where $a_{st} = a_{ts}$. The corresponding Gibbs field has density proportional to

$$\exp\left(-\frac{1}{2\sigma^2}(x-\mu)^*B(x-\mu)\right),$$

where $\mu = (\mu_s)_{s\in S}$ and B is the $|S|\times|S|$-matrix with diagonal elements 1 and off-diagonal elements $-a_{st}$ (if s and t are not neighbours then $a_{st} = 0$). Hence the field is multivariate Gaussian with covariance matrix σ^2B^{-1} (B is required to be positive definite). These fields are determined by the requirement to be Gaussian and by

$$\begin{aligned}\mathsf{E}(X_s|rest) &= \mu_s + \sum_{\langle s,t\rangle} a_{st}(X_t-\mu_t),\\ \mathsf{var}(X_s|rest) &= \sigma^2.\end{aligned}$$

Therefore they are called conditional autoregressive processes (CAR). They should not be mixed up with simultaneous autoregressive processes (SAR) where typically

$$Y_s = \mu_s + \sum_{\langle s,t\rangle} a_{st}(Y_t-\mu_t) + \eta_s$$

with white noise η of variance σ^2. The SAR field has densitiy proportional to

$$\exp\left(-\frac{1}{2\sigma^2}(x-\mu)^*B^*B(x-\mu)\right)$$

where B is defined as before. Hence the covariance matrix of the SAR process is $\sigma^2(B^*B)^{-1}$. Note that here the symmetry requirement $a_{st} = a_{ts}$ is not needed since B^*B is symmetric and the coefficients in the general form of the automodel are symmetric too. Among their various applications, CAR and SAR models are used to describe and synthesize textures and therefore are useful for classification. We refer to BESAG's papers, in particular (1974), and RIPLEY's monograph (1988).

12.3 Texture Synthesis

It is obvious how to use random field texture models for the synthesis of textures. One simply has to sample from the field running the Gibbs or some Metropolis sampler. These algorithms are easily implemented and it is fun to watch the textures evolve. A reasonable choice of the parameters ϑ_i requires some care and therefore some sets of parameters are recommended below.

Some examples for binary textures appeared in Chapter 8, where both, the Gibbs sampler and the exchange algorithm were applied to binary models of the form (12.2). Examples for the general binomial model can be found in CROSS and JAIN (1983). The Gibbs sampler for these models is particularly easy to realize: In each step compute a realization from a binomial distribution of size N and with parameter $a/(1+a)$ from (12.1). This amounts to tossing a coin with probability $a/(1+a)$ for 'head' N times independently and counting the number of 'heads' (cf. Appendix A).

To control proportions of grey values, the authors adopt the exchange algorithm which ends up in a configuration with the proportions given by the initial configuration. This amounts to sampling from the Gibbs field conditioned on fixed proportions of grey values. One updating step roughly reads:

given a configuration x DO
BEGIN
  pick sites $s \neq t$ *uniformly at random;*
  for all $u \in S\backslash\{s,t\}$ *set* $y_u := x_u; y_s := x_t; y_t := x_s;$
  $r := \Pi(y)/\Pi(x);$
  IF $r >= 1$ *THEN* $x := y$ *ELSE*
    BEGIN
      $u :=$ *uniform random number in* $(0,1);$
      IF $r > u$ *THEN* $x := y$ *ELSE retain* x
    END
END;

Fig. 12.2 shows some binary textures synthesized with different sets of ϑ-values, (a)–(d) on 64×64-lattices and (e) on a 128×128-lattice. The exchange algorithm was adopted and started from a configuration with about 50% white pixels.

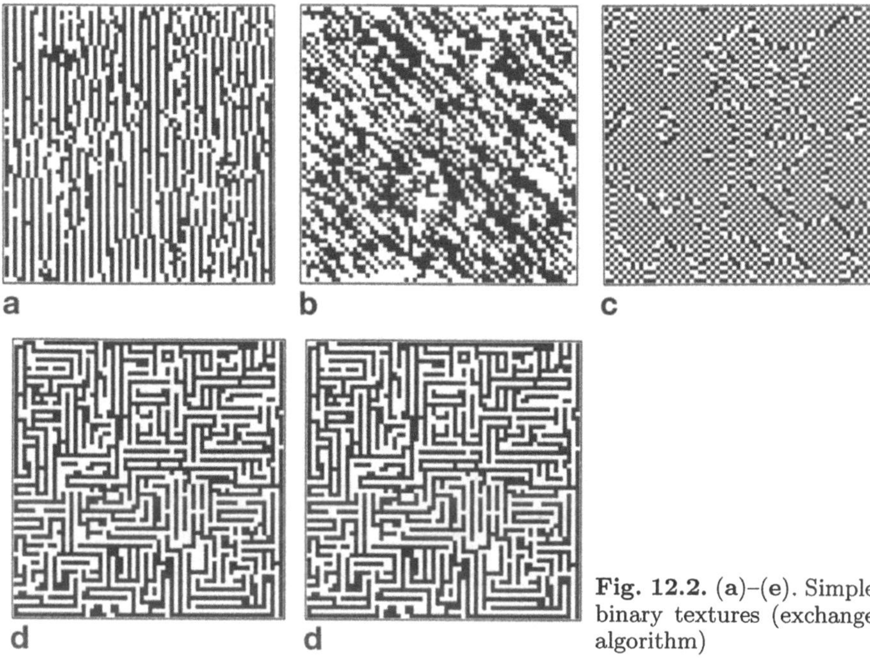

Fig. 12.2. (a)–(e). Simple binary textures (exchange algorithm)

Figs. (a) and (b) are examples of anisotropic textures, (c) is an ordered pattern, for the random labyrinths in (d) diagonals are prohibited and (e) penalizes clusters of large width. The specific parameters are:

(a) $\vartheta(0) = -0.26$, $\vartheta(1,1) = -2$, $\vartheta(1,2) = 2.1$, $\vartheta(2,1) = 0.13$, $\vartheta(2,2) = 0.015$;
(b) $\vartheta(0) = -1.9$, $\vartheta(1,1) = -0.1$, $\vartheta(2,1) = 1.9$, $\vartheta(2,2) = 0.075$;
(c) $\vartheta(0) = 5.09$, $\vartheta(1,1) = -2.16$, $\vartheta(1,2) = -2.16$;
(d) $\vartheta(0) = 0.16$, $\vartheta(1,1) = 2.06$, $\vartheta(1,2) = 2.05$, $\vartheta(2,1) = -2.03$, $\vartheta(2,2) = -2.10$;
(e) $\vartheta(0) = -4.6$, $\vartheta(1,\cdot) = 2.62$, $\vartheta(2,\cdot) = 2.17$, $\vartheta(3,\cdot) = -0.78$, $\vartheta(4,\cdot) = -0.85$.

Instead of the exchange algorithm, the Gibbs sampler can be used. In order to keep control of the histograms the prior may be shrunk towards the desired proportions of grey values using the modified prior energy $K(x) + \alpha|S|\,\|p(x) - \mu\|_2^2$ where $p(x) = (p_k(x))$, the $p_k(x)$ are the proportions of grey values in the image, and the components μ_k of μ are desired proportions (this is P. GREEN's suggestion mentioned in Chapter 8). Experiments with this prior can be found in ACUNA (1988) (cf. D. GEMAN (1990), 2.3.2). This modification is not restricted to the binomial model.

Similarly, for the other models, grey values in the sites are sampled from the normal, Poisson or other distribution, according to the form of the single-site local characteristics (for tricks to sample from these distributions cf. Appendix A).

Remark 12.3.1. Some more detailed comments on the (Gaussian) CAR-model are in order here. To run the Gibbs sampler, subsequently for each pixel s a standard Gaussian variable η_s is simulated independently of the others and

$$\tilde{x}_s = \mu_s + \sum_{\langle s,t \rangle} a_{st}(x_t - \mu_t) + \sigma\eta_s \tag{12.3}$$

is accepted as the new grey value in pixel s. In fact, the local characteristic in s is the law of this random variable. To avoid difficulties near the boundary, the image usually is wrapped around a torus.

There is a popular simulation technique derived from the well-known autoregression models. The latter are closely related to the (one-dimensional) time-series models which are studied for example in the standard text by J.E. Box and G.M. Jenkins (1970). Apparently they were initially explored for image texture analysis by Mc Cormick and Jayaramamurthy (1974); cf. also the references in Haralick and Shapiro (1992), chap. 9.11, 9.12. The corresponding algorithm is of the form (12.3). Thus the theory of Gibbs samplers reveals a close relationship between the apparently different approaches based on autoregression and random fields. The discrimination between these methods in some standard texts therefore seems to be somewhat artificial.

Frequently, the standard raster scan visiting scheme is adopted for these techniques and only previously updated neighbours of the current pixel are taken into account (i.e. those in the previous row and those on the left). The other coefficients a_{st} are temporarily set to zero. This way techniques developed for the classical one-dimensional models are carried over to the more-dimensional case. 'Such directional models are not generally regarded adequate for spatial phenomena' (Ripley (1988)).

12.4 Texture Classification

12.4.1 General Remarks

Regions of pixels will now be classified as belonging to particular texture classes. The problem may be stated as follows:

Suppose that data $y = (y_s)_{s \in S}$ are recorded – say by far remote sensing. Suppose further that a reference list of texture classes is given. Each texture class is represented by some label from a finite set L. The observation window S is covered by blocks of pixels which may overlap or not. To each of these blocks B, a label $x_B \in L$ has to be assigned expressing the belief that the grey value pattern on B represents a portion of texture type x_B. Other possible decisions or labels may be added to L like 'doubt' for 'don't know' and 'out' for 'not any of these textures'. The decision on $x = (x_B)_B$ given y follows some fixed rule.

Many conventional classifiers are based on primitive features like those mentioned in Section 11.3. For each of the reference textures the features are computed separately and represented by points P_l, $l \in L$, in a Euclidean space R^d. The space is divided into regions R_l centering around the P_l; for example, for minimum distance classifiers, R_l contains those feature vectors v for which $d(v, P_l) \le d(v, P_k)$, $k \ne l$, where d is some metric or suitable notion of distance. Now the features for a block $B \in S$ are represented by a point P and B is classified as belonging to texture class l if $P \in R_l$.

Frequently, the texture types are associated to certain densities f_l and R_l is chosen as $\{f_l \ge f_k \text{ for every } k \ne l\}$ (with ambiguity at $\{f_l = f_k\}$). If there is prior information about the relative frequency $p(l)$ of texture classes then $R_l = \{p(l)f_l \ge p(k)f_k \text{ for every } k \ne l\}$. There is a large variety of such Bayesian or non-Bayesian approaches and an almost infinite series of papers concerned with applications. The reader may consult NIEMANN (1990), NIEMANN (1983) (in German) or HARALICK and SHAPIRO (1992).

The methods sketched below are based on texture models. Basically, one may distinguish between contextual and noncontextual methods. For the former, weak constraints on the shape of texture patches are expressed by a suitable prior distribution. Hence there are label-label interactions and reasonable estimates of the true scene are provided by MAP or MMS estimators. Labeling by noncontextual methods is based on the data only and MPM estimators guarantee an optimal misclassification rate.

The classification model below is constructed from texture models like those previously discussed. Once a model is chosen – we shall take the Φ-model – different parameters correspond to different texture classes. Hence for each label $l \in L$ there is a parameter vector $\vartheta^{(l)}$. We shall write $K^{(l)}$ for the corresponding energy functions. These energy functions are combined and possibly augmented by organization terms for the labels in a prior energy function $H(y, x; \vartheta^{(l)}, l \in L)$. Note that for this approach, the labels have to be specified in advance and hence the number of texture classes one is looking for, as well.

Classification usually is carried out in three phases:

1. The learning phase. For each label $l \in L$, a training set must be available, i.e. a sufficiently large portion of the corresponding texture. Usually blocks of homogeneous texture are cut out of the picture to be classified. From these samples the parameters $\vartheta_i^{(l)}$ are estimated and thus the Gibbsian fields for the reference textures are specified. This way the textures are 'learned'. Since training sets are used, learning is supervised.
2. The training phase. Given the texture models and a parametric model for the label process, further parameters have to be estimated which depend on the whole image to be classified. This step is dropped if noncontextual methods are used.
3. The operational phase. A decision on the labeling is made which in our situation amounts to the computation of the MAP estimate (for contextual methods) or of the MPM estimate (for noncontextual models).

12.4.2 Contextual Classification

We are going now to construct the prior energy function for the pixel-label interaction. To be specific, we carry out the construction for the Φ-model. Let a set L of textures or labels be given. Assume that for each label $l \in L$ there is a Gibbs field for the associated texture class, or which amounts to the same, that the parameters $\vartheta_1^{(l)}, \ldots, \vartheta_6^{(l)}$ are given. Labels correspond to grey value configurations in blocks B of pixels. Usually the blocks center around pixels s from a subset S^L of S^P (like in the last chapter). We shall write x_s for x_{B_s} if B_s is the block around pixel s. Thus label configurations are denoted by $x = (x_s)_{S^L}$ and grey value configurations by $y = (y_s)_{S^P}$.

The energy is composed of local terms

$$K(y, l, s) = \sum_{i=1}^{6} \vartheta_i^{(l)} (\Psi(y_s - y_{s+\tau_i}) + \Psi(y_s - y_{s-\tau_i}))$$

where τ_i is the translation in S^P associated with the i-th pair clique. One might set

$$\tilde{H}_1(y, x) = \sum_s K(y, x_s, s).$$

GRAFFIGNE replaces the summands by means

$$\bar{K}(y, l, s) = \alpha_s^{-1} \sum_{t \in N_s} K(y, l, t)$$

over blocks N_s of sites around s and chooses α such that the sum of all block-based contributions reduces to $K^{(l)}$:

$$K^{(l)}(y) = \sum_s \bar{K}(y, l, s).$$

Thus each pair-clique appears exactly once. If, for example, each N_s is a 5×5-block then $\alpha_s = 50$. The modified energy is

$$H_1(y, x) = \sum_s \bar{K}(y, x, s).$$

Due to the normalization, the model is consistent with $\Pi^{(l)}$ if $x_s = l$ for all sites. Given undegraded observations y there is no label-label interaction so far and H_1 can be minimized by minimizing each local term separately which requires only one sweep. If we interpret $K(y, l, s)$ as a measure for the disparity of the actual texture around s and texture type l then this reminds us of the minimum distance methods. Other disparity measures, which are for example based on the Kolmogorov-Smirnov distance, may be more appropriate in some applications.

To organize the labels into regular patches, GRAFFIGNE adds an Ising type term

$$H_2(x) = -\eta \sum_{\langle s,t\rangle} 1_{x_s=x_t}$$

(and another correction term we shall not comment on). For data y consisting of large texture patches with smooth boundaries the Ising term organizes well (cf. the illustrations in GRAFFIGNE (1987)). On the other hand, it prefers patches of rectangular shape (cf. the discussion in Chapter 5) and destroys thin regions (cf. BESAG (1986), 2.5). This is not appropriate for real scenes like aerial photographs of 'fuzzy' landscapes. Weighting down selected configurations like in the last chapter may be more pertinent in such cases.

As soon as there are label-label interactions, computation of MAP estimation becomes time consuming. One may minimize $H = H_1 + H_2$ by annealing or sampling at low temperature, or, one may interpret $V = H_2$ as weak straints and adopt the methods from Chapter 7 HANSEN and ELLIOTT (1982) (for the binary case) and DERIN and ELLIOTT (1987) develop dynamic programming approaches giving suboptimal solutions. This requires simplifying assumptions in the model.

12.4.3 MPM Methods

So far we were concerned with MAP estimation corresponding to the $0-1$ loss function. A natural measure for the quality of classification is the misclassification rate, at least if there are no requirements on shape or organization. The Bayes estimators for this loss function are the MPM estimators (cf. Chapter 1). Separately for each $s \in S^L$, they maximize the marginal posterior distribution $\mu(x_s|y)$. Such decisions in isolation may be reasonable for tasks in land inspection but not if some underlying structure is present. Then contextual methods like those discussed above are preferable (provided sufficient computer power).

The marginal posterior distribution is given by

$$\mu(x_s|y) = Z(y)^{-1} \sum_{z_{S\backslash\{s\}}} \Pi(x_s z_{S\backslash\{s\}}, y). \qquad (12.4)$$

All data enter the model and the full prior is still present. The conditional distributions are computationally unwieldy and there are many suggestions for simplification (c.f. BESAG (1986), 2.4 and RIPLEY (1988)).

In the rest of this section, we shall indicate the relation of some conventional classification methods to (12.4).

As a common simplification, one does not care about the full prior distribution Π. Only prior knowledge about the probabilities or relative frequencies $\pi(l)$ of the texture classes is exploited. To put this into the framework above forget label-label interactions and assume that the prior does not depend on the intensities and is a product $\Pi(x) = \prod_{s\in S^L} \pi(x_s)$. Let further transition probabilities $P_s(l, y)$ for data y given label l in s be given (they are interpreted as conditional distributions $Prob(y|\text{texture } l \text{ in site } s)$ for some underlying but unknown law $Prob$). Then (12.4) boiles down to

$$\mu(x_s|y) = Z(y)^{-1}\pi(x_s)P_s(x_s, y).$$

and for the MPM estimate each $\pi(l)P_s(l, y)$ can be maximized separately. The estimation rule defines decision regions

$$A_l = \{y : \pi(l)P_s(l, y) \quad \text{exceeds others}\}$$

and l wins on A_l.

The transition probabilities $P(l, y)$ are frequently assumed to be multidimensional Gaussian, i.e.

$$P(l, y) = \frac{1}{\sqrt[2]{(2\pi)^d |\Sigma_l|}} \exp\left(-\frac{1}{2}(y - \mu_l)^* \Sigma_l^{-1}(x - \mu_l)\right)$$

with expectation vectors μ_l and covariance matrices Σ_l. Then the expectations and the covariances have to be estimated. If the labels are distributed uniformly (i.e. $\pi(l) = |L|^{-1}$) and $\Sigma_l = \Sigma$ for all l then the Bayes rule amounts to choosing the label minimizing the **Mahalanobis distance**

$$\Delta(l) = (a - \mu_l)^* \Sigma^{-1}(x - \mu_l)$$

If there are only two labels l and k then the two decision regions are separated by a hyperplane perpendicular to the line joining μ_l and μ_k.

The assumption of unimodality is inadequate if a texture is made up of several subtypes. Then semiparametric and nonparametric approaches are adopted (to get a rough idea you may consult RIPLEY and TAYLOR (1987); an introduction is given in SILVERMAN (1986)). Near the boundary of the decision regions where

$$\pi(l)P_s(l, y) \sim \pi(k)P_s(k, y), l \neq k,$$

the densities $P_s(l, \cdot)$ and $P_s(k, \cdot)$ usually both are small and one may be in doubt about correct labeling. Hence a 'doubt' label d is reserved in order to reduce the misclassification rate. A pixel s will then get the label l, if l maximizes $\pi(l)P_s(l, y)$ *and* this maximum exceeds a threshold $1 - \varepsilon$, $\varepsilon > 0$; if $\pi(l)P_s(l, y) \leq 1 - \varepsilon$ for all l then one is in doubt.

An additional label is useful also in other respects. In aerial photographs there use to be many textures like wood, damadged wood, roads, villages, ... If one is interested only in wood and damadged wood then this idea may be adopted to introduce an 'out'-label. Without such a label classification is impossible since in general the total number of actual textures is unknown and/or it is impossible to sample from each texture.

The maximization of each $\pi(l)P_s(l, y)$ may still consume too much CPU-time and many methods maximize $\pi(l)P_s(l, y_{B_s})$ for data in a set B_s around s.

Let us finally note that many commercial systems for remotely sensed data simply maximize $\pi(l)P(l, y_s)$, i.e. they only take into account the intensity at the current pixel. This method is feasible (only) if texture separation is good enough.

We stress that there is no effort to construct a closed model i.e. a probability space on which the processes of data and labels live. This is a major difference to our models. HJORT and MOHN (1987) argue (we adopt our notation):

> It is not really necessary for us to derive $P_s(l, y)$ from fully given, simultaneous probability distributions, however; we may if we wish forget the full scene and come up with realistic local models for the y_{B_s} alone, i.e. model $P_s(l, y_{B_s})$ above directly. Even if some proposed local ... model should turn out to be inconsistent with a full model for the classes, say, we are allowed to view it merely as a convenient approximation to the complex schemes nature employs when she distributes the classes over the land.

Albeit useful and important in practice, we do not study noncontextual methods in detail. The reader is referred to the papers by HJORT, MOHN and coauthors listed in the references and to RIPLEY and TAYLOR (1987), RIPLEY (1987). Let us finally mention a few of the numerous papers on Markov field models for classification: ABEND, HARLEY and KANAL (1965), HASSNER and SLANSKY (1980), COHEN and COOPER (1983), DERIN and ELLIOTT (1984), DERIN and COLE (1986), LAKSHMANAN and DERIN (1989), KHOTANZAD and CHEN (1989), KLEIN and PRESS (1989), HSIAO and SAWCHUK (1989), WRIGHT (1989), KARSSEMEIJER (1990).

Part V
Parameter Estimation

We discussed several models for Bayesian image analysis and, in particular, the choice of the corresponding energy functions. Whereas we may agree on general forms there are free parameters depending on the data to be processed. Sensitivity to such parameters was illustrated by way of several examples, like the scaling parameter in piecewise smoothing (Fig. 2.8) or the seeding parameter in edge detection (Fig. 2.10). It is even more striking in the texture models where different parameter sets characterize textures of obviously different flavour and thus critically determine the ability of the algorithms to segment and label. All these parameters should systematically be estimated from the data.

This is a hazardous problem. There are numerous problem-specific methods and few more or less general approaches. For a short discussion and references cf. GEMAN (1990), Section 6.1. We focus on the standard approach of maximum likelihood estimation or rather on modifications of this method. Recently, they received considerable interest not only in image analysis but also in the theory of neural networks and other fields of large-systems statistics.

13. Maximum Likelihood Estimators

13.1 Introduction

In this chapter, basic properties of maximum likelihood estimators are derived and a useful generalization is obtained. Only results for general finite spaces $\mathbf{X}$ are presented. Parameter estimation for Gibbs fields is discussed in the next chapter.

For the present, we do not need the special structure of the sample space $\mathbf{X}$ and hence we let $\mathbf{X}$ denote any finite set. On $\mathbf{X}$ a family

$$\Pi = \{\Pi(\cdot;\vartheta) : \vartheta \in \Theta\}$$

of distributions is considered where $\Theta \subset \mathsf{R}^d$ is a set of parameters. The 'true' or 'best' parameter $\vartheta_* \in \Theta$ is not known and needs to be determined or at least approximated. The only available information is hidden in the observation x. Hence we need a rule how to choose some $\hat{\vartheta}$ as a substitute for ϑ_* if x is picked at random from $\Pi(\cdot;\vartheta_*)$. Such a map $x \longmapsto \hat{\vartheta}(x)$ is called an **estimator** . There are two basic requirements on estimators:

(i) The estimator $\hat{\vartheta}(x)$ should tend to ϑ_* as the sample x contains more and more information.

(ii) The computation of the estimator must be feasible.

The property (i) is called **asymptotic consistency**. There is a highly developed theory providing other quality criteria and various classes of reasonable estimators. We shall focus on the popular maximum likelihood methods and their asymptotic consistency.

A **maximum likelihood** estimator $\hat{\vartheta}$ for ϑ_* is defined as follows: given a sample $x \in \mathbf{X}$, $\hat{\vartheta}(x)$ maximizes the function $\vartheta \longmapsto \Pi(x;\vartheta)$, or in formulae,

$$x \longmapsto \operatorname{argmax} \Pi(x;\cdot).$$

Plainly, there is ambiguity if the maximum is not unique.

13.2 The Likelihood Function

It is convenient to maximize the **(log-) likelihood function**

$$L(x,\cdot):\Theta\longrightarrow \mathsf{R},\quad \vartheta\longmapsto \ln\Pi(x;\vartheta)$$

instead of $\Pi(x;\cdot)$.

Example 13.2.1. (a) (independent sampling). Let us consider maximum likelihood estimation based on independent samples. There is a finite space $\mathbf{Z}$ and a family $\{\Pi(\cdot;\vartheta):\vartheta\in\Theta\}$ of distributions on $\mathbf{Z}$. Sampling n times from some $\Pi(\cdot;\vartheta)$ results in a sequence $x^{(1)},...,x^{(n)}$ in $\mathbf{Z}$ or in an element $\left(x^{(1)},...,x^{(n)}\right)$ of the n-fold product $\mathbf{X}^{(n)}$ of n copies of $\mathbf{Z}$. If independence of the single samples is assumed, then the total sample is governed by the product law

$$\Pi^{(n)}\left(\left(x^{(1)},...,x^{(n)}\right);\vartheta\right)=\Pi\left(x^{(1)};\vartheta\right)\cdot\ldots\cdot\Pi\left(x^{(n)};\vartheta\right).$$

Letting $\Pi^{(n)}=\left(\Pi^{(n)}(\cdot;\vartheta):\vartheta\in\Theta\right)$, the likelihood function is given by

$$\vartheta\longmapsto\ln\Pi^{(n)}\left((x^{(1)},...,x^{(n)});\vartheta\right)=\sum_{i=1}^{n}\ln\Pi\left(x^{(i)};\vartheta\right).$$

(b) The MAP estimators introduced in Chapter 1 were defined as maxima x of posterior distributions, i.e. of functions $x\mapsto\Pi^{post}(x\mid y)$ where y was the observed image. Note that the role of the parameters ϑ is played by the 'true' images x and the role of x here is played by the observed image y.

We shall consider distributions of Gibbsian form

$$\Pi(x;\vartheta)=Z(\vartheta)^{-1}\exp\left(-H(x;\vartheta)\right)$$

where $H(\cdot;\vartheta):\mathbf{X}\longmapsto\mathbf{R}$ is some energy function. We assume that $H(\cdot;\vartheta)$ depends linearly on the parameter ϑ, i.e. there is a vector $H=(H_1,...,H_d)$ such that $H(\cdot;\vartheta)=-\langle\vartheta,H\rangle$ ($\langle\vartheta,H\rangle=\sum_i\vartheta_iH_i$ is the usual inner product on R^d; the minus sign is introduced for convenience of notation). The distributions have the form

$$\Pi(\cdot;\vartheta)=Z(\vartheta)^{-1}\exp\left(\langle\vartheta,H\rangle\right),\vartheta\in\Theta.$$

A family Π of such distributions is an **exponential family**.

Let us derive some useful formulae and discuss basic properties of likelihood functions.

Proposition 13.2.1. *Let Θ be an open subset of R^d. The likelihood function $\vartheta\longmapsto L(x;\vartheta)$ is twice continuously differentiable for every x. The gradient is given by*

$$\frac{\partial}{\partial\vartheta_i}L(x;\vartheta)=H_i(x)-\mathsf{E}\left(H_i;\vartheta\right)$$

and the Hessean matrix is given by

$$\frac{\partial^2}{\partial\vartheta_i\partial\vartheta_j}L(x;\vartheta)=-\mathsf{cov}\left(H_i,H_j;\vartheta\right).$$

In particular, the likelihood function is concave.

Proof. Differentiation of

$$L(x;\vartheta) = \langle\vartheta, H(x)\rangle - \ln\sum_z \exp\left(\langle\vartheta, H(z)\rangle\right)$$

gives

$$\begin{aligned}\frac{\partial}{\partial\vartheta_i}L(x;\vartheta) &= H_i(x) - \frac{\sum_z H_i(z)\exp\left(\langle\vartheta, H(z)\rangle\right)}{\sum_z \exp\left(\langle\vartheta, H(z)\rangle\right)} \\ &= H_i(x) - \sum_z H_i(z)\Pi(z;\vartheta)\end{aligned}$$

and thus the partial derivative has the above form. The second partial derivative becomes

$$\begin{aligned}&\frac{\partial^2}{\partial\vartheta_i\partial\vartheta_j}L(x;\vartheta) \\ = \quad &-\frac{\sum_z H_i(z)H_j(z)\exp\left(\langle\vartheta, H(z)\rangle\right)\sum_z \exp\left(\langle\vartheta, H(z)\rangle\right)}{\left(\sum_z \exp\left(\langle\vartheta, H(z)\rangle\right)\right)^2} \\ &+\frac{\sum_z H_i(z)\exp\left(\langle\vartheta, H(z)\rangle\right)\sum_z H_j(z)\exp\left(\langle\vartheta, H(z)\rangle\right)}{\left(\sum_z \exp\left(\langle\vartheta, H(z)\rangle\right)\right)^2} \\ = \quad &-\mathsf{E}\left(H_iH_j;\vartheta\right) + \mathsf{E}\left(H_i;\vartheta\right)\mathsf{E}\left(H_j;\vartheta\right) \\ = \quad &-\mathsf{cov}\left(H_i, H_j;\vartheta\right).\end{aligned}$$

By Lemma C.4 in Appendix C, covariance matrices are positive semi-definite and by Lemma C.3 the likelihood is concave. □

One can infer the parameters from the observation only if different distributions have different parameters: a parameter $\vartheta_* \in \Theta$ is called **identifiable** if $\Pi(\cdot;\vartheta) \neq \Pi(\cdot;\vartheta_*)$ for each $\vartheta \in \Theta$, $\vartheta \neq \vartheta_*$. The following equivalent formulations will be used repeatedly.

Lemma 13.2.1. *Let Θ be an open subset of R^d. The following are equivalent:*

(a) $\Pi(\cdot;\vartheta) \neq \Pi\left(\cdot;\vartheta_*\right)$ for every $\vartheta \neq \vartheta_*$.
(b) For every $\alpha \neq 0$, the function $\langle\alpha, H(\cdot)\rangle$ is not constant.
(c) $\mathsf{var}_\mu\left(\langle\alpha, H\rangle\right) > 0$ for every strictly positive distribution μ on $\mathbf{X}$ and every $\alpha \neq 0$.

Proof. Since

$$\langle\vartheta, H\rangle - \langle\vartheta_*, H\rangle = \ln\left(\frac{\Pi(\cdot;\vartheta)}{\Pi\left(\cdot;\vartheta_*\right)}\right) + \left(\ln Z\left(\vartheta\right) - \ln Z\left(\vartheta_*\right)\right)$$

we conclude that $\langle\vartheta - \vartheta_*, H\rangle$ is constant in x if and only if $\Pi(\cdot;\vartheta) = const \cdot \Pi\left(\cdot;\vartheta_*\right)$. Since the Π's are normalized the constant equals 1. Hence part (a) is equivalent to $\langle\vartheta - \vartheta_*, H\rangle$ not being constant for every $\vartheta \neq \vartheta_*$. Plainly, it is sufficient to consider parameters ϑ in some ball $B(\vartheta_*, \varepsilon) \subset \Theta$ and we may replace the symbol $\vartheta - \vartheta_*$ by α. Hence (a) is equivalent to (b). Equivalence of (b) and (c) is obvious. □

Let us draw a simple conclusion.

Corollary 13.2.1. *Let Θ be an open subset of R^d and $\vartheta_* \in \Theta$. The map*

$$\vartheta \longmapsto \mathsf{E}\left(L(\cdot;\vartheta);\vartheta_*\right)$$

has gradient

$$\nabla \mathsf{E}\left(L(\cdot;\vartheta);\vartheta_*\right) = \mathsf{E}\left(H;\vartheta_*\right) - \mathsf{E}\left(H;\vartheta\right)$$

and Hessean matrix

$$\nabla^2 \mathsf{E}\left(L(\cdot;\vartheta);\vartheta_*\right) = -\mathsf{cov}\left(H;\vartheta\right).$$

It is concave with a maximum at ϑ_*. If ϑ_* is identifiable then it is strictly concave and the maximum is unique.

Proof. Plainly,

$$\frac{\partial}{\partial \vartheta_i}\mathsf{E}(L(\cdot;\vartheta);\vartheta_*) = \mathsf{E}(\frac{\partial}{\partial \vartheta_i}L(\cdot;\vartheta);\vartheta_*)$$

and hence by Proposition 13.2.1 gradient and Hessean have the above form. Since the Hessean is the negative of a covariance matrix the map is concave by C.4. Hence there is a maximum where the gradient vanishes, in particular at ϑ_*. By Lemma C.4,

$$\alpha\nabla^2 \mathsf{E}\left(L(\cdot;\vartheta);\vartheta_*\right)\alpha^* = \mathsf{var}\left(\langle\alpha, H\rangle;\vartheta\right).$$

If ϑ_* is identifiable this quantity is strictly negative for each $\alpha \neq 0$ by the above lemma. Hence the Hessean is negative definite and the function is strictly concave by Lemma C.3. This completes the proof. □

The last result can be extended to the case where the true distribution is not necessarily a member of the family $\Pi = (\Pi(\cdot;\vartheta) : \vartheta \in \Theta)$ (cf. the remark below).

Corollary 13.2.2. *Let $\Theta = \mathsf{R}^d$ and Γ be a probability distribution on $\mathbf{X}$. Then the function*

$$\vartheta \longmapsto \mathsf{E}(L(\cdot;\vartheta);\Gamma)$$

is concave with gradient and Hessean matrix

$$\begin{aligned} \nabla \mathsf{E}(L(\cdot;\vartheta);\Gamma) &= \mathsf{E}(H;\Gamma) - \mathsf{E}(H;\vartheta), \\ \nabla^2 \mathsf{E}(L(\cdot;\vartheta);\Gamma) &= -\mathsf{cov}(H;\vartheta). \end{aligned}$$

If some $\vartheta' \in \Theta$ is identifiable then it is strictly concave. If, moreover, Γ is strictly positive then it has a unique maximum ϑ_*. In particular, $\mathsf{E}(H;\vartheta_*) = \mathsf{E}(H;\Gamma)$.

Note that for $\Theta = \mathsf{R}^d$, Proposition 13.2.1 is the special case $\Gamma = \varepsilon_x$.

Remark 13.2.1. The corollary deals with the map

$$\vartheta \longmapsto \mathsf{E}(L(\cdot;\vartheta);\Gamma) = \sum_x \Gamma(x)\ln \Pi(x;\vartheta).$$

Subtraction of the constant

$$\mathsf{E}(\ln \Gamma(\cdot);\Gamma) = \sum_x \Gamma(x)\ln \Gamma(x)$$

and multiplication by -1 gives

$$I\left(\Pi(\cdot;\vartheta) \mid \Gamma\right) = \sum_x \Gamma(x)\ln\frac{\Gamma(x)}{\Pi(x;\vartheta)}.$$

This quantity is called **divergence, information gain** or **Kullback-Leibler information** of $\Pi(\cdot;\vartheta)$ w.r.t. Γ. Note that it is minimal for ϑ_* from Corollary 13.2.2. For general strictly positive distributions μ and ν on $\mathbf{X}$ it is defined by

$$I\left(\mu \mid \nu\right) = \sum_x \nu(x)\ln\frac{\nu(x)}{\mu(x)} = \mathsf{E}(\ln\nu;\nu) - \mathsf{E}(\ln\mu;\nu)$$

(letting $0\ln 0 = 0$ this makes sense for general ν).

It is a suitable measure for the amount of information an observer gains while realizing that the law of a random variable changes from μ to ν. The map I is no metric since it is not symmetric in μ and ν. On the other hand, it vanishes for $\nu = \mu$ and is strictly positive whenever $\mu \neq \nu$; the inequality

$$I(\mu \mid \nu) = \sum_x \nu(x)\ln\frac{\nu(x)}{\mu(x)} \geq \sum_x \nu(x)\left(1 - \frac{\mu(x)}{\nu(x)}\right) = 0$$

follows from $\ln\alpha \geq 1-\alpha^{-1}$ for $\alpha > 0$. Because equality holds for $\alpha = 1$ only, the sum in the left is strictly greater than the sum on the right whenever $\nu(x) \neq \mu(x)$. Hence $I(\mu \mid \nu) = 0$ implies $\mu = \nu$. The converse is clear.

Formally, I becomes infinite if $\nu(x) > 0$ but $\mu(x) = 0$ for some x, i.e. when 'a new event is created'. This observation is the basis of the proof for Corollary 13.2.2.

Now we can understand what is behind the last result. For example, consider parameter estimation for the binomial texture model. We should not insist that the data, i.e. a portion of a natural texture, are a sample from some binomial model. What we can do is to determine that binomial model which is closest to the unknown distribution from which 'nature' drew the data.

Proof (of Corollary 13.2.2). Gradient and Hessean matrix are computed like in the last proof. Hence strict concavity follows like there. It is not yet clear whether the gradient vanishes somewhere or not and hence existence of a maximum has to be proved.

Let $W(\vartheta) = \mathsf{E}(L(\cdot;\vartheta);\Gamma)$. We shall show that there is some ball, such that W is strictly smaller on the boundary than in the center. This yields a local maximum and the result will be proved.

(1) By Proposition 5.2.1, $\Pi(x;\beta\alpha) \longmapsto 0$ as $\beta \to \infty$, for each x not maximizing $\Pi(\cdot;\alpha)$. Such an element x exists as soon as $\Pi(\cdot;\alpha)$ is not the uniform distribution. On the other hand, $\Pi(\cdot;0)$ *is* the uniform distribution and by identifiability and Lemma 13.2.1, $\Pi(\cdot;\alpha)$ is not uniform if $\alpha \neq 0$. Since Γ is assumed to be strictly positive, we conclude that $W(\beta\alpha) \to -\infty$ as $\beta \to \infty$, for every $\alpha \neq 0$.

(2) We want to prove the existence of some ball $B(0,\varepsilon)$, $\varepsilon > 0$, such that $W(0) > W(\vartheta)$ for all ϑ on the boundary $\partial B(0,\varepsilon)$. By way of contradiction, assume that for each $k > 0$ there is $\alpha_{(k)}$, $\| \alpha_{(k)} \|= k$, such that $W\left(\alpha_{(k)}\right) \geq W(0)$. By concavity, $W(\alpha) \geq W(0)$ on the line-segments $\left\{\lambda\alpha_{(k)} : 0 \leq \lambda \leq 1\right\}$. By compactness, the sequence $\left(\gamma_{(k)}\right)$, $\gamma_{(k)} = k^{-1}\alpha_{(k)}$, in $\partial B(0,1)$ has a convergent subsequence. We may and shall assume that the sequence is convergent itself and denote the limit by γ. Choose now $n > 0$. Then $n\gamma_{(k)} \to n\gamma$ as $k \to \infty$ and $W\left(n\gamma_{(k)}\right) \geq W(0)$ for $k \geq n$. Hence $W(n\gamma) \geq W(0)$ and W is bounded from below by $W(0)$ on $\{\lambda n\gamma : 0 \leq \lambda \leq 1\}$. Since this holds for every $n \geq 0$, W is bounded from below on the ray $\{\lambda\gamma : \lambda \geq 0\}$. This contradicts (1) and completes the proof. □

13.3 Objective Functions

After these preparations we return to the basic requirements on estimators: computational feasibility and asymptotic consistency. Let us begin with the former.

By Proposition 13.2.1, a maximum likelihood estimate $\hat{\vartheta}(x)$ is a root of the equation

$$\nabla L(x;\vartheta) = H(x) - \mathsf{E}(H;\vartheta) = 0.$$

Brute force evaluation of the expectations involves summation over all $x \in \mathbf{X}$. Hence for the large discrete spaces $\mathbf{X}$ in imaging the expectation is intractable this way and analytical solution or iterative approximation by gradient ascent are practically impossible. Basically, there are two ways out of this mysery:

(i) The expectation is replaced by computationally feasible approximations, for example, adopting the Gibbs- or Metropolis sampler. On the other hand, this leads to gradient algorithms with random perturbations. Such stochastic processes are not easy to analyze. They will be addressed later.

(ii) The classical maximum likelihood estimator is replaced by a computationally feasible one.

Example 13.3.1. In this example $\mathbf{X}$ is a finite product space $\mathbf{Z}^q$. J. Besag suggests to maximize the product of conditional probabilites

$$\vartheta \longmapsto \prod_{s \in T} \Pi \left(x_s \mid x_{S \setminus s}; \vartheta \right)$$

for a subset T of the index set S instead of $\vartheta \longmapsto \Pi(x;\vartheta)$. The corresponding **pseudolikelihood function** is given by

$$\begin{aligned} PL(x;\vartheta) &= \ln \left(\prod_{s \in T} \Pi \left(x_s \mid x_{S\setminus s};\vartheta \right) \right) \\ &= \sum_{s \in T} \left(\langle \vartheta, H(x) \rangle - \ln \sum_{z_s} \exp \left(\langle \vartheta, H(z_s, x_{S\setminus s}) \rangle \right) \right). \end{aligned}$$

Application of Proposition 13.2.1 to the conditional disributions yields

$$\nabla PL(x;\vartheta) = \sum_s \left(H(x) - \mathsf{E} \left(H \mid x_{S\setminus s};\vartheta \right) \right)$$

where $\mathsf{E}\left(H \mid x_{S\setminus s};\vartheta\right)$ denotes the expectation of the function $z_s \longmapsto H\left(z_s x_{S\setminus s}\right)$ on $\mathbf{X}_s$ w.r.t. $\Pi\left(x_s \mid x_{S\setminus s};\vartheta\right)$. If Π is a Markov field with small neighbourhoods, the conditional expectations can be computed directly and hence computation of the gradient is feasible.

In the rest of this chapter we focus on asymptotic consistency. In standard estimation methods, information about the true law is accumulated by picking more and more independent samples and, for exponential models, asymptotic consistency is easily established. We shall do this as an example before long. In imaging, we are faced with several important new aspects. Firstly, estimators like the pseudolikelihood are *not* of exponential form. The second aspect is more fundamental: typical samples in imaging are *not* independent. Let us explain this by way of example. In (supervised) texture classification inference is based on a single portion of a pure texture. The samples, i.e. the grey values in the single sites, are realizations of random variables which in contextual models are correlated. This urges the question whether inference can be based on dependent observations (we shall discuss this problem in the next chapter).

In summary, various ML estimators have to be examinated. They differ in the form of the likelihood function or use independent or dependent samples. In the next sections, an abstract framework for the study of various ML estimators is introduced. Whereas it is presented in an elementary form, the underlying ideas apply in more abstract situations too (cf. Section 14.4).

Let ϑ_* be some distinguished parameter in $\Theta \subset \mathsf{R}^d$. Let for each $n \geq 1$ a finite sample space $\mathbf{X}^{(n)}$, a parametrized family

$$\Pi^{(n)} = \left\{ \Pi^{(n)}(\cdot;\vartheta) : \vartheta \in \Theta \right\}$$

and a strictly positive distribution $\Gamma^{(n)}$ on $\mathbf{X}^{(n)}$ be given. Suppose further that there are functions $g^{(n)} : \mathbf{X}^{(n)} \times \Theta \longrightarrow \mathsf{R}$ which have a common unique maximum at ϑ_* and fulfill

$$g^{(n)}(x;\vartheta) \leq -\gamma \|\vartheta - \vartheta_*\|_2^2 + g^{(n)}(x;\vartheta_*) \tag{13.1}$$

on a ball $B(\vartheta_*, r)$ in Θ for some constant $\gamma > 0$ (independent of x and n). We call a sequence $\left(G^{(n)}\right)$ of functions $G^{(n)} : \mathbf{X}^{(n)} \times \Theta \longrightarrow \mathsf{R}$ an **objective function** with reference function $\left(g^{(n)}\right)$ if each $G^{(n)}(x;\cdot)$ is concave and for all $\varepsilon > 0$ and $\delta > 0$,

$$\Gamma^{(n)}\left(\left|G^{(n)}(\vartheta) - g^{(n)}(\vartheta)\right| \leq \delta \text{ for every } \vartheta \in B(\vartheta_*, \varepsilon)\right) \longrightarrow 1$$

$$\text{as } n \longrightarrow \infty. \tag{13.2}$$

Finally, let us for every $n \geq 1$ and each $x \in \mathbf{X}^{(n)}$ denote the set of those $\vartheta \in \Theta$ which maximize $\vartheta \longmapsto G^{(n)}(x;\vartheta)$ by $\hat{\Theta}(x)$.

The $g^{(n)}(x;\cdot)$ are 'ideal' functions with maximum at the true or best possible parameter. In practice, they are not known and will be approximated by known functions $G^{(n)}(x;\cdot)$ of the samples. Basically, the G^n will be given by likelihood functions and the $g^{(n)}$ by some kind of expectation. Let us illustrate the concept by a simple example.

Example 13.3.2 (independent samples.). Let $\mathbf{Z}$ be a finite space and $\mathbf{X}^{(n)}$ the product of n copies of $\mathbf{Z}$. For each sample size n a family

$$\Pi^{(n)} = \left\{\Pi^{(n)}(\cdot;\vartheta) : \vartheta \in \Theta\right\}$$

is defined as follows: Given $\vartheta \in \Theta$ and n, under the assumption of independence, the samples are governed by the law

$$\Pi^{(n)}\left(\left(x^{(1)}, \ldots, x^{(n)}\right);\vartheta\right) = \Pi\left(x^{(1)};\vartheta\right) \cdot \ldots \cdot \Pi\left(x^{(n)};\vartheta\right).$$

Let

$$\begin{aligned} G^{(n)}\left(\left(x^{(1)}, \ldots, x^{(n)}\right);\vartheta\right) &= \frac{1}{n} \ln \Pi^{(n)}\left(\left(x^{(1)}, \ldots, x^{(n)}\right);\vartheta\right) \\ &= \frac{1}{n} \sum_{i=1}^{n} \ln \Pi\left(x^{(i)};\vartheta\right). \end{aligned}$$

Set further

$$g^{(n)}(x;\vartheta) = \mathsf{E}\left(G^{(n)}(\cdot;\vartheta); \Pi^{(n)}(\vartheta_*)\right) = \mathsf{E}\left(\ln \Pi(\cdot;\vartheta);\vartheta_*\right).$$

In this example $\left(g^{(n)}\right)$ neither depends on x nor on n. By the previous calculations, each $g^{(n)}(x;\cdot) = g(x)$ has a unique maximum at ϑ_* if and only if ϑ_* is identifiable and by lemma C.3,

$$g(\vartheta) \leq -\gamma \|\vartheta - \vartheta_*\|_2^2 + g(\vartheta_*)$$

for some $\gamma > 0$ on a ball $B(\vartheta_*;r)$ in Θ. The convergence property will be verified below.

For a general theory of objective functions the reader may consult DACUNHA-CASTELLE and DUFLO (1982), Sections 3.2 and 3.3.

13.4 Asymptotic Consistency

To justify the general concept, we show that the estimator

$$\vartheta \longmapsto \operatorname{argmax} G^{(n)}(x;\vartheta)$$

is asymptotically consistent.

Lemma 13.4.1. *Let $\Theta \subset \mathsf{R}^d$ be open and let G be an objective function with reference function g. Then for every $\varepsilon > 0$,*

$$\Gamma^{(n)}\left(\hat{\Theta}^{(n)} \subset B\left(\vartheta_*, \varepsilon\right)\right) \longrightarrow 1 \quad as \quad n \to \infty.$$

Proof. Choose $\varepsilon > 0$ such that $B(\vartheta_*, \varepsilon) \subset \Theta$. Let

$$A^{(n)}(\varepsilon, \delta) = \left\{x \in \mathbf{X}^{(n)} : \left|G^{(n)}(x;\vartheta) - g^{(n)}(x;\vartheta)\right| \leq \delta \text{ on } B(\vartheta_*, \varepsilon)\right\}.$$

We shall write g and G for $g^{(n)}(x;\cdot)$ and $G^{(n)}(x;\cdot)$, respectively, if $x \in A^{(n)}(\varepsilon, \delta)$. By assumption,

$$g(\vartheta) \leq g(\vartheta_*) - \gamma\varepsilon^2$$

for all ϑ on the boundary $\partial B(\vartheta_*, \varepsilon)$ of the ball $B(\vartheta_*, \varepsilon)$. We conclude that for sufficiently small δ,

$$G(\vartheta) < G(\vartheta_*) \quad \text{for every} \quad \vartheta \in \partial B(\vartheta_*, \varepsilon).$$

By concavity,

$$G(\vartheta) < G(\vartheta_*) \quad \text{for every} \quad \vartheta \in \Theta \backslash B(\vartheta_*, \varepsilon).$$

This is easily seen drawing a sketch. For a pedantic proof, choose $\vartheta^{out} \in \Theta \backslash B(\vartheta_*, \varepsilon)$. The line segment $[\vartheta_*, \vartheta^{out}]$ meets the boundary of $B(\vartheta_*, \varepsilon)$ in a point $\vartheta^b = \alpha\vartheta_* - (1-\alpha)\vartheta^{out}$ where $0 < \alpha < 1$. Since G is concave,

$$\alpha G(\vartheta^b) + (1-\alpha)G(\vartheta^b) = G(\vartheta^b) \geq \alpha G(\vartheta_*) + (1-\alpha)G(\vartheta^{out}).$$

Rearranging the terms gives

$$(1-\alpha)\left(G(\vartheta^b) - G(\vartheta^{out})\right) \geq \alpha\left(G(\vartheta_*) - G(\vartheta^b)\right) \quad (> 0).$$

Therefore

$$G(\vartheta_*) > G(\vartheta^b) > G(\vartheta^{out}).$$

Hence $\hat{\Theta}^{(n)}(x) \subset B(\vartheta_*, \varepsilon)$ for every $x \in A^{(n)}(\varepsilon, \delta)$. By assumption,

$$\Gamma^{(n)}\left(A^{(n)}(\varepsilon, \delta)\right) \longrightarrow 1, n \to \infty.$$

Plainly, the assertion holds for arbitrary $\varepsilon > 0$ and thus the proof is complete. □

For the verification of (13.2), the following compactness argument is useful.

Lemma 13.4.2. *Let Θ be an open subset of R^d. Suppose that all functions $G^{(n)}(x;\cdot)$ and $g^{(n)}(x;\cdot)$, $x \in \mathbf{X}^{(n)}$, $n \geq 1$, are Lipschitz continuous in ϑ with a common Lipschitz constant. Suppose further that for every $\delta > 0$ and every $\vartheta \in \Theta$,*

$$\Gamma^{(n)}\left(\left|G^{(n)}(\cdot;\vartheta) - g^{(n)}(\cdot;\vartheta)\right| \leq \delta\right) \longrightarrow 1$$

as $n \to \infty$. Then for every $\delta > 0$ and every $\varepsilon > 0$,

$$\Gamma^{(n)}\left(\left|G^{(n)}(\cdot;\vartheta) - g^{(n)}(\cdot;\vartheta)\right| \leq \delta \text{ for every } \vartheta \in B(\vartheta_*,\varepsilon) \cap \Theta\right) \longrightarrow 1.$$

Proof. Let for a finite collection $\tilde{\Theta} \subset \Theta$ of parameters

$$\begin{aligned} & A^{(n)}\left(\tilde{\Theta},\delta\right) \\ = & \left\{x \in \mathbf{X}^{(n)} : \left|G^{(n)}(x;\tilde{\vartheta}) - g^{(n)}(x;\tilde{\vartheta})\right| \leq \delta \text{ for every } \tilde{\vartheta} \in \tilde{\Theta}\right\}. \end{aligned}$$

By assumption, $\Gamma^{(n)}\left(A^{(n)}\left(\tilde{\Theta},\delta\right)\right) \longrightarrow 1$ as $n \to \infty$. Choose now $\varepsilon > 0$. By the required Lipschitz continuity, independently of n and x, there is a finite covering of $B(\vartheta_*,\varepsilon)$ by balls $B(\tilde{\vartheta},\tilde{\varepsilon})$, $\tilde{\vartheta} \in \tilde{\Theta}$, such that the oscillation of $G^{(n)}(x;\cdot)$ and $g^{(n)}(x;\cdot)$ on $B(\tilde{\vartheta},\tilde{\varepsilon}) \cap \Theta$ is bounded say by $\delta\backslash 3$. Each $\vartheta \in B(\vartheta_*,\varepsilon) \cap \Theta$ is contained in some ball $B(\tilde{\vartheta},\tilde{\varepsilon})$ and hence

$$\begin{aligned} & \left|G^{(n)}(x;\vartheta) - g^{(n)}(x;\vartheta)\right| \\ \leq & \left|G^{(n)}(x;\vartheta) - G^{(n)}(x;\tilde{\vartheta})\right| + \left|G^{(n)}(x;\tilde{\vartheta}) - g^{(n)}(x;\tilde{\vartheta})\right| \\ & + \left|g^{(n)}(x;\tilde{\vartheta}) - g^{(n)}(x;\vartheta)\right| \leq \delta \end{aligned}$$

for every $x \in A^{(n)}\left(\tilde{\Theta},\delta/3\right)$. By the introductory observation, the probability of these events converges to 1. This completes the proof. □

As an illustration how the above machinery can be set to work, we give a consistency proof for independent samples.

Theorem 13.4.1. *Let $\mathbf{X}$ be any finite space and Θ an open subset of R^d. Let further $\Pi = \{\Pi(\vartheta) : \vartheta \in \Theta\}$ be a family of distributions on $\mathbf{X}$ which have the form*

$$\Pi(x;\vartheta) = Z(\vartheta)^{-1}\exp\left(\langle\vartheta, H(x)\rangle\right).$$

Suppose that ϑ_* is identifiable. Furthermore, let $\left(\mathbf{X}^{(n)}, \Pi^{(n)}(\cdot;\vartheta)\right)$ be the n-fold product of the probability space $(\mathbf{X}, \Pi(\cdot;\vartheta))$. Then all functions

$$\vartheta \longmapsto \sum_{i=1}^{n} \ln \Pi\left(x^{(i)}\right), \quad \left(x^{(1)},...,x^{(n)}\right) \in \mathbf{X}^{(n)},$$

are strictly concave with a unique maximum $\hat{\vartheta}(x)$ and for every $\varepsilon > 0$,

$$\Pi^{(n)}\left(\hat{\vartheta}^{(n)} \in B(\vartheta_*, \varepsilon); \vartheta_*\right) \longrightarrow 1.$$

Proof. The functions $G^{(n)}$ and $g^{(n)}$ are defined in Example 13.3.2. $G^{(n)}$ is Lipschitz continuous and all functions $\vartheta \longmapsto \ln \Pi(x; \cdot)$ are Lipschitz continuous as well. Since $\mathbf{X}$ is finite and by Lemma C.1, all functions

$$G^{(n)}(x; \cdot) = \frac{1}{n} \sum_{i=1}^{n} \ln \Pi\left(x^{(i)}; \cdot\right)$$

and the $g^{(n)}$ admit a common Lipschitz constant. By the weak law of large numbers,

$$\Pi^{(n)}\left(\left|\frac{1}{n}\sum_{i=1}^{n} \ln \Pi\left(x^{(i)}; \vartheta\right) - \mathsf{E}\left(\ln \Pi(\cdot; \vartheta); \vartheta_*\right)\right| \leq \delta; \vartheta_*\right) \longrightarrow 1, n \to \infty,$$

for each $\vartheta \in \Theta$. The other hypothesis of the Lemmata 13.4.1 and 13.4.2 were checked in Example 13.3.2. Hence the assertion follows from these lemmata. □

If the true distribution Γ is not assumed to be in Π, the estimates tend to that parameter ϑ_* which minimizes the Kullback-Leibler distance between Γ and $\Pi(\vartheta_*)$.

Theorem 13.4.2. *Let $\Theta = \mathsf{R}^d$ and let Γ be a strictly positive distribution on $\mathbf{X}$. Assume the hypothesis of Theorem 13.4.1. Denote the unique maximum of $\vartheta \longmapsto \mathsf{E}\left(L(\cdot; \vartheta); \Gamma\right)$ by ϑ_*. Then for every $\varepsilon > 0$ and $n \to \infty$,*

$$\Gamma^{(n)}\left(\hat{\vartheta}^{(n)}(x) \in B(\vartheta_*, \varepsilon)\right) \longrightarrow 1.$$

Proof. The maximum exists and is unique by Corollary 13.2.2. The rest of the proof is a slight modification of the last one. □

In the next chapter, the general concept will be applied to likelihood estimators for dependent samples.

14. Spacial ML Estimation

14.1 Introduction

We focus now on maximum likelihood estimators for Markov random field models. This amounts to the study of exponential families on finite spaces $\mathbf{X}$ like in the last chapter, with the difference that the product structure of these spaces plays a crucial role.

Though independent sampling is of interest in fields like Neural Networks, it is practically useless for the estimation of texture parameters since one picture is available only. Hence methods based on correlated samples are of particular importance. We shall study families of Gibbs fields on bounded 'windows' $S \subset \mathsf{Z}^2$. The configurations x are elements of a finite product space $\mathbf{X} = \mathbf{Z}^S$. Having drawn a sample $\hat{x}$ from the unknown distribution $\Pi(\vartheta^0)$, we ask whether an estimator is close to ϑ^0. Reasonable estimates should be better for large windows than for small ones. Hence we must show that $\hat{\vartheta}(\hat{x})$ tends to ϑ^0 as S tends to Z^2, i.e. asymptotic consistency.

The indicated concepts will be made precise now. Then we shall give an elementary consistency proof for the pseudolikelihood method adopting the concept of objective functions. Finally, we shall indicate extensions to other, in particular maximum likelihood, estimators.

14.2 Increasing Observation Windows

Let the index set $S(\infty)$ be a multi-dimensional square lattice Z^q. Usually, it is two-dimensional but there are applications like motion analysis requiring higher dimension. Let further $\mathbf{X}^{(\infty)} = \mathbf{Z}^{S(\infty)}$ be the space of configurations. A neighbourhood system on $S(\infty)$ is a collection $\partial = \{\partial(s) : s \in S(\infty)\}$ of subsets of $S(\infty)$ fulfilling the axioms in definition 3.1.1. Cliques are also defined like in the finite case. The Gibbs fields on the observation windows will be induced by a neighbour potential

$$U = \{U_C : C \text{ a clique for } \partial\}$$

with real functions U_C depending on the configurations on C only (*mutatis mutandis*, the definitions are the same as for the finite case). We shall write

$U_C(x_C)$ for $U_C(x)$ if convenient. We want to apply our knowledge about finite-volume Gibbs fields and hence impose the **finite range condition**

$$|\partial(s)| < c < \infty \quad \text{for every} \quad s \in S(\infty).$$

This condition is automatically fulfilled in the finite case.

Fix now observation windows $S(n)$ in $S(\infty)$. To be definite, let the $S(n)$ be cubes $S(n) = [-n, n]^q$ in $\mathbb{Z}^q$. This is not essential; circular windows would work as well. For each cube, choose an arbitrary distribution $\mu^{(n)}$ on the boundary configurations, i.e. on $\mathbf{X}_{\partial S(n)}$. Let $clS(n) = S(n) \cup \partial(S(n))$ be the **closure** of $S(n)$ w.r.t. ∂. On $\mathbf{X}_{clS(n)}$ a Gibbs field $\Pi^{(n)}$ is defined by

$$\Pi^{(n)}\left(x_{S(n)} z_{\partial S(n)}\right) = \Pi^{(n)}\left(x_{S(n)} | z_{\partial S(n)}\right) \cdot \mu^{(n)}\left(z_{\partial S(n)}\right) \tag{14.1}$$

where the transition probability is given by

$$\Pi^{(n)}\left(x_{S(n)} | z_{\partial S(n)}\right) = Z\left(z_{\partial S(n)}\right)^{-1} \exp\left(-\sum_{C \cap S(n) \neq \emptyset} U_C\left(x_{S(n)} z_{\partial S(n)}\right)\right).$$

The slight abuse of notation for the transition probability is justified since it is the conditional distribution of $\Pi^{(n)}$ given $z_{\partial S(n)}$ on the boundary. The consistency results will depend on these local characteristics only and not on the 'boundary conditions' $\mu^{(n)}$.

The observation windows $S(n)$ will increase to $S(\infty)$, i.e.

$$S(m) \subset S(n) \quad \text{if} \quad m < n, S(\infty) = \bigcup_n S(n).$$

Let

$$I(n) = \{s \in S(n) : \partial(s) \subset S(n)\}$$

be the **interior** of $S(n)$ w.r.t. ∂.

Conditional distributions on $I(n)$ will replace the Gibbs fields on finite spaces.

Lemma 14.2.1. *Let $A \subset I(n)$. Then for every $p \geq n$,*

$$\Pi^{(p)}\left(x_A | x_{clS(n) \setminus A}\right) = \frac{\exp\left(-\sum_{C \cap A \neq \emptyset} U_C\left(x_A x_{\partial A}\right)\right)}{\sum_{z_A} \exp\left(-\sum_{C \cap A \neq \emptyset} U_C\left(z_A x_{\partial A}\right)\right)}.$$

Proof. Rewrite Proposition 3.2.1. □

By the finite range condition, the interiors $I(n)$ increase to $S(\infty)$ as the observation windows increase to $S(\infty)$. Hence a finite subset A of $S(\infty)$ will eventually be contained in all $I(n)$. The lemma shows: For all n such that $clA \subset S(n)$ the conditional probabilities w.r.t. $\Pi^{(n)}$ depend on x_{clA} only and not on n. In particular, they do not depend on the boundary conditions $\mu^{(n)}$. Therefore, we shall drop the superscript '(n)' where convenient and denote them by $\Pi\left(x_A | x_{clS(n) \setminus A}\right)$.

Remark 14.2.1. The limit theorems will not depend on the boundary distributions $\mu^{(n)}$. Canonical choices are Dirac measures $\mu^{(n)} = \varepsilon_{\omega_{\partial S(n)}}$ where ω is a fixed configuration on $S(\infty)$ or $\mu^{(n)} = \varepsilon_{z_{\partial S(n)}}$ for varying configurations $z_{\partial S(n)}$.

This corresponds to a basic fact from statistical physics: There may be a whole family of 'infinite volume Gibbs fields' on $S(\infty)$ induced by the potential, i.e. Gibbs fields with the conditional probabilities in (14.2.1) on finite sets of sites. This phenomenon is known as 'phase transition' and occurs already for the Ising model in two dimensions. In contrast to the finite volume *conditional* distributions, the finite dimensional *marginals* of these distributions do *not* agree. In fact, for every sequence $(\mu^{(n)})$ of boundary distributions there is an infinite volume Gibbs fields with marginals (14.1). For infinite volume Gibbs fields our elementary approach from Chapters 3 and 4 does not support enough theoretical background. The reader is referred to GEORGII (1988).

14.3 The Pseudolikelihood Method

We argued in the last chapter that replacing the likelihood function by the sum of likelihood functions for single-site local characteristics yields a computationally feasible estimator. We shall study this estimator in more detail now.

Let the setting of the last section be given. We consider families $\Pi^{(n)} = \{\Pi^{(n)}(\cdot;\vartheta) : \vartheta \in \Theta\}$ of distributions on $\mathbf{X}^{(n)} = \mathbf{Z}^{S(n)}$ where $\Theta \subset \mathsf{R}^d$ is some parameter set. The distributions $\Pi^{(n)}(\vartheta)$ are induced by potentials like in the last section. Fix now some finite subset T of $S(\infty)$. Recall that conditional distributions on T eventually do not depend on n. The maximum pseudolikelihood estimate of ϑ given the data x_S on $S \supset clT$ is the set $\hat{\Theta}_T(x_S)$ of those parameters ϑ which maximize the function

$$\vartheta \longmapsto \prod_{s\in T} \Pi\left(x_s | x_{S\backslash s};\vartheta\right) = \prod_{s\in T} \Pi\left(x_s|x_{\partial s};\vartheta\right).$$

If – and hopefully it is – $\hat{\Theta}_T(x_S)$ is a singleton $\{\hat{\vartheta}_T(x_S)\}$ then we call $\hat{\vartheta}_T(x_S)$ the MPLE. The estimation does not depend on the data outside $cl(T)$. Thus it is not necessary to specify the surrounding observation window.

Given some neighbour potential, the corresponding Gibbs fields were constructed in the last section. We specialize now to potentials of the form

$$U_C^{\vartheta} = -\langle\vartheta, V_C\rangle$$

where $V = (V_1, ..., V_d)$ is a vector of neighbour potentials for ∂ (V will be refered to as a d-dimensional neighbour potential). To simplify notation set for each site s,

$$V^s(x_{cl(s)}) = \sum_{C\ni s} V_C(x).$$

The definition is justified since all cliques C containing s are subsets of $\{s\} \cup \partial(s)$. With these conventions and by Lemma 14.2.1 the conditional distributions have the form

$$\Pi\left(x_s | x_{\partial(s)}; \vartheta\right) = Z(x_{\partial(s)})^{-1} \exp\left(\langle \vartheta, V^s(x_s x_{\partial(s)})\rangle\right)$$

and the pseudo- (log-) likelihood function (for T) is given by

$$PL_T(x;\vartheta) = \sum_{s \in T} \left(\langle \vartheta, V^s(x_s x_{\partial(s)})\rangle - \ln \sum_{z_s} \exp\left(\langle \vartheta, V^s(z_s x_{\partial(s)})\rangle\right) \right).$$

We must require spacial homogeneity of the potential. To define this notion let

$$\theta_u : \mathbf{X}^{(\infty)} \longrightarrow \mathbf{X}^{(\infty)}, x \longmapsto (x_{s-u})_{s \in S(\infty)}$$

be the shift by u. The potential is **shift** or **translation invariant** if

$$\begin{aligned} &t \in \partial(s) \text{ if and only if } t+u \in \partial(s+u) \\ &\text{for all } s,t,u \in S(\infty), \\ &V_{C+u}(\theta_u(x)) = V_C(x) \text{ for all cliques } C \text{ and } u \in S(\infty). \end{aligned} \tag{14.2}$$

Translation invariant potentials V are determined by the functions V_C for cliques C containing $0 \in S(\infty)$ and the finite range condition boils down to $|\partial(0)| < \infty$. The functions V^s may be rewritten in the form

$$V^s(x) = \sum_{C \ni 0} V_C \circ \theta_s(x).$$

The next condition ensures that different parameters can be told apart by the single-site local characteristics.

Definition 14.3.1. *A parameter $\vartheta^0 \in \Theta$ is called (***conditionally***)* **identifiable** *if for each $\vartheta \in \Theta$, $\vartheta \neq \vartheta^0$, there is a configuration $x_{cl(0)}$ such that*

$$\Pi\left(x_0 | x_{\partial(0)}; \vartheta\right) \neq \Pi\left(x_0 | x_{\partial(0)}; \vartheta^0\right). \tag{14.3}$$

A **maximum pseudolikelihood estimator** (MPLE) for the observation window $S(n)$ maximizes $PL_{I(n)}(x;\cdot)$. The next theorem shows that MPLE is asymptotically consistent.

Theorem 14.3.1. *Let Θ be an open subset of R^d and V a shift invariant R^d valued neighbour potential of finite range. Suppose that $\vartheta \in \Theta$ is identifiable. Then for every $\varepsilon > 0$*

$$\Pi^{(n)}\left(PL_{I(n)} \text{ is strictly concave with maximum } \hat{\vartheta} \in B(\vartheta^0, \varepsilon); \vartheta^0\right) \longrightarrow 1$$

as $n \to \infty$. The gradient of the pseudolikelihood function has the form

$$\nabla PL_{I(n)}(x;\vartheta) = \sum_{s \in I(n)} \left[V^s(x) - \mathsf{E}\left(V^s(X_s x_{\partial(s)}) | x_{\partial(s)}; \vartheta\right)\right].$$

The symbols

$$\mathsf{E}(f(X_s)|x_{\partial(s)};\vartheta), \mathsf{var}(f(X_s)|x_{\partial(s)};\vartheta), \mathsf{cov}(f(X_s),g(X_s)|x_{\partial(s)};\vartheta),$$

denote expectation, variance and covariance w.r.t. to the (conditional) distribution $\Pi(x_s|x_{\partial(s)};\vartheta)$ on $\mathbf{X}_s$. Since $s \in I(n)$ these quantities do not depend on large n.

A simple experiment should give some feeling how the pseudo-likelihood works in practice. A sample was drawn from an Ising field on a 80×80 lattice S at inverse temperature $\beta^0 = 0.3$. The sample was simulated by stochastic relaxation and the result x is displayed in Fig. 14.1(a). The pseudolikelihood function on the parameter interval $[0,1]$ is plotted in Fig. (b) with suitable scaling in the vertical direction. It is (practically) strictly concave and its maximum is a pretty good approximation of the true parameter β^0. Fig. 14.2(a) shows a 20×20 sample – in fact, the upper left part of Fig. 14.1(a). With the same scaling as in 14.1(b) the pseudolikelihood function looks like Fig. 14.1(b) and estimation is less pleasant.

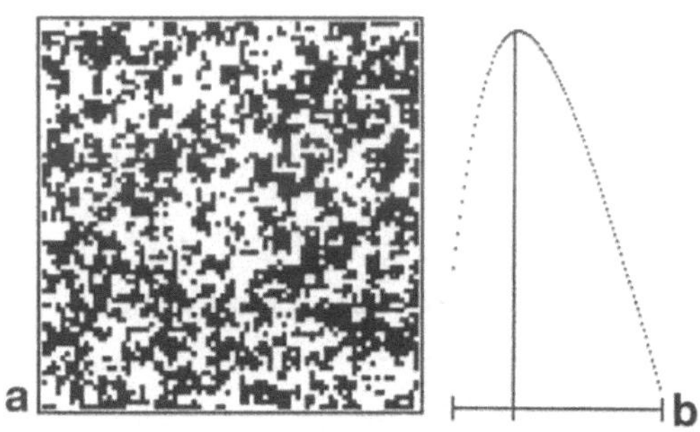

Fig. 14.1. (**a**) 80×80 sample from the Ising model; (**b**) pseudolikelihood function

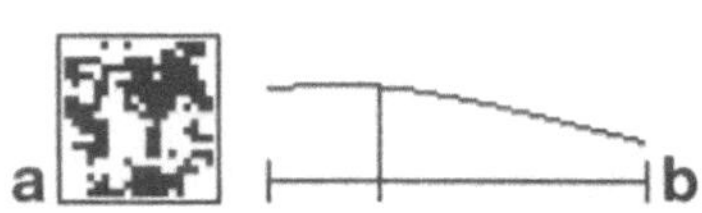

Fig. 14.2. (**a**) 20×20 sample from the Ising model; (**b**) pseudolikelihood function

CH.-CH. CHEN and R.C. DUBES (1989) apply the pseudolikelihood method to binary single-texture images modeled by discrete Markov random fields (namely to the Derin-Elliott model and to the autobinomial model) and compare them to several other techniques. Pseudolikelihood needs most CPU-time but the authors conclude that it is at least as good for the autobinomial model and significantly better for the Derin-Elliott model than the other methods.

We are going now to give an elementary proof of Theorem 14.3.1. It follows the lines sketched in Section 13.3. It is strongly recommended to have a look at the proof of Theorem 13.4.1 before working through the technically more involved proof below. Some of the lemmata are just slight modifications of the corresponding results in the last chapter.

The following basic property of conditional expectations will be used without further reference.

Lemma 14.3.1. *Let $T \subset S \subset S(\infty)$, S finite, Π a random field and f a function on $\mathbf{X}_s$. Then*

$$\mathsf{E}(f(X_S)) = \mathsf{E}(\mathsf{E}(f(X_T X_{S\setminus T})|X_{S\setminus T})).$$

Proof. This follows from the elementary identity

$$\sum_{x_S} f(x_S)\Pi(x_S) = \sum_{x_{S\setminus T}} \left(\sum_{x_T} f(x_T x_{S\setminus T})\Pi(x_T|x_{S\setminus T}) \right) \Pi(x_{S\setminus T}).$$

Independence will be replaced by conditional independence. □

Lemma 14.3.2. *Let Π be a random field w.r.t. to ∂ on $\mathbf{X}_S$, $|S| < \infty$. Let $\mathbf{T}$ be a finite family of subsets of S such that $clT \cap T' = \emptyset$ for different elements T and T' of $\mathbf{T}$. Then the family $\{X_T : T \in \mathbf{T}\}$ is independent given x_D on $D = S \setminus \cup \mathbf{T}$.*

Proof. Let

$$\mathbf{T} = (T_i)_{i=1}^k, E_i = \{X_{T_i} = x_{T_i}\}, F = \{X_{\partial T_i} = x_{\partial T_i}, 1 \le i \le k\}.$$

Then by the Markov property and a well-known factorization formula,

$$\begin{aligned} & \Pi\left(X_{T_i} = x_{T_i}, 1 \le i \le k | X_D = x_D\right) \\ = \; & \Pi\left(E_1 \cap \ldots \cap E_k | F\right) \\ = \; & \Pi(E_1|F)\Pi(E_2|E_1 \cap F)\ldots\Pi(E_k|E_1 \cap \ldots E_{k-1} \cap F). \end{aligned}$$

Again by the Markov property,

$$\begin{aligned} & \Pi(E_j|E_1 \cap \ldots \cap E_{j-1} \cap F) \\ = \; & \Pi\left(X_{T_j} = x_{T_j} | X_{\partial T_j} = x_{\partial T_j}\right) = \Pi\left(X_{T_j} = x_{T_j} | X_D = x_D\right) \end{aligned}$$

which completes the proof. □

The pseudolikelihood for a set of sites is the sum of terms corresponding to single sites. We recall the basic properties of the latter. Let $PL_s = PL_{\{s\}}$ be the pseudolikelihood for a singleton $\{s\}$ in $S(n)$.

Lemma 14.3.3. *The function $\vartheta \longmapsto PL_s(x;\vartheta)$ is twice continuously differentiable for every x with gradient*

$$\nabla PL_s(x;\vartheta) = V^s(x_{cl(s)}) - \mathsf{E}\left(V^s(X_{cl\{s\}}|x_{\partial(s)};\vartheta)\right)$$

and Hessean matrix

$$\nabla^2 PL_s(x;\vartheta) = -\mathsf{cov}\left(V_s(X_s x_{\partial(s)})|x_{\partial(s)};\vartheta\right).$$

In particular, $PL_s(x;\cdot)$ is concave. For any finite subset T of $S(\infty)$, $\alpha \in \mathsf{R}^d$ and $\vartheta \in \Theta$,

$$\alpha\nabla^2 PL_T(x;\vartheta)\alpha^* = -\sum_{s\in T}\mathsf{var}(\langle\alpha, V^s(X_s x_{\partial(s)})\rangle|x_{\partial(s)};\vartheta). \tag{14.4}$$

Proof. This is a reformulation of Proposition 13.2.1 for conditional distributions where in addition Lemma C.4 is used for (14.4). □

The version of Lemma 13.2.1 for conditional identifiability (14.3) reads:

Lemma 14.3.4. *For $s \in I(n)$ the following are equivalent:*

(i) ϑ^0 is conditionally identifiable.
(ii) For every $\alpha \neq 0$ there is $x_{\partial(0)}$ such that $x_0 \longmapsto \langle\alpha, V^s(x_0 x_{\partial(0)})\rangle$ is not constant.
(iii) For every $\alpha \neq 0$ there is $x_{\partial(0)}$ such that for every ϑ,

$$\mathsf{var}\left(\langle\alpha, V^s(X_0 x_{\partial(0)})\rangle|x_{\partial(0)};\vartheta\right) > 0 \tag{14.5}$$

Proof. Adjust Lemma 13.2.1 to conditional indentifiability. □

Since the interactions are of bounded range, in every observation window there is a sparse subset of sites which act independently of each other conditioned on the rest of the observation. This is a key observation. Let us make precise what 'sparse' means in this context:

A subset T of $S(\infty)$ enjoys the **independence property** if

$$\partial\partial(s) \cap \partial(t) = \emptyset \text{ for different sites } s \text{ and } t \text{ in } T. \tag{14.6}$$

Remark 14.3.1. The weaker property $\partial(s) \cap \partial(t) = \emptyset$ will not be sufficient since independence of variable $X_{cl(s)}$ and not of variables X_s is needed (cf. Lemma 14.3.2).

The next result shows that pseudolikelihood eventually becomes strictly concave.

Lemma 14.3.5. *There is a constant $\kappa \in [0,1)$ and a sequence $m(n) \to \infty$ such that for large n,*

$$\Pi^{(n)}\left(\vartheta \longmapsto PL_{I(n)}(x_{S(n)};\vartheta) \text{ is strictly concave}; \vartheta^0\right) \geq 1 - \kappa^{m(n)}.$$

Proof. (1) Suppose that $S \subset I(n)$ satisfies the independence property (14.6). Note that the sets $\partial(s)$, $s \in S$ are pairwise disjoint. Let $z_{\partial S}$ be a fixed configuration on ∂S. Then there is $\rho \in (0,1]$ such that

$$\Pi^{(n)}\left(X_{\partial S} = z_{\partial S};\vartheta^0\right) \geq \rho^{|S|}. \tag{14.7}$$

In fact: Since $\mathbf{X}_{\partial\partial(0)}$ is finite, for every $s \in S$,

$$\rho = \min\left\{\Pi^{(n)}(X_{\partial(s)} = z_{\partial(s)}|\theta_s(x_{\partial\partial(0)});\vartheta^0) : x_{\partial\partial(0)} \in \mathbf{X}_{\partial\partial(0)}\right\} > 0.$$

By translation invariance, the minimum is the same for all $s \in S$. By the indepence property and Lemma 14.3.2, the variables $X_{\partial(s)}$, $s \in S$, are independent conditioned on some $z_{S(n)\setminus\partial S}$. Hence (14.7) holds conditioned on $z_{S(n)\setminus\partial S}$. Since the absolute probabilities are convex combinations of the conditional ones, inequality (14.7) holds.

(2) By the finite range condition, there is an infinite sublattice T of $S(\infty)$ enjoying the independence property. Let $T(n) = T\cap I(n)$. Note that $|T(n)| \to \infty$ as $n \to \infty$.

Suppose that $T(n)$ contains a subset S with $|\mathbf{X}_{\partial(0)}|$ elements. Let $\varphi : S \to \mathbf{X}_{\partial(0)}$ be one-to-one and onto. Then $x_{\partial S} = (\theta_s(\varphi(s)))_{s\in S}$ contains a translate of every $x_{\partial(0)} \in \mathbf{X}_{\partial(0)}$ as a subconfiguration. For every configuration x on $S(n)$ with $X_{\partial S}(x) = x_{\partial S}$, the Hessean matrix of $PL_{I(n)}(x;\cdot)$ is negative definite by (14.4) and Lemma 14.3.4(iii).

By part (1),

$$\Pi^{(n)}\left(X_{\partial S} \neq x_{\partial S}\right) \leq 1 - \rho^{|S|} = \kappa < 1.$$

Similarly, if $T(n)$ contains $m(n)$ pairwise disjoint translates of S then the probability *not* to find translates of all $x_{\partial(0)}$ on $S(n)$ is less than $\kappa^{m(n)}$. Hence the probability of the Hessian being negative definite is at least $1 - \kappa^{m(n)}$ which tends to 1 as n tends to infinity. This completes the proof. □

It still has to be shown that the MPLE is close to the true parameter ϑ^0 in the limit. To this end, the general framework established in Section 13.3 is exploited. The next result suggests candidates for the reference functions.

Lemma 14.3.6. *For every $s \in I(n)$ and $x \in \mathbf{X}_{S(n)}$ the conditional expectation*

$$\vartheta \longmapsto \mathsf{E}\left(PL_s\left(X_{cl(s)};\vartheta\right)|x_{S(n)\setminus cl(s)};\vartheta^0\right)$$

is twice continuously differentiable with gradient

$$\begin{aligned}
&\nabla\mathsf{E}\left(PL_s\left(X_{cl(s)};\vartheta\right)|x_{S(n)\setminus cl(s)};\vartheta^0\right)\\
=\;&\mathsf{E}\left(V^s\left(X_{cl(s)}\right)|x_{S(n)\setminus cl(s)};\vartheta^0\right)\\
&-\mathsf{E}\left(\mathsf{E}\left(V^s\left(X_sX_{\partial(s)}\right)|X_{\partial(s)};\vartheta\right)|x_{S(n)\setminus cl(s)};\vartheta^0\right)
\end{aligned}$$

and Hessean matrix given by

$$\begin{aligned}
&\alpha\nabla^2\alpha^*\mathsf{E}\left(PL_s\left(X_{cl(s)};\vartheta\right)|x_{S(n)\setminus cl(s)};\vartheta^0\right) \qquad (14.8)\\
=\;&-\sum_{z_{\partial(s)}}\mathrm{var}\left(\langle\alpha,V^s(X_sz_{\partial(s)})\rangle|x_{\partial(s)}\vartheta\right)\Pi\left(z_{\partial(s)}|x_{S(n)\setminus cl(s)};\vartheta^0\right).
\end{aligned}$$

In particular, it is concave with maximum at ϑ^0. If ϑ^0 is conditionally identifiable then it is strictly concave.

Proof. The identities follow from those in Lemma 14.3.3 and Lemma C.4. Concavity holds by Lemma C3. The gradient vanishes at ϑ^0 by Lemma 14.3.1. Strict concavity is implied by conditional identifiability because of 14.3.4 and because the summation in (14.8) extends over all of $\mathbf{X}_{\partial(s)}$. This completes the proof. □

Let us now put things together.

Proof (of Theorem 14.3.1). Strict concavity was treated in Lemma 14.3.5. We still have to define an objective function, the corresponding reference function and to verify the required properties.

Let

$$G^{(n)}(x;\vartheta) = \frac{1}{|I(n)|} PL_{I(n)}(x;\vartheta) = \frac{1}{|I(n)|} \sum_{s\in I(n)} PL_s(x_{cl(s)};\vartheta)$$

and

$$g^{(n)}(x;\vartheta) = \frac{1}{|I(n)|} \sum_{s\in I(n)} \mathsf{E}\left(PL_s(X_{cl(s)};\vartheta)|x_{S(n)\backslash cl(s)};\vartheta^0\right).$$

By the finite range condition and translation invariance the number of different functions of ϑ in the sums is finite. Hence all summands admit a common Lipschitz constant and by Lemma C.1 all $G^{(n)}(x;\cdot)$ and $g^{(n)}(x;\cdot)$ admit a common Lipschitz constant. Similarly, there is $\gamma > 0$ such that

$$g^{(n)}(x;\vartheta) \le -\gamma\|\vartheta-\vartheta^0\|_2^2$$

on a ball $B(\vartheta^0;r) \subset \Theta$ uniformly in x and n. Choose now $\vartheta \in \Theta$ and $\delta > 0$. By the finite range condition there is a finite partition $\mathbf{T}$ of $S(\infty)$ into infinite lattices T each fulfilling the independence property. For every $T \in \mathbf{T}$ let $T(n) = T \cap I(n)$. By the independence property and by Lemma 14.3.2, the random variables $PL_s(X_{cl(s)};\vartheta)$, $s \in T(n)$, are independent w.r.t. the conditional distributions $\Pi(\cdot|x_{S(n)\backslash clT(n)};\vartheta^0)$ on $\mathbf{X}_{clT(n)}$ and by translation invariance they are identically distributed. Hence for every $T \in \mathbf{T}$, the weak law of large numbers yields for

$$\begin{aligned} &h^{(n)}(x_{clT(n)};\vartheta) \\ &= \frac{1}{|T(n)|} \sum_{s\in T(n)} \left[PL_s(x_{cl(s)};\vartheta) - \mathsf{E}\left(PL_s(X_{cl(s)};\vartheta)|x_{S(n)\backslash cl(s)};\vartheta^0\right)\right] \end{aligned}$$

that

$$\Pi^{(n)}\left(\left|h^{(n)}(x_{clT(n)};\vartheta)\right| > \delta \mid x_{S(n)\backslash cl(s)};\vartheta^0\right) \le \frac{const}{|T(n)|\delta^2}.$$

The constant $const > 0$ may be chosen uniformly in $T \in \mathbf{T}$. The same estimate holds for the absolute probabilities, since they are convex combinations of the conditional ones, which yields

$$\Pi^{(n)}\left(\left|h^{(n)}(x_{clT(n)};\vartheta)\right| > \delta;\vartheta^0\right) \leq \frac{const}{|T(n)|\delta^2}.$$

Finally, the estimate

$$\begin{aligned}&\left|G^{(n)}(x;\vartheta) - g^{(n)}(x;\vartheta)\right| \\ = &\left|\sum_{T\in\mathbf{T}} \frac{|T(n)|}{|I(n)|} h^{(n)}(x_{clT(n)};\vartheta)\right| \leq \left|\sum_{T\in\mathbf{T}} h^{(n)}(x_{clT(n)};\vartheta)\right|\end{aligned}$$

yields

$$\Pi^{(n)}\left(\left|G^{(n)}(\cdot;\vartheta) - g^{(n)}(\cdot;\vartheta)\right| \leq \delta;\vartheta^0\right) \longrightarrow 1 \text{ as } n \to \infty.$$

Hence $G^{(n)}$ is an objective function, the hypothesis of Lemma 13.4.1 and 13.4.2 are fulfilled, and the theorem is proved. □

Consistency of the pseudolikelihood is studied in GRAFFIGNE (1987) and GEMAN and GRAFFIGNE (1987), GUYON (1986), (1987), JENSEN AND MØLLER (1989), (not all proofs are correct in detail).

A modern and more elegant proof by F. COMETS (1992) is based on 'large deviations'. He also proves asymptotic consistency of spatial MLEs. These results will be sketched in the next section.

The pseudolikelohood method was introduced by J. BESAG (1974) (see also (1977)). He also introduced the **coding estimator** which maximizes some $PL_{T(n)}$ instead of $PL_{I(n)}$. The set $T(n)$ is – say a maximal – subset of $I(n)$ such that the variables $X_s, s \in T(n)$, are conditionally independent given $x_{S(n)\setminus T(n)}$. The coding estimator is computed like the MPLE.

14.4 The Maximum Likelihood Method

In the setting of Section 14.2, the spacial analogue of maximum likelihood estimators can be introduced as well. For each observation window $S(n)$ it is defined as the set $\tilde{\Theta}_{I(n)}(\mathrm{x})$ of those $\vartheta \in \Theta$ which maximize the likelihood function

$$\vartheta \longmapsto L_{I(n)}(x;\vartheta) = \ln \Pi^{(n)}(x_{I(n)} \mid x_{S(n)\setminus I(n)};\vartheta).$$

The model is identifiable if

$$\Pi^{(n)}(\cdot \mid x_{S(n)\setminus I(n)};\vartheta) \neq \Pi^{(n)}(\cdot \mid x_{S(n)\setminus I(n)};\vartheta^0)$$

for some n and $x_{S(n)\setminus I(n)}$.

For shift invariant potentials of finite range the maximum likelihood estimator is asymptotically consistent under identifiability. In principle, an elementary proof can be given along the lines of Section 14.3. In this proof, all steps but the last one would *mutatis mutandis* be like there (and even notationally simpler). We shall not carry out such a proof because of the last step. The main argument there was a law of large numbers for i.i.d. random variables. For maximum likelihood, it has to be replaced by a law of large numbers for shift invariant random fields. An elementary version – for a sequence of finite-volume random fields instead of an infinite volume Gibbs field – would have a rather unnatural form obscuring the underlying idea. We prefer to report some recent results.

F. COMETS (1992) proves asymptotic consistency for a general class of objective functions. The specializations to maximum likelihood and pseudolikelihood estimators in our setting read:

Theorem 14.4.1. *Assumme that the model is identifiable. Then for every $\varepsilon > 0$ there are $c > 0$ and $\gamma > 0$ such that*

$$\Pi^{(n)}\left(\tilde{\Theta}_{I(n)} \notin B(\vartheta^0;\varepsilon);\vartheta^0\right) \leq c \cdot \exp(-|I(n)|\gamma)$$

and

$$\Pi^{(n)}\left(\hat{\Theta}_{I(n)} \notin B(\vartheta^0;\varepsilon);\vartheta^0\right) \leq c \cdot \exp(-|I(n)|\gamma)$$

For the proof we refer to the transparent original paper.

Remark 14.4.1. The setting in COMETS (1992) is more general than ours. The configuration space $\mathbf{X}$ may be a product $\mathbf{Z}^q$ of $\mathbf{Z} = \mathsf{R}^n$ or any Polish space $\mathbf{Z}$. Moreover, finite range of potentials is not required and replaced by a summability condition. The proof is based on a large deviation principle and on the variational principle for Gibbs fields (on the infinite lattice).

Whereas pseudolikelihood estimators can be computed by classical methods, computation of maximum likelihood estimators requires new ideas. One approach will be discussed in the next section.

Remark 14.4.2. The coding estimator is a version of MLE which does not make full use of the data in the observation window.

Asymptotics of ML and MPL estimators in a general framework are also studied in GIDAS (1987), (1988), (1991a), COMETS and GIDAS (1991), ALMEIDA and GIDAS (1992). The Gaussian case is treated in KÜNSCH (1981) and GUYON (1982). An estimation framework for binary fields is developed in POSSOLO (1986). See also the pioneer work of PICKARD (cf. (1987) and the references there).

14.5 Computation of ML Estimators

BESAG's pseudolikelihood method became a popular alternative to maximum likelihood estimation in particular since the latter was not computable in the general set-up (it could be evaluated for special fields, cf. the remarks concluding this section). Only recently, suitable optimization techniques were proposed and studied. Those we have in mind are randomly perturbed gradient ascent methods. Proofs for the refined methods, for example in YOUNES (1988), require delicate estimates, and therefore, they are fairly technical. We shall not repeat the heavy formulae here, but present, a 'naive' and simple algorithm. It is based on the approximation of expectations via the law of large numbers. Hopefully, this will smooth the way to the more involved original papers.

Let us first discuss *deterministic* gradient ascent for the likelihood function. We wish to maximize a likelihood function of the type $\vartheta \mapsto \ln \Pi(x, \vartheta)$ for a fixed observation x. Generalizing slightly, we shall discuss the function

$$W : \Theta \longrightarrow \mathsf{R}, \vartheta \longmapsto \mathsf{E}(L(\cdot; \vartheta); \Gamma) \tag{14.9}$$

where

- $\Theta = \mathsf{R}^d$,
- Γ is an arbitrary probability distribution on $\mathbf{X}$.

The usual likelihood function is the case $\Gamma = \varepsilon_x$. We shall assume that

- $\mathsf{cov}(H; \vartheta)$ is positive definite for each $\vartheta \in \Theta$,
- the function W attains its (unique) maximum at $\vartheta_* \in \Theta$.

Remark 14.5.1. By Corollary 13.2.2, the last two assumptions are fulfilled, if some ϑ' is identifiable and Γ is strictly positive. Given the set-up in the last section, for likelihood functions they are fulfilled for large n with high probability.

The following rule is adopted: Choose an initial parameter vector $\vartheta_{(0)}$ and a step-size $\lambda > 0$. Define recursively

$$\vartheta_{(k+1)} = \vartheta_{(k)} + \lambda \nabla W(\vartheta_{(k)}) \tag{14.10}$$

for every $k \geq 0$. Note that λ is kept constant over all steps.

For sufficiently small step-size λ the sequence $\vartheta_{(k)}$ in (14.10) converges to ϑ_*:

Theorem 14.5.1. *Let* $\lambda \in (0, 2/(d \cdot D))$, *where*

$$D = \max\{\mathsf{var}_\mu(H_i) : 1 \leq i \leq d,\ \mu \text{ a probability distribution on } \mathbf{X}\}.$$

Then for each initial vector $\vartheta_{(0)}$, *the sequence in (14.10) converges to* ϑ_*.

Remark 14.5.2. A basic gradient ascent algorithm (which can be traced back to a paper by CAUCHY from 1847) procedes as follows: Let $W : \mathsf{R}^d \longrightarrow \mathsf{R}$ be smooth. Initialize with some $\vartheta_{(0)}$. In the k-th step - given $\vartheta_{(k)}$ - let $\vartheta_{(k+1)}$ be the maximizer of W on the ray $\{\vartheta_{(k)} + \gamma \nabla W(\vartheta_{(k)}) : \gamma \geq 0\}$. Since we need a simple expression for $\vartheta_{(k+1)}$ in terms of $\vartheta_{(k)}$ and expectations of H, we adopt the formally simpler algorithm (14.10).

Gradient ascent is ill-famed for slow convergence near the optimum. It is also numerically problematic, since it is sensitive to scaling of variables. Moreover, the step size λ above is impracticably small, and in practice, the hypothesis of the theorem will be violated.

Proof (of Theorem 14.5.1). The theorem follows from the general convergence theorem of nonlinear optimization in Appendix D. A proper specialization reads:

Lemma 14.5.1. *Let the objective function $W : \mathsf{R}^d \to \mathsf{R}$ be continuous. Consider a continuous map $a : \mathsf{R}^d \to \mathsf{R}^d$ and – given $\vartheta_{(0)}$ – let the sequence $(\vartheta_{(k)})$ be recursively defined by $\vartheta_{(k+1)} = a(\vartheta_{(k)})$, $k \geq 0$. Suppose that W has a unique maximum at ϑ_* and*

(i) the sequence $(\vartheta_{(k)})_{k\geq 0}$ is contained in a compact set;

(ii) $W(a(\vartheta)) > W(\vartheta)$ if $\vartheta \in \mathsf{R}^d$ is no maximum of W;

(iii) $W(a(\vartheta_*)) = W(\vartheta_*)$.

Then the sequence $(\vartheta_{(k)})$ converges to ϑ_* (cf. Appendix D.(c)).

The lemma will be applied to the previously defined function W and to

$$a(\vartheta) = \vartheta + \lambda \nabla W(\vartheta).$$

These maps are continuous and, by assumption, W has a unique maximum ϑ_*. The requirements (i) through (iii) will be verified now.

(iii) the gradient of W vanishes in maxima and hence (iii) holds.

(ii) Let now $\vartheta \neq \vartheta_*$, $\lambda > 0$ and $\varphi = \vartheta + \lambda \nabla W(\vartheta)$. The step-size λ has to be chosen such that $W(\varphi) > W(\vartheta)$. The latter holds if and only if the function

$$h : \mathsf{R}_+ \longrightarrow \mathsf{R}, \gamma \longmapsto W(\vartheta + \gamma \nabla W(\vartheta))$$

fulfills

$$h(\lambda) - h(0) > 0.$$

Let ∇W be represented by a row vector with transpose ∇W^*. By Corollary 13.2.1, a computation in C.3 and the Cauchy-Schwarz inequality, for every $\gamma \in [0, \lambda]$ the following estimates hold

$$\begin{aligned} h''(\gamma) &= \nabla W(\vartheta)\nabla^2 W(\vartheta + \lambda \nabla W(\vartheta))(\nabla W(\vartheta))^* \\ &= -\operatorname{var}(\langle \nabla W(\vartheta), H\rangle) \\ &\geq \|\nabla W(\vartheta)\|_2^2 \mathsf{E}(\sum_i (H_i - \mathsf{E}(H_i))^2) \\ &= -\|\nabla W(\vartheta)\|_2^2 \sum_i \operatorname{var}(H_i) \\ &\geq -\|\nabla W(\vartheta)\|_2^2 \cdot d \cdot D. \end{aligned}$$

Variance and expectations are taken w.r.t. $\Pi(\cdot; \vartheta + \gamma \nabla W(\vartheta))$, the factor D is a common bound for the variances of the functions H_i. Hence

$$\begin{aligned} h'(\gamma) &\geq h'(0) + \int_0^\gamma h''(\gamma')d\gamma' \\ &\geq \langle \nabla W(\vartheta), \nabla W(\vartheta)\rangle - \gamma \|\nabla W(\vartheta)\|_2^2 \cdot d \cdot D \\ &= (1 - \gamma \cdot d \cdot D)\|\nabla W(\vartheta)\|_2^2 \end{aligned}$$

and

$$h(\lambda) - h(0) = \int_0^\lambda h'(\gamma)d\gamma \geq \lambda(1 - \lambda \cdot d \cdot D/2)\|\nabla W(\vartheta)\|_2^2$$

which is strictly positive if $\lambda < 2/(d \cdot D)$. This proves $W(\varphi) > W(\vartheta)$ and hence (ii).

(i) Since the sequence $(W(\vartheta_{(k)}))$ never decreases, every $\vartheta_{(k)}$is contained in $L = \{\vartheta : W(\vartheta) \geq W(\vartheta_{(0)})\}$. By assumption and Lemma C.3, W is majorized by a quadratic function

$$\vartheta \longmapsto -\gamma\|\vartheta - \vartheta_*\|_2^2 + W(\vartheta_*), \gamma > 0.$$

Hence L is contained in a compact ball and (i) is fulfilled.

In summary, the lemma applies and the theorem is proved. □

The gradients

$$\nabla W(\vartheta_{(k)}) = \mathsf{E}(H; \Gamma) - \mathsf{E}(H; \vartheta_{(k)})$$

in (14.10) cannot be computed and hence will be replaced by proper estimates. Let us make this precise:

- Let $\vartheta \in \Theta$ and $n > 0$ be fixed.
- Let $\xi_1, \ldots, \xi_n$ be the random variables corresponding to the first n steps of the Gibbs sampler for $\Pi(\cdot; \vartheta)$ and set

$$\bar{H}^{(n)} = \frac{1}{n}\sum_{i=0}^{n-1} H(\xi_i).$$

- Let $\eta_1, \ldots, \eta_n$ be independent random variables with law Γ and set

$$\tilde{H}^{(n)} = \frac{1}{n}\sum_{i=0}^{n-1} H(\eta_i).$$

Note that for likelihood functions W, i.e. if $\Gamma = \varepsilon_x$ for some $x \in \mathbf{X}$, $\tilde{H}^{(n)} = H(x)$ for every n.

The 'naive' stochastic gradient algorithm is given by the rule: Choose $\varphi_{(0)} \in \Theta$. Given $\varphi_{(k)}$, let

$$\varphi_{(k+1)} = \varphi_{(k)} + \lambda\left(\tilde{H}^{(n_k)} - \bar{H}^{(n_k)}\right) \tag{14.11}$$

where for each k, n_k is a sufficiently large sample size.

The following results shows that for sufficiently precise estimates the randomly perturbated gradient ascent algorithm still converges.

Proposition 14.5.1. *Let $\varphi_{(0)} \in \Theta\backslash\{\vartheta_*\}$ and $\varepsilon > 0$ be given. Set $\lambda = (d \cdot D)^{-1}$. Then there are sample sizes n_k such that the algorithm (14.11) converges to ϑ_* with probability greater than $1-\varepsilon$.*

Sketch of a proof. We shall argue that the global convergence theorem (Appendix D) applies with high probability. The arguments of the last proof will be used without further reference.

Let us first introduce the deterministic setting. Consider $\vartheta \neq \vartheta_*$. We found that

$$W(\vartheta + \lambda\nabla W(\vartheta)) > W(\vartheta)$$

and $\nabla W(\vartheta + \lambda\nabla W(\vartheta)) \neq 0$. Hence there is a closed ball

$$A(\vartheta) = B(\vartheta + \lambda\nabla W(\vartheta), r(\vartheta))$$

such that $W(\vartheta') > W(\vartheta)$ and $\nabla W(\vartheta') \neq 0$ for every $\vartheta' \in A(\vartheta)$. In particular, $\vartheta_* \notin A(\vartheta)$. The radii $r(\vartheta)$ can be chosen continuously in ϑ. To complete the definition of A let

$$A(\vartheta_*) = \{\vartheta_*\}.$$

The set-valued map A is closed in the sense of Appendix D and, by construction of A, W is an ascent function.

Let us now turn to the probabilistic part. Let C be a compact subset of $\Theta\backslash\{\vartheta_*\}$ and $r(C) = \min\{r(\vartheta) : \vartheta \in C\}$. The maximal local oscillation $\Delta(\vartheta)$ of the energy $-\langle\vartheta, H\rangle$ depends continuously on ϑ and

$$\mathsf{P}\left(\left\|\frac{1}{n}\sum_{i=0}^{n-1}\xi_i - \mathsf{E}(\xi_i;\vartheta)\right\| > \delta;\vartheta\right) \leq \frac{1}{n\delta^2}\, const\, \exp(\sigma\Delta(\vartheta))$$

(Theorem 5.1.4). By these observations, for every $\delta > 0$ and $\gamma \in (0,1)$ there is a sample size $n(C,\gamma)$ such that uniformly in all $\vartheta \in C$,

$$\mathsf{P}\left(\left\|\vartheta + \lambda(\tilde{H}_{n(C,\gamma)} - \bar{H}_{n(C,\gamma)}) \in A(\vartheta)\right\| \leq \delta;\vartheta\right) > 1-\gamma.$$

After these preparations, the algorithm can be established. Let $\varphi_{(0)} \in \Theta\backslash\{\vartheta_*\}$ be given and set $n_0 = n(\{\varphi_{(0)}\}, \varepsilon/2)$. Then $\varphi_{(1)}$ is in the compact set $C_0 = A(\varphi_{(0)})$ with probability greater than $1-\varepsilon/2$. For the k-th step, assume that $\varphi_{(k)} \in C_k$ for some compact subset C_k of $\Theta\backslash\{\vartheta_*\}$. Let $n_k = n(C_k, \varepsilon \cdot 2^{-(k+1)})$. Then $\varphi_{(k+1)} \in A(\varphi_{(k)})$ with probability greater than $1-\varepsilon\cdot 2^{-(k+1)}$. In particular, such $\varphi_{(k+1)}$ are contained in the compact set $C_k = \bigcup\{A(\vartheta) : \vartheta \in C_{(k-1)}\}$ which does not contain ϑ_*. This induction shows that with probability greater than $1-\varepsilon$ every $\varphi_{(k+1)}$, $k > 0$, is contained in $A(\varphi_{(k)})$ and the sequence $(\varphi_{(k)})$ stays in a compact set. Hence the algorithm (14.11) converges to ϑ_* with probability greater than $1-\varepsilon$. This completes the proof.

In (14.11), gradient ascent and the Gibbs sampler alternate. It is natural to ask if both algorithms can be coupled. L. Younes (1988) answers this question in the positive. Recall that for likelihood functions W the gradient at ϑ is $H(x) - \mathsf{E}(H;\vartheta)$. YOUNES studies the algorithm

$$\begin{aligned}\vartheta_{(k+1)} &= \vartheta_{(k)} + \frac{1}{(k+1)\gamma}\left(H(x) - H(\xi_{k+1})\right) \\ \mathsf{P}(\xi_{k+1} = z|\xi_k = y) &= P_k(y,z;\vartheta)\end{aligned} \tag{14.12}$$

where γ is a large positive number and $P_k(y,z;\vartheta)$ is the transition probability of a sweep of the Gibbs sampler for $\Pi(\cdot;\vartheta_{(k)})$. For

$$\gamma > 2\Delta \cdot |S| \max\{\|H(y) - H(x)\|_2 : y \in \mathbf{X}\}$$

this algorithm converges even almost surely to the maximum ϑ_*. Again, it is a randomly perturbed gradient ascent. In fact, the difference in brackets is of the form

$$\begin{aligned}H(x) - H(\xi) &= (H(x) - \mathsf{E}(H;\vartheta)) + (\mathsf{E}(H;\vartheta) - H(\xi)) \\ &= \nabla W(\vartheta) + (\mathsf{E}(H;\vartheta) - H(\xi)).\end{aligned}$$

Let us finally turn to annealing. The goal is to minimize the true energy function

$$x \longmapsto -\langle \vartheta_*, H(x)\rangle.$$

In the standard method, one would first determine or at least approximate the true parameter ϑ_* by one of the previously discussed methods and then run annealing. YOUNES carries out estimation and annealing simultaneously. Let us state his result more precisely.

Let $(\eta_{(n)})$ be a sequence in R^d converging to ϑ_* which fulfills the following requirements:

– there are constants $C > 0$, $\varepsilon > 0$, $A > \|\vartheta_*\|$ such that

$$\begin{aligned}\|\eta_{(n+1)} - \eta_{(n)}\| &\le C/(n+1), \\ \|\eta_{(n)} - \vartheta_*\| &\le Cn^{-\varepsilon}.\end{aligned}$$

Assume further the stability condition

– For ϑ close to ϑ_* the functions $x \mapsto -\langle \vartheta, H(x)\rangle$ have the same minimizers.

Then the following holds:

Under the above hypothesis, the marginals of the annealing algorithm with schedule

$$\beta(n) = \eta_{(n)}(A\Delta|S|)^{-1}\ln n$$

converge to the uniform distribution on the minimizers of $-\langle \vartheta_*, H(\cdot)\rangle$.

YOUNES' ideas are related to those in MÉTIVIER and PRIOURET (1987) who proved convergence of 'adaptive' stochastic algorithms naturally arising in engineering. These authors, in turn, were inspired by FREIDLIN and WENTZELL (1984). The circle of such ideas is surveyed and extended in the recent monograph BENVENISTE, MÉTIVIER and PRIOURET (1990).

14.6 Partially Observed Data

In the previous sections, statistical inference was based on completely observed data x. In many applications one does not observe realizations of the Markov field X (or Π) of interest but of a random function Y of X. This was allowed for in the general setting of Chapter 1. Typical exampes are:

- data corrupted by noise,
- partially observed data.

We met both cases (and combinations): for example, $Y = X + \eta$ or an observable process $Y = X^P$ where $X = (X^P, X^L)$ with a hidden label or edge process X^L.

Inference has to be based on the data only and hence on the 'partial observations' y. The analysis is substantially more difficult than for completely observed data and therefore is beyond the scope of this text. We confine ourselves to some laconic remarks and references. At least, we wish to point out some major differences to the case of fully observed data.

Again, a family

$$\Pi = \{\Pi(\cdot;\vartheta) : \vartheta \in \Theta\}$$

of distributions on $\mathbf{X}$ is given. There is a space $\mathbf{Y}$ of data and $P(x, y)$ is the probability to observe $y \in \mathbf{Y}$ if $x \in \mathbf{X}$ is the true scene (for simplicity, we assume that $\mathbf{Y}$ is finite). The (log)likelihood function is now

$$\vartheta \longmapsto L(y;\vartheta) = \ln \Xi(y;\vartheta)$$

where $\Xi(\cdot;\vartheta)$ is the distribution of the data given parameter ϑ. Plainly,

$$\Xi(y;\vartheta) = \sum_x \Pi(x;\vartheta)P(x,y). \tag{14.13}$$

Let $\bar{\mu}(\cdot;\vartheta)$ denote the joint law of x and y, i.e.

$$\bar{\mu}(x,y;\vartheta) = \Pi(x;\vartheta)P(x,y).$$

The law of X given $Y = y$ is

$$\bar{\mu}(x|y;\vartheta) = \frac{\Pi(x;\vartheta)P(x,y)}{\sum_z \Pi(z;\vartheta)P(z,y)}.$$

In the sequel, expectations, covariance and so on will be taken w.r.t. $\bar{\mu}$; for example, the symbol $\mathsf{E}(\cdot|y;\vartheta)$ will denote the expectation w.r.t. $\bar{\mu}(x|y;\vartheta)$. To compute the gradient of $L(y;\cdot)$, we differentiate:

$$\begin{aligned}
\frac{\partial}{\partial\vartheta_i} L(y;\vartheta) &= \frac{\sum_x \frac{\partial}{\partial\vartheta_i}\Pi(x;\vartheta)P(x,y)}{\sum_x \Pi(x;\vartheta)P(x,y)} \\
&= \frac{\sum_x \frac{\partial}{\partial\vartheta_i}\ln \Pi(x;\vartheta)\bar{\mu}(x,y;\vartheta)}{\Xi(y)} \\
&= \mathsf{E}\left(\frac{\partial}{\partial\vartheta_i}\ln \Pi(\cdot;\vartheta)|y;\vartheta\right).
\end{aligned}$$

Plugging in the expressions from Proposition 13.2.1 gives

$$\nabla L(y;\vartheta) = \mathsf{E}(H|y;\vartheta) - \mathsf{E}(H;\vartheta). \tag{14.14}$$

Differentiating once more yields

$$\nabla^2 L(y;\vartheta) = \mathsf{cov}(H;\vartheta) - \mathsf{cov}(H|y;\vartheta). \tag{14.15}$$

The Hessean matrix is the difference of two covariance matrices and the likelihood in general is not concave. Taking expections does not help and therefore the natural reference functions are not concave as well. This causes considerable difficulties in two respects: (i) Consistency proofs do not follow the previous lines and require more subtle and new arguments. (ii) Even if the likelihood function has maxima, it can have numerous local maxima and stochastic gradient ascent algorithms converge to a maximum only if the initial parameter is very close to a maximizer.

If the parameter space Θ is compact, the likelihood function at least has a maximum. Recently, COMETS and GIDAS (1992) proved asymptotic consistency (under identifiability and for shift invariant potentials) in a fairly general framework and gave large deviations estimates of the type in Theorem 14.4.1.

If Θ is not compact, the nonconcavity of the likelihood function creates subtle difficulties in showing that the maximizer exists for large observation windows, and eventually stays in a compact subset of Θ (last reference, p. 145). The consistency proof in the noncompact case requires an additional condition on the behaviour of the $\Pi^{(n)}(\vartheta)$ for large $\|\vartheta\|$. The authors claim that without such an extra condition asymptotic consistency cannot hold in complete generality. We feel, that such problems are ignored in some applied fields (like applied Neural Networks). A weaker consistency result, under stronger assumptions, and by different methods, was independently obtained by YOUNES (1988a), (1989). COMETS and GIDAS remark, 'that consistency for noncompact Θ (and incomplete data) does not seem to have been treated in the literature even for i.i.d. random variables' (p. 145).

The behaviour of stochastic gradient ascent is studied in YOUNES (1989).

Besides the already mentioned papers, parameter estimation for imperfectly observed fields is addressed in CHALMOND (1988a), (1988b), (for a special model and the pseudolikelihood method), LAKSHMANAN and DERIN (1989), FRIGESSI and PICCIONI (1990) (for the two-dimensional Ising model corrupted by noise), ARMINGER and SOBEL (1990) (also for the pseudolikelihood), ALMEIDA and GIDAS (1992).

Part VI

Supplement

We inserted the examples and applications where they give reasons for the mathematical concepts to be introduced. Therefore, many important applications have not yet be touched. In the last part of the text, we collect a few in order to indicate how Markov field models can be adopted in various fields of imaging.

15. A Glance at Neural Networks

15.1 Introduction

Neural networks are becoming more and more popular. Let us comment on the particularly simple Hopfield model and its stochastic counterpart, the Boltzmann machine.

The main reason for this excursion is the close relationship between neural networks and the models considered in this text. Some neural networks even are special cases of these models. This relationship is often obscured by the specific terminology which frequently hinders the study of texts about neural networks. We show by way of example that part of the theory can be described in the language of random fields and hope thereby to smooth the way to the relevant literature. In particular, the limit theorems for sampling and annealing apply, and the consistency and convergence results for maximum likelihood estimators do as well.

While we borrow terminology from statistical physics and hence use words like energy function and Gibbs field, neural networks have their roots in biological sciences. They provide strongly idealized and simplified models for biological nervous systems. That is the reason why sites are called neurons, potentials are given by synaptic weights and so on. But what's in a name! On the other hand, recent urge of interest is to a large extent based on their possible applications to data processing tasks similar or equal to those addressed here ('neural computing') and there is no need for any reference to the biological systems which originally inspired the models (KAMP und HASLER (1990)). Moreover, ideas from statistical physics are more and more penetrating the theory. We shall not go into details and refer to texts like KAMP and HASLER (1990), HECHT-NIELSEN (1990), MÜLLER and REINHARDT (1990) or AARTS and KORST (1987). We simply illustrate the connection to dynamic Monte Carlo methods and maximum likelihood estimation.

– All results in this chapter are special cases of results in Chapters 5 and 14.

15.2 Boltzmann Machines

The neural networks we shall describe are special random fields. Hence everything we had to say is said already. The only problem is to see that this is really true, i.e. to translate statements about probabilistic neural networks into the language of random fields. Hence this section is kind of a small dictionary.

As before, there is a finite index set S. The sites $s \in S$ are now called units or neurons. Every unit may be in one of two states, usually 0 or 1 (there are good reasons to prefer ± 1). If a unit is in state 0 then it is 'off' or 'not active' if its state is 1 then it is said to be 'on', 'active' or 'it fires'. There is a neighbourhood system ∂ on S and for every pair $\{s,t\}$ of neighbours a weight ϑ_{st}. It is called synaptic weight or connection strength. One requires the symmetry condition $\vartheta_{st} = \vartheta_{ts}$. In addition, there are weights ϑ_s for some of the neurons. To simplify notation, let us introduce weights $\vartheta_{st} = 0$ and $\vartheta_s = 0$ for those neighbour pairs and neurons, which are not yet endowed with weights.

Remark 15.2.1. The synaptic weights ϑ_{st} induce pair potentials U by $U_{\{s,t\}}(x) = \vartheta_{st}x_s x_t$ (see below) and therefore symmetry is required. Networks with asymmetric connection strengths are much more difficult to analyze. From the biological point of view, symmetry definitely is not justified as experiments have shown (KAMP and HASLER (1990), p. 2).

Let us first discuss the dynamics of neural networks and then turn to learning algorithms. In the (deterministic) **Hopfield model**, for each neuron s there is a threshold ρ_s. In the sequential version, the neurons are updated one by one according to some deterministic or random visiting strategy. Given a configuration $x = (x_t)_{t\in S}$ and a current neuron s the new state y_s in s is determined by the rule

$$y_s = \left\{ \begin{matrix} 1 \\ x_s \\ 0 \end{matrix} \right\} \quad \text{if} \quad \sum_{t\in\partial(s)} \vartheta_{st}x_t + \vartheta_s \quad \left\{ \begin{matrix} > \rho_s \\ = \rho_s \\ < \rho_s \end{matrix} \right. . \tag{15.1}$$

The interpretation is as follows: Suppose unit t is on. If $\vartheta_{st} > 0$ then its contribution to the sum is positive and it pushes unit s to fire. One says that the connection between s and t is 'excitory'. Similarly, if $\vartheta_{st} < 0$ then it is 'inhibitory'. The sum $\sum_{t\in\partial(s)} \vartheta_{st}x_t + \vartheta_s$ is called the postsynaptic potential at neuron s. Updating the units in a given order by this rule amounts to coordinatewise maximal descent for the energy function

$$H(x) = -\left(\sum_{\langle s,t\rangle} \vartheta_{st}x_s x_t + \sum_s \vartheta_s x_s - \sum_t \rho_t x_t \right).$$

In fact, if s is the unit to be updated then the energy difference between the old configuration x and the new configuration $y_s x_{S\setminus\{s\}}$ is

$$H(y_s x_{S\setminus\{s\}}) - H(x) = \Delta H(x_s, y_s) = (x_s - y_s)\left(\vartheta_s + \sum_{t\in\partial(s)} \vartheta_{st}x_t - \rho_s \right)$$

since the terms with indices u and v such that $s \notin \{u, v\}$ do not change. Assume that x is fixed and the last factor is positive. Then $\Delta H(x_s, \cdot)$ becomes minimal for $y_s = 1$. Similarly, for a negative factor, one has to set $y_s = 0$. This shows that minimization of the difference amounts to the application of (15.1) (up to the ambiguity in the case $\ldots = \rho_s$).

After a finite number of steps this dynamical system will terminate in sets of local minima. Note that the above energy function has the form of the binary model in Example 3.2.1,(c).

Optimization is one of the conceivable applications of neural networks (HOPFIELD and TANK (1985)). Sampling from the Gibbs field for H also plays an important role. In either case, for a specific task there are two problems:

1. Transformation to a binary problem. The original variables must be mapped to configurations of the net and an energy function H on the net has to be designed the minima of which correspond to the minima of the original objective function. This amounts to the choice of the parameters ϑ_{st}, ϑ_s and ρ_s.
2. Finding the minima of H or sampling from the associated Gibbs field.

For (1) we refer to MÜLLER and REINHARDT (1990) and part II of AARTS and KORST (1989). Let us just mention that the transformation may lead to rather inadequate representations of the problem which result in poor performance. Concerning minimization, we already argued that functions of the above type may have lots of local minima and greedy algorithms are out of the question. Therefore, random dynamics have been suggested (HINTON and SEJNAWSKI (1983), HINTON, SEJNAWSKI and ACKLEY (1984)). For sampling, there is no alternative to Monte Carlo methods anyway.

The following sampler is popular in the neural networks community. A unit s supposed to flip its state is proposed according to a probability distribution G on S. If the current configuration is $x \in \{0,1\}^S$ then a flip results in $y = (1 - x_s)x_{S\backslash\{s\}}$. The probability to accept the flip is a sigmoid function of the gain or loss of energy. More precisely,

$$\begin{aligned} \pi(x, (1 - x_s)x_{S\backslash\{s\}}) &= G(s) \cdot (1 + \exp(\Delta H(x_s, (1 - x_s))^{-1}, \\ \pi(x, x) &= 1 - \sum_t \pi(x, (1 - x_t)x_{S\backslash\{t\}}) \\ \pi(x, y) &= 0 \quad \text{otherwise} \end{aligned} \tag{15.2}$$

Usually, G is the uniform distribution over all units. Systematic sweep strategies, given by an enumeration of the units, are used as well. In this case, the state at the current unit s is flipped with probability

$$1 + \exp(\Delta H(x_s, (1 - x_s))^{-1} \tag{15.3}$$

The sigmoid shape of the acceptance function reflects the typical response of neurons in a biological network to the stimulus of their environment. The random dynamics given by (15.2) or (15.3) define **Boltzmann machines** .

The fraction in (15.2) or (15.3) may be rewritten in the form

$$\begin{aligned}\frac{1}{1+\exp(\Delta H(x_s,y_s))} &= \frac{\exp(-H(y))}{\exp(-H(y))+\exp(-H((1-y_s)x_{S\setminus\{s\}}))}\\ &= \Pi_s(y|x)\end{aligned}$$

where Π_s is the single-site local characteristic of the Gibbs field Π associated with H. Hence Boltzmann dynamics are special cases of Gibbs samplers. Plainly, one may adopt Metropolis type samplers as well.

Remark 15.2.2. If one insists on states $x \in \{-1,1\}$, a flip in s results in $y=(-x_s)x_{S\setminus\{s\}}$. In this case the local Gibbs sampler is frequently written in the form

$$\Pi_s(y|x) = \frac{1}{2}\left(1-\tanh\left(x_s h_s(x)\right)\right)$$

with

$$h_s(x) = \sum_{t\in\partial(s)} \vartheta_{st} + \vartheta_{ss} - \rho_s.$$

The corresponding Markov process is called **Glauber dynamics**.

For convenience, let us repeat the essentials. The results are formulated for the random sweep strategy in (15.2) only. Analoguous results hold for systematic sweep strategies.

Proposition 15.2.1. *The Gibbs field for H is invariant under the kernel in (15.2).*

For a cooling schedule $\beta(n)$ let $\pi^{(n)}$ be the sampler in (15.2) for the energy function $\beta(n)H$, let $\sigma = |S|$ and Δ the maximal local oscillation of H.

Theorem 15.2.1. *If the proposal matrix G is strictly positive and if the cooling schedule $\beta(n)$ increases to infinity not faster than $(\sigma\Delta)^{-1}\ln n$ then for every initial distribution ν the distributions $\nu\pi^{(1)}\ldots\pi^{(n)}$ converge to the uniform distribution on the minimizers of H.*

Remark 15.2.3. Note that the theorem covers sequential dynamics only. The limit distribution for synchroneous updating was computed in Chapter 10.

Example 15.2.1. Boltzmann machines have been applied to various problems in combinatorial optimization and imaging. AARTS and KORST (1989), Chapter 9.7.2, carried out simulations for the 10 and 30 cities travelling salesman problems (cf. Chapter 8) on Boltzmann machines and by Metropolis annealing. We give a sketch of the method but the reader should not get lost in details.

The underlying space is $\mathbf{X} = \{0,1\}^{N^2}$, where N is the number of cities, the cities have numbers $0,\ldots,N-1$ and the configurations are (x_{ip}) where $x_{ip} = 1$ if and only if the tour visits city i at the p-th position. In fact, a configuration x represents a tour if and only if for each i one has $x_{ip} = 1$ for precisely one p and for each p one has $x_{ip} = 1$ for precisely one i. Note that most configurations do not correspond to feasible tours. Hence constraints are imposed in order to drive the output of the machine towards a feasible solution. This is similar to constraint optimization in Chapter 7.

One tries to

$$\text{minimize} \quad G(x) = \sum_{i,j,p,q=0}^{N-1} a_{ijpq} x_{ip} x_{jq},$$

where

$$\begin{array}{ll} a_{ijpq} = d(i,j) & \text{if} \quad q = (p+1) \bmod \sigma\,, \\ a_{ijpq} = 0 & \text{otherwise,} \end{array}$$

under the constraints

$$\begin{array}{rcl} \sum_i x_{ip} & = & 1, \quad p = 0, \ldots, N-1 \\ \sum_p x_{ip} & = & 1, \quad i = 0 \ldots, N-1. \end{array}$$

The Boltzmann machine has units (ip) and the following weights:

$$\begin{array}{rcl} \vartheta_{ip,jq} & = & -d(i,j) \quad \text{if} \quad i \neq j, q = (p+1)\text{mod}N, \\ \vartheta_{ip,ip} & > & \max\{d(i,k) + d(i,l) : k \neq l\}, \\ \vartheta_{ip,jq} & < & -\min\{\vartheta_{ip,ip}, \vartheta_{jq,jq}\}, \text{ if } (i = j \text{ and } p \neq q) \text{ or } (i \neq j \text{ and } p = q). \end{array}$$

Wereas the concrete form of the energy presently is not of too much interest, note that the constraints are introduced as weak constraints getting stricter and stricter as temperature decreases (similar to Chapter 7). The authors found that 'the Boltzmann machine cannot obtain results that are comparable to the results obtained by simulated annealing'. Whereas for these small problems the Metropolis method found near optimal solutions in few seconds, the Boltzmann machine needed computation times ranging from few minutes for the 10 cities problem up to hours for the 30 cities problem to compute the final output. Moreover, the results were not too reliable. Frequently, the machine produced non-tours and the mean final tour length considerably exceeded the smallest known value of the tour length. For details cf. the above reference. MÜLLER and REINHARDT (1990), 10.3.1., draw similar conclusions.

Because of the poor performance of Boltzmann machines in this and other applications, modifications are envisaged. It is natural to allow larger state spaces and more general interactions. This amounts to a reinterpretation of the Markov field approach in terms of Boltzmann machines. This coalescence will not surprise the reader of a text like this. In fact, the reason for the past discrimination between the two concepts has historical and not intrinsic reasons (cf. AZENCOTT (1990)–(1992)).

For sampling, note that $\pi^{|S|}$ is strictly positive and hence Theorems 5.1.2, 5.1.3 and 5.1.4 and Proposition 15.2.1 imply

Theorem 15.2.2. *If the proposal matrix G is strictly positive then $\nu\pi^n$ converges to the Gibbs field Π with energy function H. Similarly,*

$$\frac{1}{n}\sum_{i=0}^{n-1} f(\xi_i) \longrightarrow \mathsf{E}(f;\Pi)$$

in probability.

15.3 A Learning Rule

A most challenging application of neural networks is to use them as (auto-) associative memories. To illustrate this concept let us consider classification of patterns as belonging to certain classes. Basically, one proceeds along the lines sketched in Chapter 12. Let us start with a simple example.

Example 15.3.1. The Boltzmann machine is supposed to classify incoming patterns as representing one of the 26 characters $a, \ldots, z$. Let the characters be enumerated by the numbers $1, \ldots, 26$. These numbers (or labels) are represented by binary patterns $10\ldots0, \ldots, 0\ldots01$ of length 26, i.e. configurations in the space $\{0,1\}^{S^{out}}$ where $S^{out} = \{1, \ldots, 26\}$. Let S^{in} be a - say - 64×64-square lattice and $\{0,1\}^{S^{in}}$ the space of binary patterns on S^{in}. Some of these patterns resemble a character a, others resemble a character p and most configurations do not resemble any character at all (perhaps cats or dogs or noise). If for instance a noisy version $x_{in} = x_{S^{in}}$ of the character a is 'clamped' to the units in S^{in} the Boltzmann machine should show the code $x_{out} = x_{S^{out}}$ of a, i.e. the configuration $10\ldots0$, on the 'display' S^{out}. More precisely: A Gibbs field Π on $\{0,1\}^S$, where S is the disjoint union of S^{in} and S^{out} has to be constructed such that the conditional distribution $\Pi(x_{out}|x_{in})$ is maximal for the code x_{out} of the noisy character x_{in}. Given such a Gibbs field, the label can be found maximizing $\Pi(\cdot|x_{in})$. In other words, x_{out} is the MAP estimate given x_{in}. The actual value $\Pi(x_{out}|x_{in})$ is a measure for the credibility of the classification. Hence $\pi(10\ldots0|x_{in})$ should be close to 1 if x_{in} really is a (perhaps noisy) version of the character a and very small if x_{in} is some pepper and salt pattern.

Since the binary configurations in $\{0,1\}^{S^{in}}$ are 'inputs' for the 'machine' the elements of S^{in} are called **input neurons** . The patterns in $\{0,1\}^{S^{out}}$ are the possible outputs and hence an $s \in S^{out}$ is called an **output neuron.**

An algorithm for the construction of a Boltzmann machine for a specific task is called a **learning algorithm**. 'Learning' is synonymous for estimation of parameters. The parameters to be estimated are the connection strenghts ϑ_{st}.

Consider the following set-up: An outer source produces binary patterns on S as samples from some random field Γ on $\{0,1\}^S$. Learning from Γ means that the Boltzmann machine adjusts its parameters ϑ in such a way that its outputs resemble the outputs of the outer source Γ. The machine learns from a series of samples from Γ and hence learning amounts to estimation in the statistical sense. In the neural network literature samples are called **examples**. Here again the question of computability arises and leads to additional requirements on the estimators. In neural networks, the neighbourhood systems typically are large. All neurons of a subsystem may interact. For instance, the output neurons in the above example typically should display configurations with precisely one figure 1 and 25 figures 0. Hence it is reasonable to connect all output neurons with inhibitory, i.e. negative, weights. Since each output neuron should interact with additional units it has more than 26 neighbours. In more involved applications the neighbourhood systems are even larger. Hence even pseudolikelihood estimation may become computationally too expensive. This leads to the requirement, that estimation should be **local**. This means that a weight ϑ_{st} has to be estimated from the values x_s and x_t of the examples only. A local estimation algorithm requires one additional processor for each neighbour pair only and these processors work independently. We shall find that the stochastic gradient algorithms in Sections 14.5 and 14.6 fulfill the locality requirement. We are going now to spezialize this method to Boltzmann machines.

To fix the setting, let a finite set S of units and a neighbourhood system ∂ on S be given. Moreover, let $S' \subset S$ be a set of distinguished sites. The energy function of a Boltzmann machine has the form

$$H(x) = -\left(\sum_{\langle s,t\rangle} \vartheta_{st} x_s x_t + \sum_{s\in S'} \vartheta_s x_s\right).$$

To simplify notation, let $\vartheta_{ss} = \vartheta_s$ and

$$J = \{\{s,t\} \in S \times S : t \in \partial(s) \quad \text{or} \quad s = t \in S'\}.$$

Since $x_s^2 = x_s$ the energy function can be rewritten in the form

$$H(x) = -\sum_{\{s,t\}\in J} \vartheta_{st} x_s x_t.$$

The law of a Boltzmann machine then becomes

$$\Pi(x;\vartheta) = Z^{-1} \exp\left(\sum_{\{s,t\}\in J} \vartheta_{st} x_s x_t\right).$$

Only probability distributions on $\mathbf{X} = \{0,1\}^S$ of this type can be learned perfectly. We shall call them **Boltzmann fields** on $\mathbf{X}$.

Recall that we wish to construct a 'Boltzmann approximation' $\Pi(\cdot;\vartheta_*)$ to a given random field Γ on $\mathbf{X} = \{0,1\}^S$. In principle, this is the problem discussed in the last two chapters since a Boltzmann field is of the exponential form considered there: Let $\Theta = \mathsf{R}^J$, $H_{st}(x) = X_sX_t(x)$ and $H = (H_{st})_{\{s,t\}\in J}$. Then

$$\Pi(\cdot;\vartheta) = Z(\vartheta)^{-1}\exp(\langle\vartheta, H\rangle).$$

The weights ϑ_{st} play the role of the former parameters ϑ_i and the variables X_sX_t play the role of the functions H_i.

The family of these Boltzmann fields is identifiable.

Proposition 15.3.1. *Two Boltzmann fields on* $\mathbf{X}$ *coincide if and only if they have the same connection strengths.*

Proof. Two Boltzmann fields with equal weights coincide. Let us show the converse.

The weights ϑ_{st} define a potential V by

$$\begin{array}{lllll} V_{st}(x) = \vartheta_{ss}x_sx_t & \text{if} & \{s,t\} & \in & J, \\ V_{st}(x) = 0 & \text{if} & \{s,t\} & \notin & J, \\ V_A(x) = 0 & \text{if} & |A| & \geq & 3. \end{array}$$

which is normalized for the 'vacuum' $o \equiv 0$. By Theorem 3.3.3, the V_A are uniquely determined by the Boltzmann field and if one insists to write them in the above form, the ϑ_{st} are uniquely determined as well.

For a direct proof, one can spezialize from Chapter 3: Let $\Pi(\cdot;\vartheta) = \Pi(\cdot;\tilde{\vartheta})$. Then

$$\sum \tilde{\vartheta}_{st}x_sx_t - \sum \vartheta_{st}x_sx_t = \ln Z(\tilde{\vartheta}) - \ln Z(\vartheta) = C$$

and the difference does not depend on x. Plugging in $x \equiv 0$ shows $C = 0$ and hence the sums are equal. For sets $\{s,t\}$ of one or two sites plug in x with $x_s = 1 = x_t$ and $x_r = 0$ for all $r \notin \{s,t\}$, which yields

$$\vartheta_{st} = \sum \vartheta_{uv}x_ux_v = \sum \tilde{\vartheta}_{st}x_ux_v = \tilde{\vartheta}_{st}. \qquad \square$$

The quality of the Boltzmann approximation usually is gauged by the Kullback-Leibler distance. Recall that the Kullback-Leibler information is the negative of the properly normalized expectation of the likelihood defined in Corollary 13.2.1. Gradient and Hessean matrix have conspicuous interpretations as the following specialization of Proposition 13.2.1 shows.

Lemma 15.3.1. *Let* Γ *be a random field on* $\mathbf{X}$ *and let* $\vartheta \in \Theta$. *Then*

$$\begin{aligned} \frac{\partial I(\Pi(\vartheta)|\Gamma)}{\partial\vartheta_{st}} &= \mathsf{E}(X_sX_t;\vartheta) - \mathsf{E}(X_sX_t;\Gamma), \\ \frac{\partial^2 I(\Pi(\vartheta)|\Gamma)}{\partial\vartheta_{st}\partial\vartheta_{uv}} &= \mathsf{cov}(X_sX_t, X_uX_v;\vartheta). \end{aligned}$$

The random variables X_sX_t equal 1 if $x_s = 1 = x_t$ and vanish otherwise. Hence they indicate whether the connection between s and t is active or not. The expectations $\mathsf{E}(X_sX_t;\vartheta) = \Pi(X_s = 1 = X_t;\vartheta)$ or $\mathsf{E}(X_sX_t;\Gamma) = \Gamma(X_s = 1 = X_t)$ are the probabilities that s and t both are on. Hence they are called the **activation probabilities** for the connections $\langle s,t\rangle$.

Remark 15.3.1. For $s \in S'$ the activation probability is $\Pi(X_s = 1)$. Since $\Pi(X_s = 0) = 1 - \Pi(X_s = 1)$ the activation probabilities determine the one-dimensional marginal distributions of Π for $s \in S'$. Similarly, the two-dimensional marginals can easily be computed from the one-dimensional marginals and the activation probabilities. In summary, random fields on $\mathbf{X}$ have the same one- and two-dimensional marginals (for $s \in S'$ and neighbour pairs, respectively) if and only if they have the same activation probabilities.

Proof (of Lemma 15.3.1). The lemma is a reformulation of the first part of Corollary 13.2.2. □

The second part of Corollary 13.2.2 reads:

Theorem 15.3.1. *Γ be a random field on $\mathbf{X}$. Then the map*

$$\Theta \longrightarrow \mathsf{R}, \vartheta \longmapsto I(\Pi(\cdot;\vartheta)|\Gamma)$$

is strictly convex and has a unique global minimum ϑ_*. $\Pi(\cdot;\vartheta_*)$ is the only Boltzmann field with the same activation probabilities on J as Γ.

Gradient descent with fixed step-size $\lambda > 0$ (like (14.10)) amounts to the rule: Choose initial weights $\vartheta_{(0)}$ and define recursively

$$\vartheta_{(k+1)} = \vartheta_{(k)} - \lambda \nabla I(\Pi(\vartheta_{(k)})|\Gamma) \tag{15.4}$$

for every $k \geq 0$. Hence the individual weights are changed according to

$$\begin{aligned} & \vartheta_{(k+1),st} \\ = \quad & \vartheta_{(k),st} - \lambda\left(\Pi(X_s = 1 = X_t;\vartheta_{(k)}) - \Gamma(X_s = 1 = X_t)\right). \end{aligned} \tag{15.5}$$

This algorithm respects the locality requirement which unfortunately outrules better algorithms. The convergence Theorem 14.5.1 for this algorithm reads:

Theorem 15.3.2. *Let Γ be a random field on $\mathbf{X}$. Choose a real number $\lambda \in (0, 8\cdot|J|^{-1})$. Then for each vector $\vartheta_{(0)}$ of initial weights, the sequence $(\vartheta_{(k)})$ in (15.4) converges to the unique minimizer of the function $\vartheta \mapsto I(\Pi(\cdot;\vartheta)|\Gamma)$.*

Proof. The theorem is a special case of Theorem 14.5.1. The upper bound for λ there was $2/(d\cdot D)$ where d was the dimension of the parameter space and D an upper bound for the variances of the H_i. Presently, $d = |J|$ and, since each X_sX_t is a Bernouilli variable, one can choose $D = 1/4$. This proves the result. □

In summary: if $\Gamma = \Pi(\cdot;\vartheta)$ is a Boltzmann field then

$$W(\vartheta) = I\left(\Pi(\cdot;\vartheta)|\Pi(\cdot;\vartheta_*)\right)$$

has a unique minimum at ϑ_* which theoretically, but not in practice, can be approximated by gradient descent (15.4). If Γ is no Boltzmann field then gradient descent results in the Boltzmann field with the same activation probabilites as Γ.

The **learning rule** for Boltzmann machines usually is stated as follows (cf. AARTS and KORST (1987)): Let $\varphi_{(0)}$ be a vector of initial weights and λ a small positive number. Determine recursively new parameters $\varphi_{(k+1)}$ according to the rule:

(i) Observe independent samples $\eta_1, \ldots, \eta_{n_k}$ from Γ and compute the empirical means

$$M_{k,st} = \frac{1}{n_k} \sum_{i=1}^{n_k} \eta_{i,s}\eta_{i,t}.$$

(ii) Run the Gibbs sampler for $\Pi(\cdot;\varphi_{(k)})$, observe samples $\xi_1, \ldots, \xi_{m_k}$ and compute relative frequencies

$$H_{m_k} = \frac{1}{m_k} \sum_{i=1}^{m_k} \xi_{i,s}\xi_{i,t}.$$

(iii) Let

$$\varphi_{(k+1),st} = \varphi_{(k),st} - \lambda\left(H_{m_k} - M_{n_k}\right). \tag{15.6}$$

Basically, this is stochastic gradient descent discussed in Section 14.5. To be in accordance with the neural networks literature, we must learn some technical jargon.

Part (i) is called the **clamped phase** since the samples from Γ are 'clamped' to the neurons. Part (ii) is the **free phase** since the Boltzmann machine freely adjusts its states according to its own dynamics.

Convergence for sufficiently large sample sizes n_k and m_k follows easily from Proposition 14.5.1.

Proposition 15.3.2. *Let $\varphi_{(0)} \in \mathbb{R}^{|J|}\backslash\{\vartheta_*\}$ and $\varepsilon > 0$ be given. Set $\lambda = 4\cdot|J|^{-1}$. Then there are sample sizes $n_k = m_k$ such that the algorithm (15.6) converges to ϑ_* with probability greater than $1-\varepsilon$.*

For suitable constants the algorithm

$$\varphi_{(k+1)} = \varphi_{(k)} - ((k+1)\gamma)^{-1}\left(\xi_{k+1} - \eta_{k+1}\right) \tag{15.7}$$

converges almost surely. The proof is a straightforward modification of YOUNES (1988). For further comments cf. Section 14.5.

The following generalization of the above concept receives considerable interest. One observes that adding neurons to a network gives more flexibility. Hence the enlarged set $T = S \cup R$ of neurons, $R \cap S = \emptyset$, is considered. As before, there is a random field Γ on $\{0,1\}^S$ and one asks for a Boltzmann field $\Pi(\cdot;\vartheta)$ on $\{0,1\}^T$ with marginal distribution $\Pi^S(\cdot;\vartheta)$ on $\{0,1\}^S$ close to Γ in the Kullback-Leibler distance. Like in (14.13) the marginal is given by

$$\Pi^S(x_S;\vartheta) = \sum_{x_R} \Pi(x_R x_S;\vartheta).$$

Remark 15.3.2. A neuron $s \in S$ is called **visible** since in most application it is either an input or an output neuron. The neurons $s \in R$ are neither observed nor clamped and hence they are called **hidden neurons**. The Boltzmann field on T has now to be determined from the observations on S only.

Like in Section 14.6 inference is based on partially observed data and hence is unpleasant. Let us note the explicit expressions for the gradient and the Hessean matrix. To this end we introduce the distribution

$$\tilde{\Pi}(x;\vartheta) = \Gamma(x_S)\Pi(x_R|x_S;\vartheta)$$

and denote expectations and covariance matrices w.r.t. $\tilde{\Pi}(\cdot;\vartheta)$ by $\tilde{\mathsf{E}}(\cdot;\vartheta)$ and $\widetilde{\mathrm{cov}}(\cdot;\vartheta)$.

Lemma 15.3.2. *The map $\vartheta \mapsto I(\Pi^S(\cdot;\vartheta)|\Gamma)$ has first partial derivatives*

$$\frac{\partial}{\partial \vartheta_{st}} I(\Pi^S(\cdot;\vartheta)|\Gamma) = \mathsf{E}(X_s X_t;\vartheta) - \tilde{\mathsf{E}}(X_s X_t;\vartheta)$$

and second partial derivatives

$$\frac{\partial^2}{\partial \vartheta_{st}\partial \vartheta_{uv}} I(\Pi^S(\cdot;\vartheta)|\Gamma) = \mathrm{cov}(X_s X_t, X_u X_v;\vartheta) - \widetilde{\mathrm{cov}}(X_s X_t, X_u X_v;\vartheta).$$

Proof. Integrate in (14.14) and (14.15) w.r.t. Γ. □

Hence the Kullback-Leibler distance in general is not convex and (stochastic) gradient descent (15.6) converges to a (possibly poor) local minimum, except it is started close to an optimum.

There is a lot of research on such and related problems (cf. VAN HEMMEN and KÜHN (1991) and the references therein) but they are not yet sufficiently well understood. For some promising attempts cf. the papers by R. AZENCOTT (1990)–(1992). He addresses in particular learning rules for synchroneous Boltzmann machines.

16. Mixed Applications

We conclude this text with a sample of further typical applications. They once more illustrate the flexibility of the Bayesian framework. The first example concerns the analysis of motion. It shows how the ideas developed in the context of piecewise smoothing can be transfered to a problem of appearently different flavour. In single photon emission tomography – the second example – a similar approach is adopted. In contrast to former applications, shot noise is predominant here. The third example is different from the others. The basic elements are no longer pixel based like grey levels, labels or edge elements. They have an own structure and thereby a higher level of interpretation may be achieved. This is a hint along which lines middle or even high level image analysis might evolve. Part of the applications recently studied by leading researchers is presented in CHELLAPA and JAIN (1993).

16.1 Motion

The analysis of image sequences has received considerable interest, in particular the recovery of visual motion. We shall shortly comment on two-dimensional motion. We shall neither discuss the reconstruction of motion in real three-dimensional scenes (TSAI and HUANG (1984), WENG, HUANG and AHUJA (1987), NAGEL (1981)) nor the background of motion analysis (JÄHNE (1991), MUSMANN, PIRSCH and GALLERT (1985), NAGEL (1985), AGGARWAL and NANDHAKUMAR (1988)).

Motion in an image sequence may be indicated by displacement vectors connecting corresponding picture elements in subsequent images. These vectors constitute the **displacement vector field**. The associated field of velocity vectors is called **optical flow**. There are several classes of methods to determine optical flow; most popular are feature based and gradient based methods. The former are related to texture segmentation: Around a pixel an observation window is selected and compared to windows in the next image. One decides that the pixel has moved to that place where the 'texture' in the window resembles the texture in the original window most. Gradient based methods infer optical flow from the change of grey values. These two approaches are compared in AGGARWAL (1988) and NAGEL and ENKELMANN (1986). A third approach are image transform methods using spatiotemporal frequency filters (HEEGER (1988)). We shall shortly comment on a gradient based approach primarily proposed by B.K.P. HORN and B.G. SCHUNCK (1981) (cf. also SCHUNCK (1986)) and its Bayesian version, examined and applied by HEITZ and BOUTHEMY (1990a), (1992) (cf. also HEITZ and BOUTHEMY (1990b)). Let us note in advance that the transformation of the classical method into a Bayesian one follows essentially the lines sketched in Chapter 2 in the context of smoothing and piecewise smoothing.

For simplicity, we start with continuous images described by an intensity function $f(u,v,t)$ where $(u,v) \in D \subset \mathrm{R}^2$ are the spacial coordinates and $t \in \mathrm{R}_+$ is the time parameter. We assume that the changes of f in t are caused by two-dimensional motion alone. Let us follow a picture element travelling across the plane during a time interval $T = (t_0 - \Delta\tau, \tau + \Delta\tau_0)$. It runs along a path $(u(t), v(t))_{\tau \in T}$. By assumption, the function

$$\tau \longmapsto g(\tau) = f(u(\tau), v(\tau), \tau)$$

is constant and hence its derivative w.r.t τ vanishes:

$$\begin{aligned} 0 = \frac{d}{d\tau} g(\tau) &= \frac{d}{d\tau} f \circ (u(\cdot), v(\cdot))(\tau) \\ &= \frac{\partial f(u(\tau), v(\tau), \tau)}{\partial u} \frac{du(\tau)}{d\tau} + \frac{\partial f(u(\tau), v(\tau), \tau)}{\partial v} \frac{dv(\tau)}{d\tau} \\ &\quad + \frac{\partial f(u(\tau), v(\tau), \tau)}{\partial t} \frac{d\tau}{d\tau}, \end{aligned}$$

or, in short-hand notation,

$$\frac{\partial f}{\partial u}\frac{du}{dv} + \frac{\partial f}{\partial v}\frac{dv}{dt} = -\frac{\partial f}{\partial t}.$$

Denoting the velocity vector $\left(\frac{du}{d\tau}, \frac{dv}{d\tau}\right)$ by ω, the spacial gradient $\left(\frac{\partial f}{\partial u}, \frac{\partial f}{\partial v}\right)$ by ∇f and the partial derivatives by f_z the equation reads

$$\langle \nabla f, \omega \rangle = -f_t.$$

It is called the **image flow** or **motion constraint equation**. It does not determine uniquely the optical flow ω and one looks for further constraints. Consider now the vector field ω for fixed time τ. Then ω depends on u and v only. Since in most points of the scene motion will not change abruply, a first requirement is smoothness of optical flow i.e. spatial differentiability of ω and, moreover, that $\|\nabla\omega\|$ should be small on the spatial average. Image flow constraints and smoothness requirements for optical flow are combined in the requirement that optical flow minimizes the functional

$$\omega \longmapsto \int_D \alpha^2(\langle \nabla f, \omega \rangle + f_t)^2 + \|\nabla \omega\|_2^2 du\, dv$$

for some constant α. Given smooth functions, this is the standard problem in calculus of variations usually solved by means of the Euler-Lagrange equations. There are several obvious shortcomings. Plainly, the motion constraint equation does not hold in occlusion areas or on discontinuities of motion. On the other hand, these locations are of particular interest. Moreover, velocity fields in real word images tend to be piecewise continuous rather than globally continuous. The Bayesian method to be described takes this into account.

Let us first describe the prior distribution. It is similar to that used for piecewise smoothing in Example 2.3.1. The energy function has the form

$$H(\omega, b) = \sum_{\langle s,t \rangle} \Psi(\omega_s - \omega_t)(1 - b_{\langle s,t \rangle}) + H_2(b)$$

where b is an edge field coupled to the velocity field ω. HEITZ and BOUTHEMY use the disparity function

$$\Psi(\Delta) = \begin{cases} \gamma^{-2}(\|\Delta\|_2 - \gamma)^2 & \text{if} \quad \|\Delta\|_2 > \gamma \\ -\gamma^{-2}(\|\Delta\|_2 - \gamma)^2 & \text{if} \quad \|\Delta\|_2 \le \gamma \end{cases}.$$

There is a smoothing effect whenever $\|\omega_s - \omega_t\|_2 \le \gamma$. A motion discontinuity, i.e. a boundary element, is favoured for large $\|\omega_s - \omega_t\|_2$ presumably corresponding to a real motion discontinuity. The term H_2 is used to organize the boundaries, for example, to weight down unpleasant local edge configurations like isolated edges, blind endings, double edges and others, or to reduce the total contour length.

Next, the observations must be given as a random function of (ω, b). One observes the (discrete) partial derivatives f_u, f_v and f_t. The motion constraint equation is statistically interpreted and the following model is spezified:

$$-f_t(s) = \langle \nabla f(s), \omega \rangle + \eta_s$$

with noise η accounting for the deviations from the theoretical model. The authors choose white noise and hence arrive at the transition density

$$h_{\omega_s} = Z_1^{-1} \exp\left(-\frac{1}{2\sigma^2} (f_t(s) + \langle \nabla f(s), \omega \rangle)^2 \right).$$

Plainly, this makes sense only at those sites where the motion constraint equation holds. The set SC of such sites is determined in the following way: The intensity function is written in the form

$$f(\omega, t) = \langle a_t, \omega \rangle + c_t.$$

A necessary condition for the image flow constraint to hold is that $a_t \sim a_{t+\Delta t}$ for small Δt. A statistical test for this hypothesis is set to work and the site s is included in SC if the hypothesis is not rejected. The law of f_t given (ω, b) becomes

$$h(f_t | \omega, b) = \prod_{s \in SC} h_{\omega_s}(f_t(s)).$$

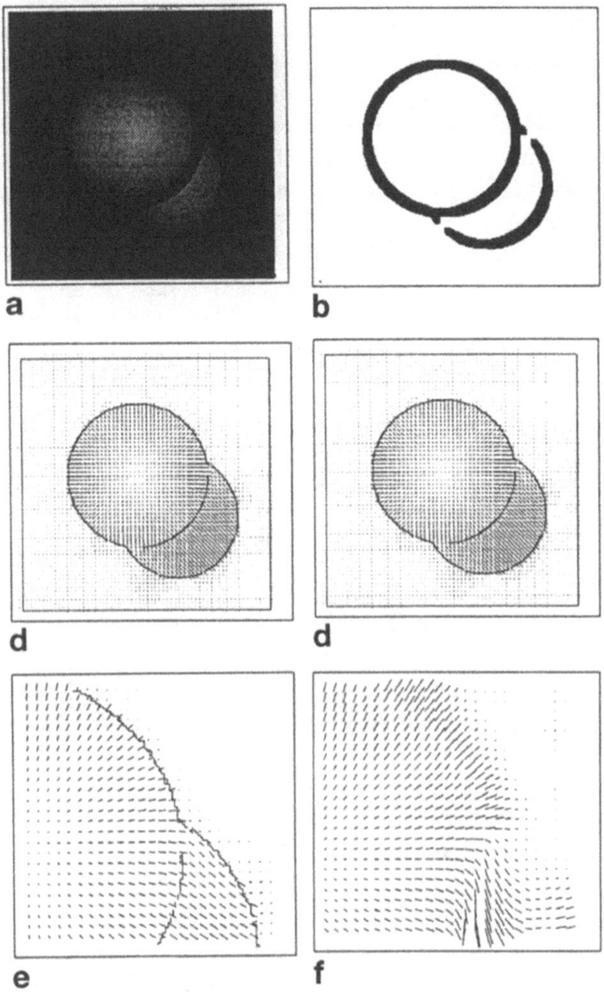

Fig. 16.1. (a)–(f). Moving balls. By courtesy of F. HEITZ, IRISA

This model may be refined taking into account that motion discontinuities are likely to contribute to intensity discontinuities. Hence motion discontinuities should have low probability if there is no corresponding intensity edge. The latter are 'observed' setting an edge detector to work (the authors use CANNY's criterion, cf. DERICHE (1987)). It gives edge configurations $(\beta_{\langle s,t\rangle})$ and the corresponding transition probability is

$$g_{b_{\langle s,t\rangle}}(\beta_{\langle s,t\rangle}) = Z_2^{-1}\exp(-\vartheta(1-\beta_{\langle s,t\rangle})b_{\langle s,t\rangle})$$

where ϑ is a large positive parameter. In summary, the law of the observations (f_t, β) given (ω, b) is

$$h_{\omega,b}(f_t,\beta) = \prod_{s\in SC} h_{\omega_s}(f_t(s)) \prod_{\langle s,t\rangle} g_{b_{\langle s,t\rangle}}(\beta_{\langle s,t\rangle}).$$

Combination with the prior yields an energy function for the posterior distribution:

$$\begin{aligned} H(\omega, b|f_t, b) &= \sum_{\langle s,t\rangle} \Psi(\omega_s - \omega_t)(1 - b_{\langle s,t\rangle}) + H_2(b) \\ &\quad + \sum_s \frac{1}{2\sigma^2}(f_t(s) + \langle \nabla f(s), \omega\rangle)^2 + \sum_{\langle s,t\rangle} \vartheta(1 - \beta_{\langle s,t\rangle}) b_{\langle s,t\rangle}). \end{aligned}$$

The model is refined further including a feature based term (LALANDE and BOUTHEMY (1990), HEITZ and BOUTHEMY (1990b) and (1992)). Locations and velocities of 'moving edges' are estimated by a moving edge estimator (BOUTHEMY (1989)) and related to optical flow thus further improving the performance near occlusions.

To minimize the posterior energy the authors adopt the ICM algorithm first initialized with zero motion vectors and the intensitity edges β for b. For processing further frames, the last estimated fields were used as initialization. The first step needed between 250 and 400 iterations whereas only half of this number of iterations were needed in the subsequent steps. Plainly, this method fails at cuts. These must be detected and the algorithm must be initialized anew.

In Fig. 16.1, for a synthetic scene the Bayesian method is contrasted with the method of Horn and Schunck. The foreground disk in (a) is dilated while the background disk is translated. White noise is added to the background. The state of the motion discontinuity process after 183 iterations of ICM is displayed in Fig. (c) and the corresponding velocity field in Fig. (d). Fig. (e) is the upper right part of (e) and Fig. (f) shows the result of the Horn-Schunck algorithm. As expected, the resulting motion field is blurred across the motion discontinuities. In Fig. (b) the white region corresponds to the set SC whereas in the black region the motion constraint equation was supposed not to hold.

For Fig. 16.2, frames of an everyday TV sequence were processed: the woman on the right moves up and the camera follows her motion. Fig (b) shows the intensity edges extracted from (a). In (c) the estimated motion boundaries (after 400 iterations) are displayed and (d) shows the associated optical flow estimation. Fig. (e) is a detail of (d) showing the woman's head. It is contrasted with the result of the Horn-Schunck method in (f). The Bayesian method gives a considerably sharper velocity field.

Figs. 16.1 and 16.2 appear in HEITZ and BOUTHEMY (1992) and are reproduced by kind permission of F. HEITZ, IRISA. Motion detection and segmentation in the Bayesian framework is a field of current research.

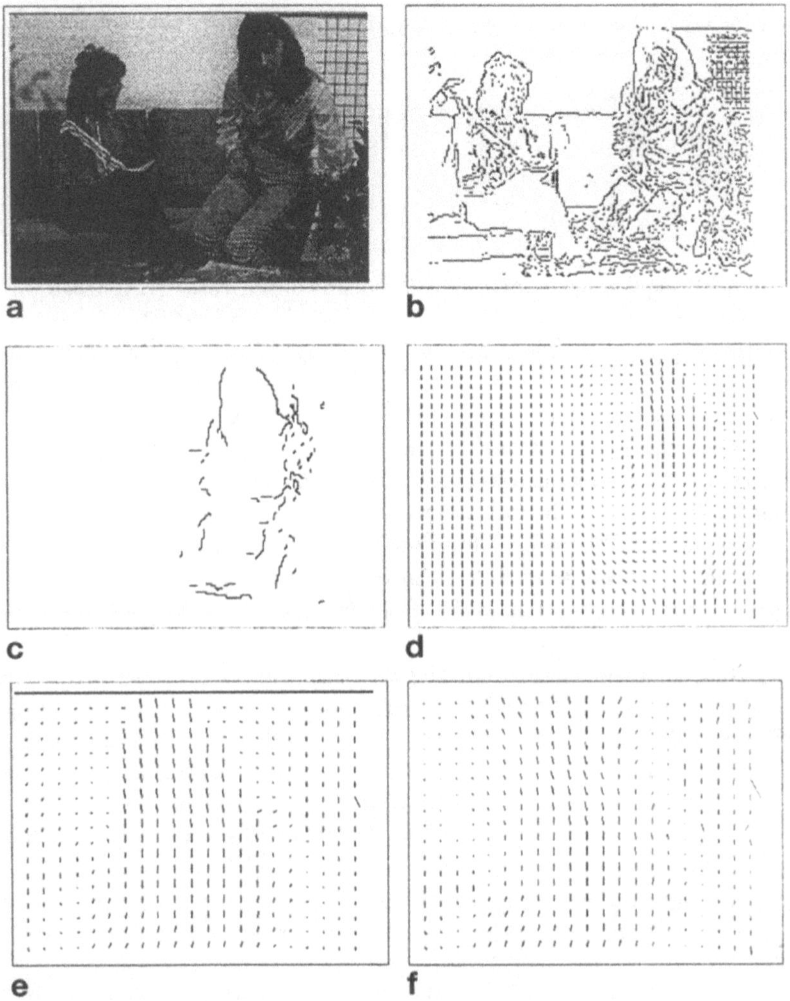

Fig. 16.2. (a)–(f). Rising woman. By courtesy of F. HEITZ, IRISA

16.2 Tomographic Image Reconstruction

Computer tomography is a radio-diagnostic method for the representation of a cross section of a part of the body or objects of industrial inspection. The 3-dimensional structure can be reconstructed from a pile of cross sections.

In **transmission tomography**, the object is bombarded with atomic particles part of which is absorbed. The inner structure is reconstructed from counts of those particles which pass through the object. In **emission tomography** the objective is to determine the distribution of a radio-pharmaceutical in a part of the body. The concentration is an indicator for say existence of cancer or metabolic activity. Detectors are placed around the region of interest counting for example photons emitted by radioactive decay of isotopes contained in the pharmaceutical and which are not absorbed on their way to the detectors. From these counts the distribution has to be reconstructed. A variety of reconstruction algorithms for emission tomography are described in BUDINGER, GULLBERG and HUESMAN (1979). S. GEMAN and D.E. MC CLURE (1987) studied this problem in the Bayesian framework.

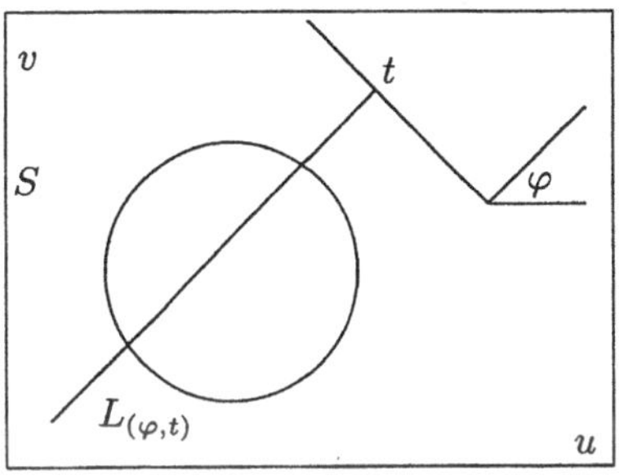

Fig. 16.3

Let us first give a rough idea of the degradation mechanism in single photon emission tomography (SPECT). Let $S \subset \mathrm{R}^2$ be the region of interest. The probability that a photon emitted at $s \in S$ towards a detector at $t \in \mathrm{R}^2$ is given by

$$p(s,t) = \exp(-\int_{L(s,t)} \mu)$$

where $\mu(r)$ is the attenuation coefficient at r and the integral is taken along the line segment $L(s,t)$ between s and t. The exponential basically comes in since the differential loss dI of intensity along a line element dl at $t \in \mathrm{R}^2$ is proportional to I, dl and μ, i.e. $dI = -\mu(l)I(l)dl$. An idealized detector counts photons from a single direction φ only. The number of photons emitted at s is proportional to the density x_s. The number $Y_{(\varphi,t)}$ of photons reaching this detector is a Poisson random variable with mean

$$R_x(\varphi,t) = \tau \int_{L(\varphi,t)} x.p(\cdot,t)$$

where the integral is taken along the line $L(\varphi,t)$ through t with orientation φ and $\tau > 0$ is proportional to the duration of exposure. R_x is called the **attenuated Radon transform** (ART) of x. In practice, the collector has finite size and hence counts photons along lines $L(\varphi',t')$ for (φ',t') in some neighbourhood $D(\varphi,t)$ of (φ,t). Hence the actual mean of $Y(\varphi,t)$ is

$$\lambda(\varphi,t) = \int_{D(\varphi,t)} R_x(\varphi',t')d\varphi' dt'.$$

There is a finite number of collectors located around S. Given $x = (x_s)_{s \in S}$, the counts in these collectors are independent and hence realizations from a finite family $Y = (Y_{(\varphi,t)})_{(\varphi,t)\in T}$ of independent Poisson variables $Y_{(\varphi,t)}$ with mean $\lambda(\varphi,t)$ are observed. Given the density of x, the probability of the family y of counts is

$$P(x,y) = \prod_{(\varphi,t)\in T} \mathrm{e}^{-\lambda(\varphi,t)} \frac{\lambda(\varphi,t)^{y(\varphi,t)}}{y(\varphi,t)!}$$

Remark 16.2.1. Only the predominant shot noise has been included so far. The model is adaptable to other effects like photon scattering, background radiation or sensor effects (cf. Chapter 2).

Theoretically, the MLE can be computed from $P(\cdot,y)$. In fact, the mathematical foundations for this approach are laid in SHEPP and VARDI (1982). These authors adopt an EM algorithm for the implementation of ML reconstructions (cf. also VARDI, SHEPP and KAUFMAN (1985)). ML reconstructions in general are too rough and therefore it is natural to adopt piecewise smoothing techniques like those in Chapter 2. This amounts to the choice of a prior energy function. The set S will be assumed to be digitized and the sites are arranged on part of a square grid. S. GEMAN and D. MC CLURE used a prior of the simple form

$$H(x) = \beta \sum_{\langle s,t\rangle_p} \Psi(x_s - x_t) + \frac{\beta}{\sqrt{2}} \sum_{\langle s,t\rangle_d} \Psi(x_s - x_t)$$

with the disparity function Ψ in (2.4) and a coupling constant $\beta > 0$. The symbol $\langle s,t\rangle_p$ indicates that s and t are nearest neighbours in the vertical or horizontal direction and, similarly, $\langle s,t\rangle_d$ corresponds to nearest neighbours on the diagonals (which explains the factor $\sqrt{2}$). One might couple an edge process to the density process x like in Example 2.3.1.

In summary, the posterior distribution is Gibbsian with energy function

$$H(x|y) = \sum_{(\varphi,t)\in T} \lambda(\varphi,t) + \ln(y(\varphi,t)!) - y(\varphi,t)\ln(\lambda(\varphi,t)).$$

MAP and MMS estimates may now be approximated by annealing or sampling and the law of large numbers. The reconstructions based on the MAP estimator turned out to be more satisfactory than those based on the ML estimator. For illustrations see S. GEMAN and MCCLURE (1987) and D. GEMAN and GIDAS (1991).

16.3 Biological Shape

The concepts presented in this text may be modified and developed in order to tackle problems more complex than those in the previous examples. In the following few lines we try to impart a rough idea of the pattern theoretical study 'Hands' by U. GRENANDER, Y. CHOW and D.M. KEENAN (1991) and GRENANDER (1989). These authors develop a global shape model and apply it to the analysis of real pictures of hands. They focus on restoration of the shape in two dimensions from noisy observations. It is assumed that the relevant information about shape is contained in the boundary. The general ideas apply to other types of (biological) shape as well.

Let us first consider two extreme 'classical' approaches to the restoration of boundaries from noisy digital pictures: general purpose methods and tailor made methods. We illustrate these techniques by way of simple examples (taken from 'Hands'):

1. General techniques from the tool box of image processing may be combined for instance in the following way (cf. HARALICK and SHAPIRO (1992)):
   a) Remove part of the noise by filtering the picture by some moving average or median filter.
   b) Reduce noise further filling small holes and removing small isolated regions.
   c) Threshold the picture.
   d) Extract the boundary.
   e) Smooth the boundary closing small gaps or removing blind ends.
   f) Detect the connected components and keep the largest as an estimate of the hand contour.
2. Templates may be fitted to the data: Construct a template - for example by averaging the boundaries of several hands - and fit it to the data by least squares or other criteria. Three parameters have to be estimated, two for location and one for orientation. If a scale change is included there is another parameter for scale.

The first method has some technical disadvantages like sensitivity to non uniform lighting etc.. More important in the present context is the following: the technique applies to any kind of picture. The algorithm does not have any knowledge about the characteristic features of a human hand (similar to the edge detector in Example 2.4.1). Therefore it does not care if, for example, the restoration lost a finger. The second algorithm knows exactly how an ideal hand looks like but does not take into account variability of smaller features like the proportions of individual hands or relative positions of fingers. The Bayesian approach developed in 'Hands' is based on the second method but relaxing the rigid constraints (that the restoration is a linear transform of the template) incorporates both, ideal shape *and* variability.

'Ideal boundaries' are assumed to be closed, nonintersecting and continuous. Hence the space $\mathbf{X}$ should be a subset of the space of closed Jordan curves in the plane. This subset – or rather an isomorphic space – is constructed in the following way: The boundaries of interest are supposed to be the union of a fixed number σ of arcs. Hence $S = \{1, \dots, \sigma\}$ is the set of 'sites' and for each $s \in S$ there is a space $\mathbf{Z}_s$ of smooth arcs in R^2. To be definite, let each $\mathbf{Z}_s$ be the set of all straight line segments. The symbol $\mathbf{Z}$ denotes the set of all σ-tuples of line segments forming (closed nonintersecting) polygons. By such polygons, the shapes of hands may be well approximated but also the shapes of houses or other objects. Most polygons in $\mathbf{Z}$ will not correspond to the shape of any object. Hence the space of reasonable boundaries is reduced further: A template $t = (t_1, \ldots, t_\sigma)$ representing the typical features of interest is constructed. For biological shapes it is reasonable to chose an approximation from $\mathbf{Z}$ to an average of several objects (hands). The space $\mathbf{X}$ of possible restorations is a set of deformed t's. It should be rich enough to contain (approximations of the) contours of most individual hands. The authors introduce a group G of similarity transformations on $\mathbf{Z}_s$ and let X be the set of those elements in $\mathbf{Z}$ composed of σ arcs $g_i(t_i)$, $1 \leq i \leq \sigma$, i.e. the nonintersecting closed polygons $\cup_{1 \leq i \leq \sigma} g_i(t_i)$ where the endpoint of $g_i(t_i)$ is the initial point of $g_{i+1}(t_{i+1})$ ($\sigma+1$ is identified with 1). The transformations in G are induced by linear transformations $\tilde{g}$ on the plane via

$$g(\tau) = \{\tilde{g}(u,v) : (u,v) \in \tau\}, \tau \in \mathbf{Z}_s.$$

The planar transformations $\tilde{g}$ are members of low-dimensional Lie groups, for example:

- The group $US(2)$ of uniform scale changes g:

$$g(u,v) = (cu, cv), c > 0.$$

- The general linear group $GL(2)$, where each $g \in G$ is a linear transformation

$$g(u,v) = \Gamma \begin{pmatrix} u \\ v \end{pmatrix}$$

  with a 2×2-matrix G of full rank.
- The product of $US(2)$ and the orthogonal group $O(2)$.

Note that $(g_1(t_1), \ldots, g_\sigma(t_\sigma))$ in general cannot be uniquely reconstructed from the associated polygon.

The prior distribution on $\mathbf{X}$ is constructed from a Gibbs field on G^n (here our construction of Gibbs fields on discrete spaces is not sufficient any more). First a measure m on G and a Gibbsian density

$$f(g_1, \ldots, g_\sigma) = Z^{-1} \exp\left(-\sum_{i=1}^{\sigma} H_{i,i+1}(g_i, g_{i+1}) - \sum_{i=1}^{\sigma} H_i(g_i) \right)$$

are selected (again $\sigma + 1$ is identified with 1). The Gibbs field on G is given by the formula

$$\Gamma(B) = \int_B f(g_1, \ldots, g_\sigma) dm \otimes m$$

for Borel sets B in G^n. To obtain a prior distribution on $\mathbf{X}$ the image distribution of Γ under the map

$$(g_1, \ldots, g_\sigma) \longmapsto (g_1(t_1), \ldots, g_\sigma(t_\sigma))$$

is conditioned on $\mathbf{X}$. Since all spaces in question are continuous, conditioning requires some subtle limit arguments. In the 'Hands' study various priors of this kind are examinated.

Finally, the space of observations and the degradation mechanism must be specified. Suppose we are given a noisy monochrome picture of a hand in front of a light background. The picture is thresholded and thus divided into two regions – one correponding to the hand and one to the background. We want to restore the boundary from the former set and thus the observations are the random subsets of the observation window. A 'real' boundary $x \in \mathbf{X}$ is degraded in a deterministic and a random way. Any boundary x defines a set $I(x)$, its 'interiour'. It is found giving an orientation to the Jordan curve x – say clockwise – and letting $I(x)$ the set on the right hand of the curve. This set is then deformed into the random set $y = I^{deg}(x)$ by some kind of noise. The specific form of the transition density $f_x(y)$ depends upon the technology used to acquire the digital picture.

Given all ingredients, the Bayesian machinery can be set to work. One may either approximate the MAP estimate by Metropolis annealing or the least squares estimate, i.e. the mean of the posterior, via the law of large numbers and a sampling algorithm. Due to the continuous state spaces and the form of the degradation mechanism and the prior, the formerly introduced methods have to be modified and refined which amounts to considerable technical problems. We refer to the authoritative treatment by GRENANDER, CHOW and KEENAN (1991).

U. GRENANDER developed a fairly general framework in which such problems can be studied. In GRENANDER (1989) he presents applications from various fields like the theory of shape or the theory of formal languages.

Several algorithms for simulation and basic results from linear algebra and analysis are collected. Nothing is new and most results can be found in standard texts. For simulation, a standard reference is KNUTH (1969); RIPLEY (1987a) perhaps is more adapted to our needs. On the other hand, some of the remarks we found illuminating are scattered over the literature. For the Perron-Frobenius theorem, we refer to the excellent treatment by SENETA (1981) and, similarly, for convex analysis to ROCKAFELLAR (1970). But there is not much of the theory really needed here and sometimes short proves can be given for these special cases. Moreover, it often requires considerable effort to get along with specific notation. For convenience of the reader, we therefore collect the results we need and present them in the language the reader hopefully is familiar with now.

Part VII

Appendix

A. Simulation of Random Variables

This appendix provides some background for the simulation of random variables and illustrates their practical use for stochastic algorithms. Basic versions of some standard procedures are given explicitely (they are written in PASCAL but should easily be translated to other languages like MODULA or FORTRAN). There is no fine-tuning. For more involved techniques we refer to KNUTH (1981) and RIPLEY (1987).

Most algorithms in this text are based on the outcomes of random mechanisms and hence we need a source of randomness. Hopefully, there is no random component in our computer. Importing randomness from external physical sources is expensive and gives data which are not easy to control. Therefore, *deterministic* sequences of numbers which *behave* like random ones are generated. More precisely, they share important statistical properties of ideal random numbers, or, they pass statistical tests applied to finite parts which aim to detect relevant departures from randomness.

Independent uniformly distributed variables are a useful source of randomness and can be turned into almost everything else. Thus simulation is performed in two steps:

(i) simulation of i.i.d. random variables uniformly distributed on $[0, 1)$,
(ii) transformation into variables with desired distribution.

A.1 Pseudo-random Numbers

We shortly comment on the generation of **pseudo-random numbers.** Among others, the following requirements are essential:

(1) a good approximation to a uniform distribution on $[0, 1)$,
(2) close to independency,
(3) easy, fast and exact to generate.

Complex algorithms for the generation are by no means necessarily 'more random' than simple ones and there are good arguments that it is better to choose a simple and well-understood class of algorithms and to use a generator from this class good enough for the prespecified purposes.

Remark A.1.1. We cautionarily abstain from an own judgement and quote from RIPLEY (1988), §5:

> The whole history of pseudo-random numbers is riddled with myths and extrapolations from inadequate examples. A healthy scepticism is needed in reading the literature.

and from §1 in the same reference:

> PARK and MILLER (1988) comment that examples of good generators are hard to find .... Their search was, however, in the computer science literature, and mainly in texts at that; random number generation seems to be one of the most misunderstood subjects in computer science!

Therefore, we restrict attention to the familiar linear congruential method. To meet (3), we consider sequences $(u_k)_{k\geq 0}$ in $[0,1)$ which are defined recursively, a member of the sequence depending only on its predecessor:

$$u_0 = seed, \;\; u_{k+1} = f(u_k)$$

for some initial value $seed \in [0,1)$ and a function $f : [0,1) \to [0,1)$. One may choose a fixed seed and then the sequence can be repeated. One may also bring pure chance into the game and, for instance, couple the seed to the internal clock of the computer. We shall consider functions f given by

$$f(u) = (au + b) \bmod 1 \tag{A.1}$$

for natural numbers a and b ($v \bmod 1$ is the difference of v and its integer part). Hence the graph of f consists of a straight lines with gradient a. The choice of the number a is somewhat tricky, which stems from the finite-precision arithmetic in which $f(u)$ is computed in practice.

We give now some informal arguments that (1) and (2) are met. We claim: Let intervals I and J in $[0,1)$ be given with length $\lambda(I)$ and $\lambda(J)$ considerably greater than a^{-1}. *Assume* that u_k is uniformly distributed on $[0,1)$. Then

$$\text{Prob}\,(u_{k+1} \in J \mid u_k \in I) \sim \text{Prob}\,(u_{k+1} \in J) \sim \lambda(J).$$

This means that u_{k+1} is approximately uniformly distributed over $[0,1)$ and that this distribution is not affected by the location of u_k. The function f is linear on the a elementary intervals $[k/a,(k+1)/a)$, $0 \leq k < a$. An interval J is scattered by f^{-1} over the elementary intervals and

$$\lambda(f^{-1} \cap I_e) = \frac{n}{a}\lambda(J) = \lambda(I_e)\lambda(f^{-1}(J))$$

if I_e is the union of n elementary intervals. If I is any interval in $[0,1)$ let I_e be the maximal union of n elementary intervals. Then

$$\frac{n}{a} \leq \lambda(I) < \frac{n+2}{a}, \frac{n}{a}\lambda(J) \leq \lambda(I \cap f^{-1}(J)) < \frac{n+2}{a}\lambda(J).$$

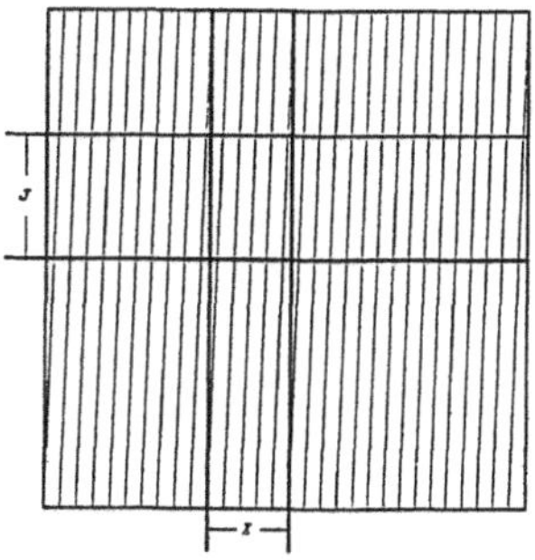

Fig. A.1. $f(u) = au + b \bmod 1$

If u_k is uniformly distributed over $[0,1)$ then

$$\frac{n}{n+2}\lambda(J) < \text{Prob}(u_{k+1}|u_k \in I) < \frac{n+2}{n}\lambda(J).$$

Hence the above assertion holds for large n (which implies that a has to be large). Such considerations are closely related to the concept of 'mixing' in ergodic theory (cf. BILLINGSLEY (1965), in particular Examples 1.1 and 1.6 and the section on mixing in Chapter 1.1).

In practice, we manipulate integer values and not real numbers. The **linear congruential generator** is given by

$$v_0 = seed, \;\; v_{k+1} = (av_k + b) \bmod c$$

for a multiplier a, a shift b and a modulus c, all natural numbers, and $seed \in \{0, 1, \ldots, c-1\}$ ($n \bmod c$ is the difference of n and the largest integer multiple of c less or equal to n). This generates a sequence in $\{0, 1, \ldots, c-1\}$ which is transformed into a sequence of pseudo-random numbers in $[0,1)$ by

$$u_k = \frac{v_k}{c}.$$

Plainly, (u_k) and (v_k) are periodic with period at most c. The full period can always be achieved, for example with $a = b = 1$ (which does not make sense). It is necessary to choose a, b and c properly, according to some principles which are supported by detailed theoretical and practical investigations (KNUTH (1981), ch. 3): (i) The computation of $(av + b) \bmod c$ must be done exact, with no round off errors. (ii) The *modulus* should be large – about 2^{32} or more – to allow large (not necessarily maximal) period and the function mod should be easy to evaluate. If integers are represented in binary form then for powers $c = 2^p$ one gets $n \bmod c$ by simply keeping the p lowest bits of n. (iii) The *shift* is of minor importance: basically, $b \neq 0$ prevents 0 automatically to be mapped to 0. If c is a power of 2 then b should be an odd number; $b = 1$ seems to be a reasonable choice. Hence the search for good generators reduces to the choice of the *multiplier*. (iv) If c is a power of 2 then the multiplier a should be picked such that $a \bmod 8 = 5$. A weak form of the requirements (1) and (2) is that the k-tuples $(u_i, \ldots, u_{i+k-1})$, $i \geq 0$, evenly fill a fine lattice in $[0,1)^k$ at least for k-values up to 8; the latter is by no means self-evident as the examples below illustrate. For this one needs many different values in the sequence and hence large period. B. RIPLEY tested a series of generators on various machines (RIPLEY (1987a), (1989b)). Among other choices, he and others advocate

$$a = 69069,\ b = 1,\ c = 2^{32}$$

from MARSAGLIA (1972) (e.g. used for the VAX compilers). This generator has period 2^{32} and 69069 mod 8 = 5. Good generators are available through internet. Ask an expert!

Examples. In Fig. A.2, pairs (u_k, u_{k+1}) for several generators are plotted. The examples are somewhat artificial but, unfortunately, similar phenomena occur with some generators integrated into widely used commercial systems; a well-known example is IBM's notoriously bad and once very popular generator RANDU, where $v_{k+1} = (2^{16} + 3)v_k \bmod 2^{31}$; successive triples (v_k, v_{k+1}, v_{k+2}) lie on 15 hyperplanes, cf. RIPLEY (1987a), p. 23, MARSAGLIA (1968) or HUBER (1985)). The modulus is 2048 in all examples. In (a) we used $a = 65$ and $b = 1$ for 2048 pairs, (b) is a plot of the first 512 pairs of the same generator; in (c) we had $a = 1229$ and $b = 1$ and in (d) $a = 3$ and $b = 0$, both for 2048 pairs. The individual form of the plots depends on the seed. For more examples and a thorough discussion see RIPLEY (1987a).

Particularly easy to implement in hardware are the **shift register generators**. They generate 0-1-sequences (b_i) according to the rule

$$b = (a_1 b_{i-1} + \ldots + a_d b_{i-d}) \bmod 2,$$

with $a_j \in \{0,1\}$. If $a_{j_1} = \ldots = a_{i_k} = 1$ and $a_j = 0$ otherwise then

$$b_i = b_{i-j_1} EOR\, b_{i-j_2} EOR \ldots EOR\, b_{i-j_k}$$

where EOR is the exclusive or function which has the same truth table as addition mod 2 (cf. RIPLEY (1987), 2.3 ff).

For theoretical background – mostly based on number theoretic arguments – we refer to RIPLEY's monograph, 2.2 and 2.7.

A.2 Discrete Random Variables

Besides the various kinds of noise, we need realizations of random variables X with a finite number of states $x_1, \ldots, x_N$. We assume that there is function *RND* which – if called repeatedly – generates independent samples from a uniform distribution on $\{1, \ldots, \text{maxrand}\}$; for example:

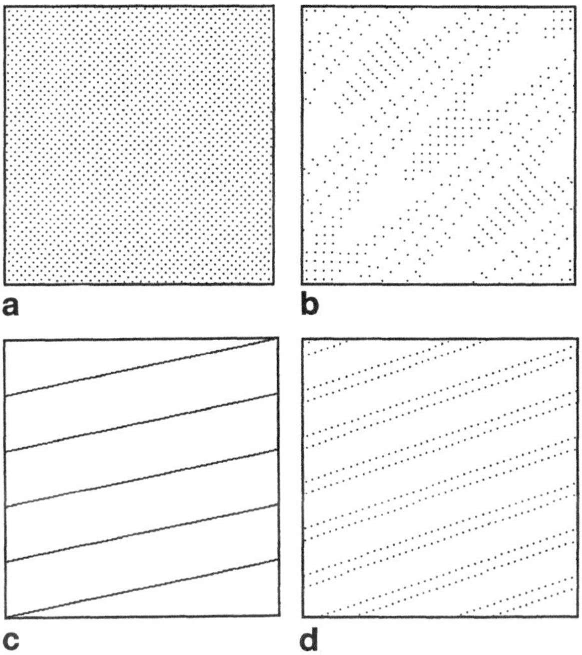

Fig. A.2. (a)–(d)

```
CONST maxrand=$ffffff;
FUNCTION RND: LONG-INTEGER;
{returns a random variable RND uniformly distributed on the num-
   bers 0,...,maxrand}
($ffffff is 16^6 - 1 = 2^24 - 1).
```

With the function

```
FUNCTION UCRV: REAL;
{returns a Uniform (Continuous) Random Variable UCRV on [0,N]}
BEGIN UCRV:=RND/maxrand*N END; {UCRV}
```

one samples uniformly from $\{0, 1/maxrand, \ldots, N\}$ or approximately uniformly from $[0, N]$. In particular,

```
FUNCTION U : REAL;
BEGIN U:=rnd/maxrand END; {U}
```

samples from $[0, 1]$. To sample uniformly from $\{k, \ldots, m\}$ set

```
FUNCTION UDRV (k,m:INTEGER): INTEGER;
{returns a Uniform Discrete Random Variable UDRV on k,...,m,
   uses FUNCTION U}
BEGIN UDRV:=TRUNC(U*(m - k)) + k END; {UDRV}
```

where *TRUNC* computes the integer part. Random visiting schedules for Metropolis algorithms on $N \times N$ grids need two such lines, one for each coordinate. For a Bernoulli variable B with $\mathsf{P}(B = 1) = p = 1 - \mathsf{P}(B = 0)$, let $B = 1$ if $U \leq p$ and zero otherwise:

```
FUNCTION BERNOULLI (p:REAL):INTEGER:
{returns a Bernoulli variable with values 0 and 1 and prob(1) = p,
   uses FUNCTION U}
BEGIN IF (U<=p) THEN BERNOULLI:=1 ELSE BERNOULLI:=0
   END; {BERNOULLI}
```

This way one generates channel noise or samples locally from an Ising field. Let, more generally, X take values $1, \ldots, N$ with probabilities $p_1, \ldots, p_N$. A straightforward method to simulate X is to partition the unit interval into subintervals $I_i = (c_{i-1}, c_i], 0 = c_o \leq c_1 \leq \ldots \leq c_n$ of length p_i. Then one generates U, looks for the index i with $u \in I_i$ and sets $X = i$. In fact,

$$\mathsf{P}(X - i) = \mathsf{P}(U \in I_i) = p_i.$$

This may be rephrased as follows: compute the cumulative distribution function $F(i) = \sum_{k \leq i} p_k$ and find i such that

$$F(i-1) < U \leq F(i).$$

The following procedure does this:

```
TYPE lut_type {vectors (p_1,...,p_N) usually representing look-up
   tables}
    : ARRAY[1...N] OF REAL;
FUNCTION DRV(p {vector of probabilities}:lut_type) : INTEGER;
{returns a Discrete Random Variable with prob(i)=p[i], uses FUNC-
   TION U}
VAR i : INTEGER; cdv {values of the cumulative distribution
   function} :REAL;
BEGIN
  i:=1; cdf:=0;
  WHILE (cdf<U) DO BEGIN i:=SUCC(i); cdf:=cdf+p[i]) END;
  DRV:=i
END; {DRV}
```

(where SUCC(i) = i+1). If U is in I_i then it is found after i steps and hence the expected number of steps is $\sum ip_i = \mathsf{E}(X)$. We do not loose anything by rearranging the states. Then the expected number of steps becomes minimal if they are arranged in order of decreasing p_i. On the other hand, there is a tradeoff between computing time for search and ordering and the latter only pays off if X is needed for several times with the same p_i. Sometimes the problem itself suggests a natural order of search. If (p_i) is unimodal (i.e. increasing on $[1, \ldots, m]$ and decreasing on $[m+1, \ldots, N]$) one should search left or right from the mode m. Similarly, in restoration started with the degraded image, one may search left and right of the current grey value.

For larger N a binary search becomes more efficient: One checks if U is in the first or second half of the I_i and repeats until k with $U \in I_k$ is found. For small N it does not pay off since all values of the cumulative distribution function are needed in advance.

```
VAR
  p {a probability vector} :lut_type;
  cdf {a cumulative distribution function} :lut_type;
PROCEDURE addup (p:lut_type;N:INTEGER;
  VAR cdf {cdf[i]=p[1]+ ... +p[i] is the c.d.f.} :lut_type);
{returns the complete c.d.f. cdf=(cdf[1],...,cdf[N])}
VAR i:INTEGER;
BEGIN cdf[1]:=p[1]; FOR i:=2 TO N DO cdf[i]:=cdf[i-1]+p[i] END;
   {addup}
FUNCTION DRV(p:lut-type; N:INTEGER;cdf:lut_type) :INTEGER;
{returns a Discrete Random Variable DRV, uses FUNCTION U}
VAR i : INTEGER;
BEGIN
  l:=0; r:=N;
  REPEAT
    i:=TRUNC((l+r)/2);
    IF (U>=r) THEN l:=i ELSE r:=i;
  UNTIL (l>=r);
  DRV:=i
END; {DRV}
BEGIN READ(p,N); addup(p,N,cdf); X:=DRV(p,N,cdf) END; {DRV}
```

More involved methods exploit the internal representation of numbers, cf. Marsaglia's method (KNUTH (1981)).

A.3 Local Gibbs Samplers

Frequently it is cheaper to compute multiples cp_k or $cF(k)$ of the probabilities or the c.d.f. than to compute the quantities p_k or $F(k)$, respectively. Let, for instance, a local Gibbs sampler be given in the form

$$p_g = Z^{-1} \exp\left(-\beta h(g)\right)$$

for $g \in G = \{0, \ldots, g\_\max\}$. Then we recursively compute $G = Z \cdot F$ by

$$G(-1) = 0, G(g+1) = G(g) + \exp\left(-\beta h(g+1)\right),$$

realize $V = G(g\_\max) * U$ (uniform in $(0, G(g\_max)) = (0, Z)$) and choose g such that $G(g-1) < V \leq G(g)$. This amounts to a minor ffmodification in the last two procedures. As long as the energy does not change the values of G or $\exp(-\beta h(\cdot))$ should be computed in advance and stored in a look-up table. In sampling, this can be done once and forever, whereas in annealing a new look-up table has to be computed for every sweep.

Computation time increases with increasing number of states. Time can be saved by sampling only from a subset of states with high probability. One has to be careful in doing so since in general the resulting algorithm is no longer in accordance with the theoretical findings. For local samplers an argument of the following type helps to find the 'negligible' subset.

Lemma A.3.1. *Let $\varepsilon > 0$ and set*

$$h_\beta^* = h_{\min} + (\ln r - \ln \varepsilon)/\beta,$$

where $h_{\min} = \min\{h(g) : g \in G\}$. Then the set

$$G_\beta = \{g \in G : h(g) > h_\beta^*\}$$

has probability less or equal to ε.

Proof. Setting $r = p\_\max$,

$$\begin{aligned} G_\beta &= \{g \in G : h(g) > h_\beta^*\} = \{g \in G : h(g) - h_{\min} > \beta^{-1} \ln(r \cdot \varepsilon^{-1})\} \\ &= \{g \in G : \exp(-\beta(h(g) - h_{\min})) \leq \varepsilon \cdot r^{-1}\} \\ &= \{g \in G : \exp(-\beta \cdot h(g)) \leq \exp(-\beta \cdot h_{\min}) \cdot \varepsilon \cdot r^{-1}\}. \end{aligned}$$

G_β has at most r elements and thus

$$\mu(G_\beta) \leq r \cdot \varepsilon \cdot r^{-1} \cdot Z_s^{-1} \cdot \exp(-\beta \cdot h_{\min}) \leq \varepsilon$$

which proves the result. □

A simpler alternative is the Metropolis sampler.

A.4 Further Distributions

We can generate approximations to all kinds of random variables by the above general method. On the other hand, various constructions from probability theory may be exploited to design decent algorithms.

A.4.1 Binomial Variables

They are finite sums of i.i.d. Bernoulli variables. To be specific, let $X = X_1 + \ldots + X_N$ for independent variables with $\mathsf{P}(X_i = 1) = p = 1 - \mathsf{P}(X_i = 0)$. X is realized generating U for N times and counting the number X of U_i less (or equal to) p.

```
FUNCTION BINOMIAL (N:INTEGER;p:REAL):INTEGER;
{uses FUNCTION U}
VAR i:INTEGER;
BEGIN
  BINOMIAL:=0;
  FOR i:=1 TO N DO IF (U<=p) THEN BINOMIAL:=SUCC(BINOMIAL)
END; {BINOMIAL}
```

If you insist on the general method you may compute the probabilities

$$p_k = \mathsf{P}(X = k) = \binom{N}{k} p^k (1-p)^{N-k}$$

recursively by

$$p_k = p_{k-1}\left(1 + \frac{(N+1)p - k}{k(1-p)}\right).$$

A useful general principle is the **inversion method**.

Theorem A.4.1. *Let Y be a real-valued random variable with c.d.f. $F(t) = \mathsf{P}(Y \le t)$. Set*

$$F^-(u) = \min\{t : F(t) \ge u\}.$$

Then $X = F^-(U)$ has c.d.f. F.

Corollary A.4.1. *Let X be a real-valued random variable with invertible c.d.f. F. Then $X = F^{-1}(U)$ has c.d.f. F.*

Example A.4.1. (a) The general method (p. 288) is a special case. In fact, if X takes values $x_1, \ldots, x_N$ with probabilities $p_1, \ldots, p_N$, respectively, then

$$F = \sum_{k=1}^{N} p_k \mathbf{1}_{[x_k,\infty)}.$$

For $u \in (0,1)$, we have $F^-(u) = x_k$ if and only if $F(x_{k-1}) < u \le F(x_k)$.

(b) An **exponential distribution** has density $\alpha e^{-\alpha t}$, $\alpha > 0$ on R_+ (and 0 on the negative axis). We have:

The random variable $X = -\frac{1}{\alpha}\ln U$ is exponentially distributed for parameter α.

Proof. The exponential c.d.f. is $F(t) = 1 - e^{-\alpha t}$ with inverse $F^{-1}(u) = -\frac{1}{\alpha}\ln(1-u)$. By the corollary, $Y = -\frac{1}{\alpha}\ln(1-U)$ has an exponential distribution and – since $1 - U$ has the same distribution as U – the result is proved. □

Hence we may use

```
FUNCTION E (alpha:REAL):REAL;
{returns an exponentially distributed variable; the parameter alpha
   must be strictly positive; uses FUNCTION U}
BEGIN E:=-ln(U)/alpha END; {E}
```

Proof (of the theorem). By right-continuity of F the minima in F^- exist. First we observe that the supergraph of F^- and the subgraph of F coincide:

$$\{(u,t) : F^-(u) \le t\} = \{(u,t) : u \le F(t)\}.$$

In fact, for an element (u,t) from the left set, $F^-(u) \le t$, hence

$$F(t) \ge F\left(F^-(u)\right) = F\left(\min\{t : F(t) \ge u\}\right) \ge u$$

and (u,t) is contained in the right set. Conversely, let $u \le F(t)$. Since F^- increases,

$$F^-(u) \le F^-(F(t)) = \min\{r : F(r) \ge F(t)\} = t$$

again by right-continuity. We conclude

$$\begin{aligned} \mathsf{P}(X \le t) &= \mathsf{P}\left(F^-(U) \le t\right) \\ &= \mathsf{P}\left(U \le F(t)\right) = F(t). \end{aligned}$$

This completes the proof. □

A.4.2 Poisson Variables

They have countable state space $\{0, 1, \ldots\}$ and law

$$\mathsf{P}(X = k) = \frac{\alpha^k}{k!} e^{-\alpha}, \ \alpha > 0.$$

One gets approximate Poisson variables either by

(i) truncating to get a finite approximation and using the general method, or by

(ii) binomial approximation: for $N \cdot p_N \to \alpha$ one has

$$\binom{N}{k} p_N^k \left(1 - p_N\right)^{N-k} \to \frac{\alpha k}{k!} e^{-\alpha}$$

and hence for large N and $p = \alpha N^{-1}$ the binomial distribution is close to the Poisson distribution.

A direct method is derived from the Poisson process: Let $E_1, \ldots, E_n, \ldots$ be i.i.d. exponentially distributed for parameter 1. By induction, $S_n = E_1 + \ldots + E_n$ has an Erlang distribution (which is a special Γ-distribution) with c.d.f.

$$G_n(t) = \sum_{k=n}^{\infty} e^{-t} \frac{t^k}{k!}, \ t \ge 0,$$

and $G_n(t) = 0$ for $t < 0$. Set

$$N(\alpha) = \max\{k : S_k \le \alpha\}.$$

It can be shown that this makes sense with probability 1 and on this set $N(\alpha) \geq n$ if and only if $S_n \leq \alpha$ (for details cf. BILLINGSLEY (1979)). This event has probability

$$\begin{aligned} \mathsf{P}(N(\alpha) = n) &= \mathsf{P}(N(\alpha) \geq n) - \mathsf{P}(N(\alpha) \geq n+1) \\ &= G_n(\alpha) - G_{n+1}(a) = \frac{\alpha^n}{n!} e^{-\alpha} \end{aligned}$$

as desired. To get a suitable form for simulation, recall that $E = -\ln U$ is exponential with parameter 1. For such E_i, $S_n \leq \alpha < S_{n+1}$ if and only if

$$U_1 \cdot \ldots \cdot U_n \geq e^{-\alpha} > U_1 \cdot \ldots \cdot U_{n+1}.$$

Hence one generates U's until their product is less than $e^{-\alpha}$ for the first time and lets X be the last index. This method is fast for small α. For large α many U's have to be realized and other methods are faster.

```
FUNCTION POISSON(alpha:REAL):INTEGER;
{returns a Poisson variable; the parameter alpha must be strictly
   positive; uses function U}
VAR i:INTEGER; y,c:REAL;
BEGIN
  c:=exp(-alpha);
  i:=0; y:=1;
  WHILE (y>=c) DO BEGIN y:=y*U; i:=SUCC(i) END;
  POISSON:=i
END; {POISSON}
```

A.4.3 Gaussian Variables

The importance of the normal distribution is mirrored by the variety of sampling methods.

Plainly, it is sufficient to generate standard Gaussian (normal) variables N, since variables

$$Y = \sigma N + \mu$$

are Gaussian with mean μ and variance σ^2.

The inversion method does not apply directly since the c.d.f. is not available in closed form; hence the method has to be applied to approximations.

Frequently, one finds the somewhat cryptic formula

$$X = \sum_{i=1}^{12} U_i - 6.$$

It is based on the **central limit theorem** which states: Given a sequence of real i.i.d. random variables Y_i with finite variance σ^2 (and hence finite expectation μ), the c.d.f. of the normalized partial sums

$$S_n^* = \frac{1}{n^{1/2}\sigma}\left(\sum_{i=1}^{n} Y_i - n\mu\right)$$

tend to the c.d.f. of a standard Gaussian variable (i.e. with expectation 0 and variance 1) uniformly. Since $\mathsf{E}(U) = 1/2$ and $\mathsf{var}(U) = 1/12$ the variable X above is such a normalized sum for $Y_i = U_i$ and $n = 12$.

These are approximative methods.

There is an appealing 'exact method' given by BOX and MULLER (1958) which we report now. It is very easy to write a program if the subroutines for the squareroot, the logarithm, sinus and cosinus are available. It is slow but has essentially perfect accuracy. The generation of N is based on the following elementary result:

Theorem A.4.2 (The Box-Muller Method). *Let U_1 and U_2 be i.i.d. uniformly distributed random variables on $(0,1)$. Then the random variables*

$$\begin{aligned} N_1 &= (-2\cdot\ln U_1)^{1/2}\cdot\cos(2\pi U_2)\,, \\ N_2 &= (-2\cdot\ln U_1)^{1/2}\cdot\sin(2\pi U_2)\,, \end{aligned}$$

are independent standard Gaussian.

To give a complete and selfcontained proof recall from analysis:

Theorem A.4.3 (Integral Transformation Theorem). *Let D_1 and D_2 be open subsets of R^2, $\varphi : D_1 \mapsto D_2$ a one-to-one continuously differentiable map with continuously differentiable inverse φ^{-1} and $f : D_2 \mapsto \mathsf{R}$ some real function. Then f is (Lebesgue-) integrable on D_2 if and only if $f\circ\varphi$ is integrable on D_1 and then*

$$\int_{D_2} f(x)dx = \int_{D_1} f\circ\varphi\,|\det J_\varphi(x)|\,dx,$$

where $\det J_\varphi(x)$ is the determinant of the Jakobian $J_\varphi(x)$ of φ at x.

A simple corollary is the

Theorem A.4.4 (Transformation Theorem for Densities). *Let Z_1, Z_2, U_1 and U_2 be random variables. Assume that the random vector (U_1, U_2) takes values in the open subset G' of R^2 and has density f on G'. Assume further that (Z_1, Z_2) takes values in the open subset G of R^2. Let $\varphi : G \to G'$ be a continuously differentiable bijection with continuously differentiable inverse $\varphi^{-1} : G' = \varphi(G) \to G$. Given*

$$\begin{pmatrix} U_1 \\ U_2 \end{pmatrix} = \varphi\begin{pmatrix} Z_1 \\ Z_2 \end{pmatrix},$$

the random vector (Z_1, Z_2) on g has density

$$g(z) = f\circ\varphi(z)\,|J_\varphi(z)|\,.$$

Proof. Let D be an open subset of G. By the transformation theorem,

$$\begin{aligned} \mathsf{P}((Z_1, Z_2) \in D) &= \mathsf{P}\left(\varphi^{-1}(U_1, U_2) \in D\right) = \mathsf{P}((U_1, U_2) \in \varphi(D)) \\ &= \int_{\varphi(D)} f(x)dx = \int_D f \circ \varphi(x) \left|J_\varphi(x)\right| dx. \end{aligned}$$

Since this identity holds for each open subset D of G the density of (Z_1, Z_2) has the desired form. □

Proof (for the Box-Muller method). Let us first determine the map φ from the last theorem. We have

$$N_1^2 = -2 \cdot \ln(U_1) \cdot \cos^2(2\pi U_2),\ N_2^2 = -2 \cdot \ln(U_1) \cdot \sin^2(2\pi U_2),$$

hence $N_1^2 + N_2^2 = -2 \cdot \ln(U_1)$ and

$$U_1 = \exp\left(-(N_1^2 + N_2^2)/2\right).$$

Moreover $N_2/N_1 = \tan(2\pi U_2)$, i.e.

$$U_2 = (2\pi)^{-1} \cdot \arctan\left(N_2/N_1\right).$$

Hence φ is defined on an open subset of R^2 with full Lebesgue measure and has the form

$$\varphi(z_1, z_2) = \begin{pmatrix} \varphi_1(z_1, z_2) \\ \varphi_2(z_1, z_2) \end{pmatrix} = \begin{pmatrix} \exp(-(z_1^2 + z_2^2)/2) \\ (2\pi)^{-1} \arctan(z_2/z_1) \end{pmatrix}.$$

The partial derivatives of φ are

$$\frac{\partial\varphi_1}{\partial z_1}(z) = -z_1 \cdot \exp\left(-(z_1^2 + z_2^2)/2\right), \quad \frac{\partial\varphi_1}{\partial z_2}(z) = -z_2 \cdot \exp\left(-(z_1^2 + z_2^2)/2\right),$$

$$\frac{\partial\varphi_2}{\partial z_1}(z) = \frac{1}{2\pi} \cdot \frac{-z_2}{z_1^2 + z_2^2}, \qquad \frac{\partial\varphi_2}{\partial z_2}(z) = \frac{1}{2\pi} \cdot \frac{z_1}{z_1^2 + z_2^2}$$

which implies

$$\begin{aligned} \left|\det J_\varphi(z)\right| &= \frac{1}{2\pi} \exp\left(-(z^2 + z^2)/2\right) \\ &= \frac{1}{(2\pi)^{1/2}} \exp\left(-z_1^2/2\right) \cdot \frac{1}{(2\pi)^{1/2}} \exp\left(-z_2^2/2\right). \end{aligned}$$

Since (U_1, U_2) has density $\mathbf{1}_{(0,1)\times(0,1)}$ the transformation formula holds. □

Here is a procedure for the Box-Muller method in PASCAL:

```
PROCEDURE BOXMULLER (VAR N1,N2:REAL);
{returns a pair N1, N2 of independent standard Gaussian variables}
{uses FUNCTION U}
CONST pi=3.1415927
VAR U1, U2:REAL;
BEGIN
  U1:=U; U2:=U;
  N1:=SQRT(-2*ln(U1))*cos(2*pi*U2);
  N2:=SQRT(-2*ln(U1))*sin(2*pi*U2)
END; {BOXMULLER}
```

A single standard Gaussian deviate is obtained similarly. For the generation of degraded images this method is quick enough since it is needed only once for each pixel. On the other hand, we cannot resist to describe another algorithm which avoids the time-consuming computation of the trigonometric functions sin and/or cos. It is based on a general principle, perhaps even more flexible than the inversion method.

A.4.4 The Rejection Method

Sampling from a density f is equivalent to sampling from its subgraph: Given (X, Y) uniformly distributed on $\mathcal{F} = \{(s,u) : f(s) \le u\}$, the X-coordinate has density f:

$$\mathsf{P}(X \le t) = \iint_{\mathcal{F}} du\, ds = \int_{-\infty}^{t} \int_{0}^{f(s)} du\, ds = \int_{-\infty}^{t} f(s)\, ds.$$

Uniform samples from $\mathcal{F}$ may be obtained from uniform samples from a larger area $\mathcal{G}$ *conditional* on $\mathcal{F}$: sample (V, W) uniformly from $\mathcal{G}$, reject until $(V, W) \in \mathcal{F}$ and then let $X = V$. In most applications, the larger set $\mathcal{G}$ is the subgraph of $M \cdot g$ for another density g. Note that the arguments hold also for multi-dimensional X.

For the **general rejection method** let f and g be probability densities such that $f/g \le M < \infty$. To sample from f, generate V from g and, independently, $W = MU$ uniformly from $[0, M]$. Repeat this until $W \le f(V)/g(V)$ and then let $X = V$.

The formal justification is easy:

$$\begin{aligned}\mathsf{P}\,(V \le t\,, V \text{ is accepted}) &= \mathsf{P}\,(\mathsf{V} \le \mathsf{t}, \mathsf{U} \le \mathsf{f(V)/(g(V) \cdot M)}) \\ &= \int_{-\infty}^{t} \int_{0}^{f(s)/(g(s)M)} du\, g(s)\, ds = \frac{1}{M} \int_{-\infty}^{t} f(s)\, ds.\end{aligned}$$

Hence V is accepted with probability M^{-1} and

$$\mathsf{P}\,(V \le t \mid V \text{ is accepted}) = \int_{-\infty}^{t} f(s)\, ds$$

as desired.

A.4.5 The Polar Method

This is a variant of the Box-Muller method to generate standard normal deviates. It is due to G. MARSAGLIA. It is easy to write a program if the square-root and logarithm subroutines are available. It is substantially faster than the Box-Muller method since it avoids the calculation of the trigonometric functions (but still slower than some other methods, cf. KNUTH (1981), 3.4.1) and it has essentially perfect accuracy.

The Box-Muller theorem may be rephrased as follows: given (W, Θ) uniformly distributed on $[0,1] \times [0, 2\pi)$, the variables $N_1 = (-2 \ln W)^{1/2} \sin \Theta$ and $N_2 = (-2 \ln W)^{1/2} \cos \Theta$ are independent standard Gaussian. The rejection method allows to sample directly from $(W, \cos \Theta)$ and $(W, \sin \Theta)$ thus avoiding to calculate the sinus and cosinus:

Given (Z_1, Z_2) uniformly distributed on the unit disc and the polar coordinates R, Θ, i.e. $Z_1 = R \cos \Theta$ and $Z_2 = R \sin \Theta$, $W = R^2$ and Θ have joint density $\frac{1}{2\pi}$ on $[0,1] \times [0, 2\pi)$ and hence are uniform and independent. Plainly, $W = Z_1^2 + Z_2^2$, $\cos \Theta = W^{-1/2} Z_1$ and $\sin \Theta = W^{-1/2} Z_2$ and we may set

$$N_1 = \left(\frac{-2 \ln W}{W} \right)^{1/2} Z_1, \; N_2 = \left(\frac{-2 \ln W}{W} \right)^{1/2} Z_2.$$

To sample from the unit disk, we adopt the rejection method: sample (V_1, V_2) uniformly from the square $[-1, 1]^2$ until $V_1^2 + V_2^2 \leq 1$ and then set $(Z_1, Z_2) = (V_1, V_2)$.

```
PROCEDURE POLAR (VAR N1,N2:REAL);
{returns a pair N1, N2 of standard Gaussian deviates}
{uses FUNCTION U}
VAR V1, V2, W, D : REAL;
BEGIN
  REPEAT
    BEGIN V1:=2*U; V2:=2*U; W:=SQR(V1)+SQR(V2) END
  UNTIL (0<W<=1);
  D:=SQRT(-2*ln(W)/W);
  N1:=D*V1; N2:=D*V2
END; {POLAR}
```

Remark A.4.1. The outcomes of the random number generator are transformed by these algorithms in a nonlinear way. Fig. A.3 shows plots of subsequent pairs from the Box-Muller algorithm (a) and the polar algorithm (b) applied to the generator from Fig. A.2 (a) and from the polar method applied to the (unspecified) generator from ST PASCAL plus version 2.00.

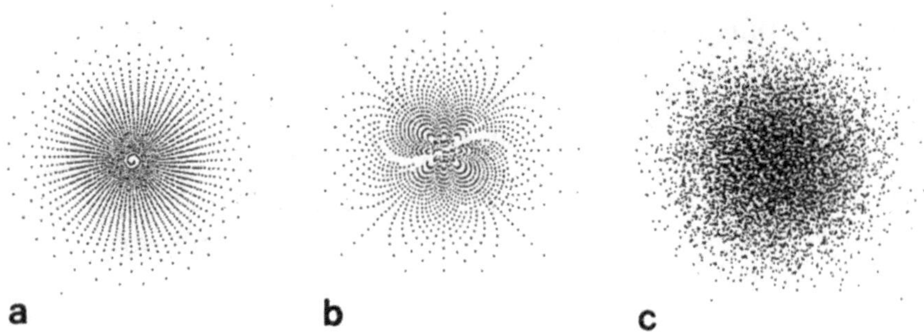

Fig. A.3. (a–c)

B. The Perron-Frobenius Theorem

Let $\mathbf{X}$ denote a finite set. A Markov kernel or transition matrix $P = (P(x,y))_{x,y\in\mathbf{X}}$ is **primitive** if some power P^τ is strictly positive, i.e. $P^\tau(x,y) > 0$ for all $x, y \in \mathbf{X}$.

Theorem B.0.5. *Let P be a primitive Markov kernel. Then $\gamma = 1$ is an eigenvalue of P. The corresponding right eigenvectors are constant and the left eigenspace is spanned by a distribution μ. This distribution μ is the unique invariant distribution of P and strictly positive. Moreover, $\gamma > |\lambda|$ for any eigenvalue $\lambda \neq \gamma$.*

The eigenvalue $\gamma = 1$ is the **Perron-Frobenius eigenvalue** of P. X

Proof. We assume first that P is strictly positive. Let C be the cone $\mathsf{R}_+^{\mathbf{X}}\backslash\{0\}$. Define the continuous function h on C by

$$h(\nu) = \min\left\{\frac{\nu P(x)}{\nu(x)} : x \in \mathbf{X}\right\}.$$

Plainly, $h(C)$ coincides with the image under h of the set of probability vectors. Hence $h(C)$ is compact and has a greatest element γ. Let $\mu \in C$ be a maximizer. By way of contradiction we show that μ is a left eigenvector for γ. By the choice of γ, $\mu P(x) \geq \gamma\mu(x)$. If $\mu P \neq \gamma\mu$ then this inequality is strict for at least one x and since P is strictly positive this implies that $(\mu P - \gamma\mu)\, P$ is strictly positive. But then $h(\mu P) > \gamma$ which contradicts the choice of γ. Hence $\mu P = \gamma\mu$. Note that for each x the component $\mu(x) = \gamma^{-1}\mu P(x)$ is strictly positive. We may assume that μ is normalized, i.e. $\sum_x \mu(x) = 1$. Then

$$\sum_x \mu(x)P(x,y) = \mu P(y) = \gamma\mu(y).$$

Since the sum over the rows of P is 1, summation over y yields $\gamma = 1$. Hence $\mu P = \mu$ and μ is an invariant distribution for P.

To see that γ is a simple eigenvalue choose any real left eigenvector ν for γ (if ν were complex we could consider the real and imaginary parts separately). Let

$$c = \min\left\{\frac{\nu(x)}{\mu(x)} : x \in \mathbf{X}\right\}.$$

Then we have always $\nu(z) \geq c \cdot \mu(z)$. If this inequality were strict for a single z, then it were strict for every $x \in \mathbf{X}$ since

$$\nu(x) - c\mu(x) = \frac{1}{\gamma} \sum_z (\nu(z) - c\mu(z))\, P(z,x) > 0.$$

This contradicts the choice of c. Hence $\nu = c \cdot \mu$ which shows that the left eigenspace of γ has dimension 1.

Consider any eigenvalue λ of P. Let ν be a left eigenvector for λ and $t = \min\{P(x,x) : x \in \mathbf{X}\} > 0$. Since

$$\nu(P - tI) = \nu(\lambda - t)$$

we have for every $y \in \mathbf{X}$

$$\sum_x |\nu(x)|\,(P(x,y) - tI(x,y)) \geq |\lambda - t||\nu(y)|$$

and hence

$$\sum_x |\nu(x)| P(x,y) \geq (|\lambda - t| + t)\, |\nu(y)|.$$

Recalling the definitions of h and γ, we conclude

$$\gamma = \max h(C) \geq (|\lambda - t| + t).$$

This shows that either $\lambda = \gamma$ or $|\lambda| < \gamma$.

These arguments can be repeated for right eigenvalues (except the proof of $\gamma = 1$). The γ produced is the same since $|\lambda| < 1$ for $\lambda \neq \gamma$ is a statement about eigenvalues only.

Assume now that P is nonnegative and the power P^τ is strictly positive. Observe: (i) For every eigenvalue λ of P the power λ^τ is an eigenvalue of P^τ and the eigenvectors of P for λ are eigenvectors of P^τ for λ^τ. (ii) For a stochastic matrix the number $\gamma = 1$ is always an eigenvalue. Hence P inherits the stated properties from P^τ. □

C. Concave Functions

A subset C of a linear space E is called **convex** if for all $x, y \in C$ the line-segment

$$[x, y] = \{\lambda x + (1 - \lambda)y : 0 \leq \lambda \leq 1\}$$

is contained in C. For $x^{(1)}, \ldots, x^{(n)} \in E$ and $\lambda^{(1)}, \ldots, \lambda^{(n)} \geq 0$, $\sum_i \lambda^{(i)} = 1$, the element $x = \sum_i \lambda^{(i)} x^{(i)}$ is called a **convex combination** of the elements $x^{(i)}$. For $x = (x_1, \ldots, x_d)$, $y = (x_1, \ldots, y_d) \in \mathsf{R}^d$, the symbol $\langle x, y \rangle$ denotes the Euclidean scalar product $\sum_i x_i y_i$ and $\| \cdot \|$ denote Euclidean norm. A real-valued function g on a subset Θ of R^d is called **Lipschitz continuous** if there is $\lambda > 0$ such that

$$|g(x) - g(y)| \leq \lambda \|x - y\| \quad \text{for all} \quad x, y \in \Theta.$$

If $g : \Theta \to \mathsf{R}$ is differentiable the gradient of g at x is given by

$$\nabla g(x) = \left(\frac{\partial}{\partial x_1} g(x), \ldots, \frac{\partial}{\partial x_d} g(x) \right)$$

where $\frac{\partial}{\partial x_1} g(x)$ is the partial derivative w.r.t. x_i of g at x.

Lemma C.0.1. *Let Θ be an open subset of R^d.*

(a) Every continuously differentiable function on Θ is Lipschitz continuous on every compact subset of Θ.

(b) A convex combination of functions on Θ with common Lipschitz constant is Lipschitz continuous admitting the same constant.

Proof. (a) Let g be continuously differentiable on Θ. The map $x \mapsto \|\nabla g(x)\|$ is continuous and hence bounded on a compact subset C of Θ by some constant $\gamma > 0$. By the mean value theorem, for $x, y \in C$ there is some z on $[x, y]$ such that

$$g(y) - g(x) = \langle \nabla g(z), y - x \rangle.$$

Hence

$$|g(y) - g(x)| \leq \gamma \|y - x\|.$$

(b) Let $g^{(1)}, \ldots, g^{(n)}$ be Lipschitz continuous with constant γ and $\lambda^{(1)}, \ldots, \lambda^{(n)} \geq 0$, $\sum_i \lambda^{(i)} = 1$. Then

$$\left|\sum_i \lambda^{(i)} g^{(i)}(y) - \sum_i \lambda^{(i)} g^{(i)}(x)\right| \le \sum_i \lambda^{(i)} \left|g^{(i)}(y) - g^{(i)}(x)\right| \le \gamma \|y - x\|.$$

□

A real-valued function g on a convex subset Θ of R^d is called **concave** if

$$g(\lambda x + (1-\lambda)y) \ge \lambda g(x) + (1-\lambda)g(y) \quad \text{for all} \quad x, y \in \Theta \text{ and } 0 \le \lambda \le 1.$$

If the inequality is strict then g is called **strictly concave**. The function g is **(strictly) convex** if $-g$ is (strictly) concave.

Lemma C.0.2. *Let g be a twice continuously differentiable function on an open interval on the real line. If the second derivative g'' is (strictly) negative then g is (strictly) concave.*

The converse holds also true.

Proof. Denote the end points of the interval by a and b and let $a < x < y < b$, $0 < \lambda < 1$ and $z = \lambda x + (1-\lambda)y$. If the second derivative g'' is negative then the first derivative g' decreases and

$$\begin{aligned} g(z) - g(x) &= \int_x^z g'(u)\,du \ge g'(z)(z-x), \\ g(y) - g(z) &= \int_z^y g'(u)\,du \le g'(z)(y-z). \end{aligned}$$

Using $z - x = (1-\lambda)(y-x)$ and $y - z = \lambda(y-x)$ this may be rewritten as

$$\begin{aligned} g(z) &\ge g(x) + (1-\lambda)g'(y-x), \\ g(z) &\ge g(y) - \lambda g'(z)(y-x). \end{aligned}$$

Hence

$$g(z) \ge \lambda g(x) + (1-\lambda)g(y)$$

which proves concavity of g. If the second derivative of g is strictly negative then the inequalities are strict and g is strictly concave. □

We shall write

$$\nabla^2 g(x) = \left(\frac{\partial^2}{\partial x_i \partial x_j} g(x)\right)_{i,j=1}^n$$

for the Hessean matrix. A $d \times d$-matrix A is called **negative semi-definite** if $\alpha A \alpha^* \le 0$ for every $\alpha \in \mathsf{R}^d \backslash \{0\}$ (where x is a row vector and x^* its transpose). It is **negative definite** if these inequalities are strict. Plainly, it is sufficient to require the conditions for $\alpha \in U \backslash \{0\}$, where U contains a ball around $0 \in \mathsf{R}^d$. A is called **positive (semi-) definite** if $-A$ is negative (semi-) definite. Recall further, that the directional derivative of a function g on R^d at x in direction $z \in \mathsf{R}^d$ is $\langle z, \nabla g(x) \rangle$.

Lemma C.0.3. *Let g be a twice continuously differentiable real-valued function on a convex open subset Θ of R^d. Then*

(a) If the Hessean of g is negative semi-definite then g is concave on θ (and conversely). If it is negative definite then g is strictly concave (and conversely).

(b) Let $g(x^{(0)}) = 0$ be a maximum of g and $B(x^{(0)}, r)$ a closed ball in Θ. If $\nabla^2 g$ is negative definite on Θ then there is $\gamma > 0$ such that

$$g(x) \leq -\gamma \|x - x^{(0)}\| \quad \textit{for every} \quad x \in B(x^{(0)}, r).$$

Proof. (a) The function g is concave on Θ if and only if for every $x^{(0)}$ in Θ and z with norm 1 it is concave on the line segment $\{x^{(0)} + \lambda z : \lambda \in L\}$ where

$$L = \left\{\lambda \in \mathsf{R} : x^{(0)} + \lambda z \in \Theta\right\}.$$

Set

$$h : L \to \mathsf{R}\,, \lambda \mapsto g\left(x^{(0)} + \lambda z\right).$$

Then

$$\begin{aligned} h''(\lambda) &= \frac{d}{d\lambda}\left\langle z, \nabla g\left(x^{(0)} + \lambda z\right)\right\rangle \\ &= \sum_{i=1}^{d} z_i \frac{d}{d\lambda}\frac{\partial}{\partial x_i} g(x^{(0)} + \lambda z) = \sum_{i=1}^{d} z_i \sum_{j=1}^{d} z_j \frac{\partial^2}{\partial x_i \partial x_j} g(x^{(0)} + \lambda z) \\ &= z \nabla^2 g(x^{(0)} + \lambda z) z^* \leq 0. \end{aligned} \tag{C.1}$$

Hence h is concave by Lemma C.2 and so is g. Similarly, g is strictly concave if the Hessean is negative definite.

(b) We continue with just introduced notation. Let

$$\left\{x^{(0)} + \lambda z : -\alpha \leq \lambda \leq \alpha\right\}$$

be the intersection of a line through $x^{(0)}$ with $B(x^{(0)}, r)$. By assumption, the last inequality in the proof of (b) is strict. By continuity and compactness, $-h'' < -\gamma'$ for some $\gamma' > 0$ which is independent of λ and z. Integrating twice yields the assertion. □

The Hessean matrices in this text have the form of covariance matrices and thus share some useful properties. Let ξ and η be real-valued random variables on a (finite) probability space. The covariance of x and η is defined as $\mathsf{cov}(\xi, \eta) = \mathsf{E}\left((\xi - \mathsf{E}(\xi))(\eta - \mathsf{E}(\eta))\right)$. A straightforward computation shows $\mathsf{cov}(\xi, \eta) = \mathsf{E}(\xi\eta) - \mathsf{E}(\xi)\mathsf{E}(\eta)$. The **variance** $\mathsf{var}(\xi)$ is $\mathsf{cov}(\xi, \xi)$. If $\xi = (\xi_1, \ldots, \xi_x)$ takes values in R^n then $\mathsf{cov}(\xi) = \left(\mathsf{cov}(\xi_i, \xi_j)\right)_{i,j}$ is the **covariance matrix** of ξ.

Lemma C.0.4. *Let* $\xi = (\xi_1, \ldots, \xi_n)$ *be a* R^n*-valued random vector on a (finite) probability space. Then for every* $\alpha \in \mathsf{R}^n$

$$\alpha \mathsf{cov}(\xi)\alpha^* = \mathsf{var}\left(\langle \alpha, \xi \rangle\right).$$

In particular, covariance matrices are positive semi-definite.

Proof. This follows from

$$\sum_{i,j} \alpha_i \alpha_j \mathsf{E}\left((\xi_i - \mathsf{E}(\xi_i))(\xi_j - \mathsf{E}(\xi_j))\right) = \mathsf{E}\left(\left[\sum_i \alpha_i(\xi_i - \mathsf{E}(\xi_i))\right]^2\right). \qquad \square$$

D. A Global Convergence Theorem for Descent Algorithms

Let A be a mapping defined on R^d assigning to every point $\vartheta \in \mathsf{R}^d$ a subset $A(\vartheta) \subset \mathsf{R}^d$. It is called **closed at** ϑ if $\vartheta_{(k)} \to \vartheta$ and $\varphi_{(k)} \in A\left(\vartheta_{(k)}\right)$, $\varphi_{(k)} \to \varphi$, imply $\varphi \in A(\vartheta)$. Given some **solution set** $R \subset \mathsf{R}^d$, the mapping A is said to be **closed** if it is closed at every $\vartheta \in \mathsf{R}$. A continuous real-valued function W is called a **descent function** for R and A if it satisfies

(i) if $\vartheta \notin R$ and $\varphi \in A(\vartheta)$ then $W(\varphi) < W(\vartheta)$
(ii) if $\vartheta \in R$ and $\varphi \in A(\vartheta)$ then $W(\varphi) \leq W(\vartheta)$.

Theorem D.0.6 (Global Convergence Theorem). *Let R be a solution set, A be closed and W a descent function for R and A. Suppose that given $\vartheta_{(0)}$ the sequence $\left(\vartheta_{(k)}\right)_{k\geq 0}$ is generated satisfying $\vartheta_{(k+1)} \in A(\vartheta_{(k)})$ and being contained in a compact subset of R^d. Then the limit of any convergent subsequence of $\left(\vartheta_{(k)}\right)_{k\geq 0}$ is an element of R.*

The simple proof can be found in LUENBERGER (1989), p. 187.

In our applications, the solution set is given by the global minima of W. The following special cases are needed:

(a) A is given by a continuous point-to-point map $a : \mathsf{R}^d \to \mathsf{R}^d$ via $A(\vartheta) = \{a(\vartheta)\}$. Plainly, A is closed.

(b) There are a continuous map $a : \mathsf{R}^d \to \mathsf{R}^d$ and a continuous function $r : \mathsf{R}^d \to \mathsf{R}_+$. A is defined by $A(\vartheta) = B\left(a(\vartheta), r(\vartheta)\right)$ where $B(\vartheta, r)$ is the closed ball with radius r centering around ϑ. Again, A is closed: Let $\vartheta_{(k)} \to \vartheta$ and $\varphi_{(k)} \to \varphi$. Then

$$\left\|a\left(\vartheta_{(k)}\right) - \varphi_{(k)}\right\| \to \|a(\vartheta) - \varphi\| .$$

($\|\cdot\|$ is any norm on R^d). If $\varphi_{(k)} \in A\left(\vartheta_{(k)}\right)$ then the left side is bounded from above by $r\left(\vartheta_{(k)}\right)$ and thus the limit is less or equal to $\lim_{k\to\infty} r(\vartheta_k) = r(\vartheta)$. Hence $\varphi \in B\left(a(\vartheta), r(\vartheta)\right) = A(\vartheta)$ which proves the assertion.

(c) If there is a unique minimum ϑ_* then $\vartheta_{(k)} \to \vartheta_*$. In fact, by compactness there is a convergent subsequence (with limit ϑ_*) and every subsequence converges. Otherwise – again by compactness – there would be a clusterpoint $\vartheta_c \neq \vartheta_*$.

References

[1] AARTS E. and KORST J. (1987): Simulated Annealing and Boltzmann Machines. Wiley & Sons, Chichester New York Brisbane Toronto Singapore

[2] ABEND K., HARLEY T. and KANAL L.N. (1965): Classification of binary patterns. IEEE Trans. Inform. Theory **IT-11**, 538–544

[3] ACUNA C. (1988): Parameter estimation for stochastic texture models. Ph.D. thesis, Dept. of Mathematics and Statistics, University of Massachusetts

[4] AGGARWAL J.K. and NANDHAKUMAR N. (1988): On the computation of motion from sequences of images. A review. Proc. IEEE **76**, 917–935

[5] ALMEIDA P.M. and GIDAS B. (1992): A variational method for estimating the parameters of MRF from complete or noncomplete data. To appear in: Ann. Applied Prob., 46 pp

[6] ALUFFI-PENTINI F., PARISI V. and ZIRILLI F. (1985): Global optimization and stochastic differential equations. J. Optim. Theory Appl. **47**, 1–16

[7] AMIT Y. and GRENANDER U. (1989): Compare sweeping strategies for stochastic relaxation. Div. Appl. Math., Brown University

[8] ARMINGER G. and SOBEL M.E. (1990): Pseudo-maximum likelihood estimation of mean and covariance structures with missing data. J. Amer. Statist. Assoc. **85**, 195–103

[9] AVERINTSEV M.B. (1978): On some classes of Gibbsian random fields. In: Dobrushin, R.L., Kryukov, V.I., Toom, A.L. (eds.) Locally Interacting Systems and their Applications in Biology. Proceedings held in Pushchino, Moscow region. Lecture Notes in Mathematics, vol. 653. Springer, Berlin Heidelberg New York, pp. 91–98

[10] AZENCOTT R. (1988): Simulated Annealing. Séminaire Bourbaki, no. 697

[11] AZENCOTT R. (1990a): Synchroneous Boltzmann machines and Gibbs fields: Learning algorithms. In: Foglman Soulié, F. and Hérault, J. (eds.) Neurocomputing, NATO ASI Series, vol. F68. Springer, Berlin Heidelberg New York, pp. 51–62

[12] AZENCOTT R. (1990b): Synchroneous Boltzmann machines and artificial learning. In: Les Entrétiens de Lyon, Neural Networks Biological Computers or Electronic Brains. Springer, Berlin Heidelberg New York, pp. 135–143

[13] AZENCOTT R. (1991): Extraction of smooth contour lines in images by synchroneous Boltzmann machine. Procedings Int. J. Cong. Neural Nets, Singapore

[14] AZENCOTT R. (1992a): Simulated Annealing: Parallelization techniques. Edited by R. Azencott. Wiley & Sons

[15] AZENCOTT R. (1992b): Boltzmann machines: high-order interactions and synchroneous learning. In: Barone P., Frigessi A., Piccioni M. (eds) Stochastic models, statistical methods, and algorithms in image analysis. Lecture Notes in Statistics, vol. 74. Springer, Berlin Heidelberg New York, pp. 17–45

[16] BADDELEY A.J. and SILVERMAN B.W (1984): A cautionary example on the use of second order methods for analyzing point patterns. Biometrics **40**, 1089–1093

[17] BALDI P. (1986): Limit set of homogeneous Ornstein-Uhlenbeck processes, destabilization and annealing. Stochastic Process. Appl. **23**, 153–167

[18] BARKER A.A. (1965): Monte Carlo calculations of the radial distribution functions for a proton-electron plasma. Aust. J. Phys. **18**, 119–133

[19] BARONE P. and FRIGESSI A. (1989): Improving stochastic relaxation for Gaussian random fields. Probability in the Engineering and Informational Sciences **4**, 369–389

[20] BEARDWOOD J., HALTON J.H. and HAMMERSLEY J.M. (1959): The shortest path through many points. Proc. Cambridge Phil. Soc. **55**, 299–327

[21] BENVENISTE A., MÉTIVIER M. and PRIOURET P. (1990): Adaptive algorithms and stochastic approximations. Springer, Berlin Heidelberg New York London Paris Tokyo HongKong Barcelona

[22] BESAG J. (1974): Spatial interaction and the statistical analysis of lattice systems (with discussion). J. of the Royal Statist. Soc., series B, **36**, 192–236

[23] BESAG J. (1977): Efficiency of pseudolikelihood for simple Gaussian field. Biometrika **64**, 616–619

[24] BESAG J. (1986): On the statistical analysis of dirty pictures (with discussion). J. of the Royal Statist. Soc., series B, **48**, 259–302

[25] BESAG J. (1989): Towards Bayesian image analysis. J. Appl. Stat. **16**, 395–407

[26] BESAG J. and MORAN P.A.P. (1975): On the estimation and testing of spatial interaction in Gaussian lattice processes. Biometrika **62**, 555–562

[27] BESAG J., YORK J. and MOLLIÉ A. (1991): Bayesian image restoration with two applications in spatial statistics. Ann. Inst. Statist. Math. **43**, 1–59

[28] BIBERMAN L.M. and NUDELMAN S. (1971): Photoelectronic imaging devices, vol. 1, 2. Plenum, New York

[29] BILLINGSLEY P. (1965): Ergodic theory and information. Wiley & Sons, New York London Sidney

[30] BILLINGSLEY P. (1979): Probability and measure. Wiley & Sons, New York Chichester Brisbane Toronto

[31] BINDER K. (1978): Monte Carlo methods in Statistical Physics. Springer, Berlin Heidelberg New York

[32] BLAKE A. (1983): The least disturbance principle and weak constraints. Pattern Recognition Lett. **1**, 393–399

[33] BLAKE A. (1989): Comparison of the efficiency of deterministic and stochastic algorithms for visual reconstruction. IEEE Trans. PAMI **11**(1), 2–12

[34] BLAKE A. and ZISSERMAN A. (1987): Visual reconstruction. MIT Press, Cambridge (Massachusetts) London (England)

[35] BONOMI E. and LUTTON J.-L. (1984): The N-city travelling salesman problem: Statistical mechanics and the Metropolis algorithm. SIAM Rev. **26**, 551–568

[36] BOX G.E.P. and MULLER M.E. (1958): A note on the generation of random normal deviates. Ann. Math. Statist. **29**, 610–611

[37] BOX J.E. and JENKINS G.M. (1970): Time series analysis. Holden-Day, San Francisco

[38] BUDINGER T., GULLBERG G. and HUESMAN R. (1979): Emission computed tomography. In: Herman G. (ed.) Image Reconstruction from Projections: Implementation and Application. Springer, Berlin Heidelberg New York

[39] CATONI O. (1991a): Applications of sharp large deviations estimates to optimal cooling schedules. Ann. Inst. H. Poincaré **27**, 463–518

[40] CATONI O. (1991b): Sharp large deviations estimates for simulated annealing algorithms. Ann. Inst. H. Poincaré **27**, 291–383

[41] CATONI O. (1992): Rough large deviations estimates for simulated annealing. Application to exponential schedules. Ann. Probab. **20**, 109–146

[42] ČERNY V. (1985): Thermodynamical approach to the travelling salesman problem: an efficient simulation algorithm. JOTA **45**, 41–51

[43] CHALMOND B. (1988a): Image restoration using an estimated Markov model. Prepublications Université de Paris-Sud, Departement de Mathematique, Bat. 425, 91405 Orsay, France

[44] CHALMOND B. (1988b): Image restoration using an estimated Markov model. Signal Processing **15**, 115–129

[45] CHELLAPA R. and JAIN A. ((eds.) (1993): Markov random fields: theory and application. Academic Press, Boston San Diego

[46] CHEN C.-C. and DUBES R.C. (1989): Experiments in fitting discrete Markov random fields to textures. IEEE Computer Vision and Pattern Recognition, pp. 298–303

[47] CHIANG T.-S. and CHOW Y. (1988): On the convergence rate of the annealing algorithm. SIAM J. Control and Optimization **26**, 1455–1470

[48] CHIANG T.-S. and CHOW Y. (1989): A limit theorem for a class of inhomogeneous Markov processes. Ann. Probab. **17**, 1483–1502

[49] CHIANG T.-S. and CHOW Y. (1990): The asymptotic behaviour of simulated annealing processes with absorption. Report Institute of Mathematics, Academia Sinica, Taipei, Taiwan

[50] CHIANG T.-S, HWANG HH.-R. and SHEU SH.-J. (1987): Diffusions for global optimization in R^n. SIAM J. Control Optim. **25**, 737–753

[51] CHOW Y, GRENANDER U. and KEENAN D.M (1987): Hands. A pattern theoretic study of biological shapes. Division of Applied Mathematics, Brown University, Providence, Rhode Island 02912, USA

[52] CHOW Y. and HSIEH J. (1990): On occupation times of annealing processes. Institute of Mathematics, Academia Sinica, Taipei, Taiwan

[53] COHEN F.S. and COOPER D.B. (1983): Real time textured image segmentation based on noncausal Markovian random field methods. In: Proc. SPIE Conf. Intell. Robots, Cambridge, MA

[54] COMETS F. (1992): On consistency of a class of estimators for exponential families of Markov random fields on the lattice. Ann. Statist. **20**, 455–486

[55] COMETS F. and GIDAS B. (1991): Asymptotics of maximum likelihood estimators for the Curie-Weiss model. Ann. Statist. **19**, 557–578

[56] COMETS F. and GIDAS B. (1992): Parameter estimation for Gibbs distributions from partially observed data. Ann. Appl. Probab. **2**, 142–170

[57] CROSS G.R. and JAIN A.K. (1983): Markov random field texture models. IEEE Trans. PAMI **5**, 25–39

[58] DACUNHA-CASTELLE D. and DUFLO M. (1982): Probabilité et Statistique 2. Masson, Paris

[59] DAWSON D.A. (1975): Synchroneous and asynchroneous reversible Markov systems. Canad. Math Bull. **17**, 633–649

[60] DENNIS J.E. and SCHNABEL R.B. (1983): Numerical methods for unconstrained optimization and nonlinear equations. Prentice Hall, Inc., Englewood Cliffs, New Jersey

[61] DERICHE R. (1987): Using Canny's criteria to derive a recursively implemented optimal edge detector. Int. J. Computer Vision, pp. 1167–187

[62] DERIN H. (1985): The use of Gibbs distributions in image processing. In: Blake I. and Poor V. (eds.) Communications and Networks: A Survey of Recent Advances. Springer, New York

[63] Derin H. and Cole W.S. (1986): Segmentation of textured images using Gibbs random fields. Comput. Vision, Graphics, Image Processing **35**, 72–98
[64] Derin H. and Elliott H. (1987): Modeling and segmentation of noisy and textured images using random fields. IEEE Trans. PAMI **9**, 39–55
[65] Derin H., Elliott H., Christi R. and Geman D. (1984): Bayes smoothing algorithms for segmentation of binary images modeled by Markov random fields. IEEE Trans. PAMI **6**, no. 6, 707–720
[66] Devijver P.A. and Dekesel M.M. (1987): Learning the parameters of a hidden Markov random field image model: a simple example. In: Devijver P.A. and Kittler J. (eds.) Pattern Recognition Theory and Applications, NATO ASI Series, vol. F30. Springer, Berlin Heidelberg New York, pp. 141–163
[67] Diaconis P. and Stroock D. (1991): Geometric bounds for eigenvalues of Markov chains. Ann. Appl. Probab. **1**, 36–61
[68] Dinic E.A. (1970): Algorithm for solution of a problem of maximal flow in a network with power estimation. Soviet. Math. Dokl. **11**, 1277–1280
[69] Dobrushin R.L. (1956): Central Limit Theorem for Non-Stationary Markov Chains I, II. Theo. Prob. Appl. **1**, pp. 65–80; Theo. Prob. Appl. **1**, 329–383
[70] Dress A. and Krüger M. (1987): Parsimonious phylogenic trees in metric spaces and simulated annealing. Adv. Appl. Math. **8**, 8–37
[71] Edwards R.G. and Sokal A.D. (1988): Generalization of the Fortuin-Kasteleyn-Swendson-Wang representation and Monte-Carlo algorithm. Phys. Rev. **D 38**, 2009–2012
[72] Edwards R.G. and Sokal A.D. (1989): Dynamic critical behavior of Wolff's collective-mode Monte Carlo algorithm for the two-dimensional O(n) nonlinear σ-model. Phys. Rev. **D 40**, 1374–1377
[73] Fill J.A. (1991) Eigenvalue bounds on convergence to stationarity for nonreversible Markov chains, with an application to the exclusion process. Ann. Appl. Probab. **1**, 62–87
[74] Föllmer H. (1988): Random fields and diffusion processes. In: Hennequin R.L. (ed.), École d'Été de Probabilités de Saint Flour XV-XVII, 1985–87. Lecture Notes in Mathematicss, vol. 1362. Springer, Berlin Heidelberg New York
[75] Ford L.R. and Fulkerson D.R. (1962): Flows in networks. Princeton University Press, Princeton
[76] Fortuin C.M. and Kasteleyn P.W. (1972): On the random cluster model. Physica (Utrecht) **57**
[77] Freidlin M.I. and Wentzell A.D. (1984): Random perturbations of dynamical systems. Springer, Berlin Heidelberg New York
[78] Frigessi A., Hwang Ch.-R., Sheu Sh.-J. and di Stefano P. (1993): Convergence rates of the Gibbs sampler, the Metropolis algorithm and other single site updating dynamics. J. of the Royal Statist. Soc., Series B **55**, 205–219
[79] Frigessi A., Hwang Ch.-R. and Younes L. (1992): Optimal spectral structure of reversible stochastic matrices, Monte Carlo methods and the simulation of Markov random fields. Ann. Appl. Probab. **2**, 610–628
[80] Frigessi A. and Piccioni M. (1990): Parameter estimation for two-dimensional Ising fields corrupted by noise. Stochastic Process. Appl. **34**, 297–311
[81] Gantert N. (1989): Laws of Large Numbers for the Annealing Algorithm. Stochastic Process. Appl **35**, 309–313
[82] Gelfand S.B. and Mitter S.K. (1985): Analysis of simulated annealing for optimization. Proc. of the Conference on Decision and Control, Ft. Lauderdale, FL., pp. 779–786

[83] GELFAND S.B. and MITTER S.K. (1991): Weak convergence of Markov chain sampling methods and annealing algorithms to diffusions. J. Optimization Theory Appl. **68**, 483–498

[84] GELFAND S.B. and MITTER S.K. (1992): Simulated annealing-type algorithms for multivariate optimization. Algorithmica (in press)

[85] GEMAN D. (1987): Stochastic model for boundary detection. Image and Vision Computing **5**, 61–65

[86] GEMAN D. (1990): Random fields and and inverse problems in imaging. In: Hennequin P.L. (ed.) École d'Été de Probabilité de Saint-Flour XVII-1988. Lecture Notes in Mathematics, vol. 1427. Springer, Berlin Heidelberg New York London Paris Tokyo Hong Kong Barcelona, pp. 113–193

[87] GEMAN D. and GEMAN S. (1987): Relaxation and annealing with constraints. Complex Systems Technical Report no. 35, Div. of Applied Mathematics, Brown University

[88] GEMAN D. and GEMAN S. (1991): Discussion on the paper by Besag J., York J. and Mollié A.: Bayesian image restauration with two applications in spatial statistics. Ann. Inst. Statist. Math., vol. 43

[89] GEMAN S. and GEMAN D. (1984): Stochastic relaxation, Gibbs distributions, and the Bayesian restoration of images. IEEE Trans. PAMI **6**, 721–741

[90] GEMAN D., GEMAN S. and GRAFFIGNE CHR. (1987): Locating texture and object boundaries. In: Devijer P.A. and Kittler J. (eds.) Proceedings of the NATO Advanced Study Institute on Pattern Recognition Theory and Applications, NASA ASI Series. Springer, Berlin Heidelberg New York

[91] GEMAN D., GEMAN S., GRAFFIGNE CHR. and PING DONG (1990): Boundary detection by constrained optimization. IEEE Trans. PAMI **12**, 609–628

[92] GEMAN D. and GIDAS B. (1991): Image analysis and computer vision. NRC Report. Spatial Statistics and Image Processing, 43 pp

[93] GEMAN S. and GRAFFIGNE CHR. (1987): Markov random field models and their applications to computer vision. In: Gleason M. (ed.) Proceedings of the International Congress of Mathematicians (1986). Amer. Math. Soc. Providence, pp. 1496–1517

[94] GEMAN S. and HWANG CH.-R. (1986): Diffusions for global optimization. SIAM J. Control Optim. **24**, 1031–1043

[95] GEMAN S. and MCCLURE D.E. (1987): Statistical methods for tomographic image reconstruction. In: Proceedings of the 46th Session of the ISI, Bulletin of the ISI, vol. 52

[96] GEMAN S., MCCLURE D., MANBECK K. and MERTUS J. (1990): Comprehensive statistical model for single photon emission computed tomography. Brown University

[97] GEORGII H.-O. (1988): Gibbs measures and phase transition. In: De Gruyter Studies in Mathematics, vol. 9. de Gruyter, Berlin New York

[98] GIDAS B. (1985a): Nonstationary Markov chains and convergence of the annealing algorithm. J. Stat. Phys. **39**, 73–131

[99] GIDAS B. (1985b): Global optimization via the Langevin equation. Proceedings of the 24th Conference on Decision and Control, Ft. Lauderdale, FL, Dec. 1985, pp. 774–786

[100] GIDAS B. (1987): Consistency of maximum likelihood and pseudolikelihood estimators for Gibbs distributions. Proceedings of the Wokshop on Stochastic Differential Systems with Applications. In: Electronical/Computer Engineering, Control Theory and Operations Research, IMS, University of Minnesota. Springer, Berlin Heidelberg New York

[101] Gidas B. (1988): Consistency of maximum likelihood and pseudolikelihood estimators for Gibbs distributions. In: Fleming W., Lions P.L. (eds.) Stochastic Differential Systems, Stochastic Control Theory and Applications, Springer, New York, pp. 129–145

[102] Gidas B. (1989): A renormalization group approach to image processing problems. IEEE Trans. PAMI **11**, 164–180

[103] Gidas B. (1991a): Parameter estimation for Gibbs distributions I: fully observed data. In: Chellapa R., Jain R. (eds.) Markov Random Fields: Theory and Applications. Academic Press, New York

[104] Gidas B. (1991b): Metropolis-type Monte Carlo simulation algorithms and simulated annealing. Trends in Contemporary Probability, 88 pp

[105] Gidas B. and Hudson. H.M. (1991): A non-linear multi-grid EM algorithm for emission tomography. Preprint, 45 pp

[106] Gidas B. and Torreao J. (1989): A Bayesian/geometric framework for reconstructing 3-D shapes in robot vision. SPIE vol. 1058, High Speed Computing II, 86–93

[107] Goldstein L. (1988): Mean square rates of convergence in the continuous time simulated annealing algorithm on R^d. Adv. Appl. Math. **9**, 35–39

[108] Goldstein L. and Waterman M.S. (1987): Mapping DNA by stochastic relaxation. Adv. Appl. Math. **8**, 194–207

[109] Gonzalez R.C. and Wintz P. (1987); Digital image processing, second edition. Addison and Wesley, Reading, Massachusetts

[110] Goodman J. and Sokal A.D. (1989): Multigrid Monte Carlo method. Conceptual foundations. Phys. Rev. D **40**, 2035–2071

[111] Graffigne Chr. (1987): Experiments in texture analysis and segmentation. Thesis, Brown University

[112] Green P.J. (1986): Discussion on the paper by J. Besag: On the statistical analysis of dirty pictures. J. R. Statist. Soc. B **48**, 284–285

[113] Green P.J. (1991): Discussion on the paper by Besag J., York J. and Mollié A.: Bayesian image restoration with two applications in spatial statistics. Ann. Inst. Statist. Math. vol. 43

[114] Green P.J. and Han Xiao-liang (1992) Metropolis methods, Gaussian proposals and antithetic variables. In: Barone P., Frigessi A., Piccioni M. (eds) Stochastic models, statistical methods, and algorithms in image analysis. Lecture Notes in Statistics, vol. 74. Springer, Berlin Heidelberg New York, pp. 142–164

[115] Greig D.M., Porteous B.T. and Seheult A.H. (1986): Discussion on the paper by J. Besag: On the statistical analysis of dirty pictures. J. R. Statist. Soc. B **48**, 282–284

[116] Greig D.M., Porteous B.T. and Seheult A.H. (1989): Exact maximum a posteriori estimation for binary images. J. R. Statist. Soc. B **51**, 271–279

[117] Grenander U. (1976, 1978, 1981): Lectures on pattern theory (3 vols.). Springer, Berlin Heidelberg New York

[118] Grenander U. (1983): Tutorial in pattern theory. Technical Report, Division of Applied Mathematics, Brown University, Providence, Rhode Island 02912, USA

[119] Grenander U. (1989): Advances in pattern theory. Ann. Statist. **17**, 1–30

[120] Grenander U., Chow Y. and Keenan D. (1991): A pattern theoretic study of biological shapes (Research Notes in Neural Computing, vol. 2). Springer, Berlin Heidelberg New York

[121] Griffeath D. (1976): Introduction to random fields, chapter 12. In: Kemeney J.G., Snell J.L. and Knapp A.W.: Denumerable Markov Chains. Graduate Texts in Mathematics, vol. 40. Springer, New York Heidelberg Berlin

[122] GRIMMETT G.R. (1973): A theorem about random fields. Bull. London Math. Soc. **5**, 81–84

[123] GUYON X. (1982): Parameter estimation for a stationary process on a d-dimensional lattice. Biometrika **69**, 95–105

[124] GUYON X. (1986): Estimation d'un champ de Gibbs. Preprint Univ. Paris-I

[125] GUYON X. (1987): Estimation d'un champ par pseudo-vraisemblance conditionelle: Étude asymptotique et application au cas markovien. In: Droesbeke F. (ed.) Spatial processes and Spatial time Series Analysis. Publ. Fac. Univ. St Louis, Bruxelles, pp. 15–62

[126] HAARIO H. and SAKSMAN E. (1991) Simulated annealing process in general state space. Adv. Appl. Prob. **23**, 866–893

[127] HAJEK B. (1985): A tutorial survey of theory and applications of simulated annealing. Proc of the 24th Conference on Decision and Control, Ft. Lauderdale, FL, Dec. 1985, pp. 755–760

[128] HAJEK B. (1988): Cooling schedules for optimal annealing. Math. Oper. Res. **13**, pp. 311–329

[129] HAJEK B. and SASAKI G. (1989): Simulated annealing – to cool or not. Systems and Control Letters **12**, 443–447

[130] HAMMERSLEY J.M. and CLIFFORD P. (1968): Markov fields on finite graphs and lattices. Preprint Univ. of CAL, Berkeley

[131] HANSEN F.R. and ELLIOTT H. (1982): Image segmentation using simple random field models. Computer Graphics and Image Processing **20**, 101–132

[132] HARALICK R.M. (1979): Statistical and structural approaches to texture. Proc. 4th Int. Joint Conf. Pattern Recog., pp. 45–60

[133] HARALICK R.M., SHANMUGAN R. and DINSTEIN I. (1973): Textural features for image classification. IEEE Trans. Syst. Man Cyb., vol. SMC-3, no. 6, 610–621

[134] HARALICK R.M. and SHAPIRO L.G. (1992): Computer and robot vision, volume 1. Addison-Wesley, Reading, Massachusetts

[135] HASSNER M. and SLANSKY J. (1980): The use of Markov random fields as models of textures. Comput. Graphics Image Processing **12**, 357–370

[136] HASTINGS W.K. (1970): Monte Carlo sampling methods using Markov chains and their applications. Biometrika **57**, 97–109

[137] HECHT-NIELSEN R. (1990): Neurocomputing. Addison-Wesley, Reading, Massachusetts

[138] HEEGER D.J. (1988): Optical flow using spatiotemporal filters. Int. Comp. Vis. **1**, 279–302

[139] HEITZ F. and BOUTHEMY (1990a): Motion estimation and segmentation using a global Bayesian approach. IEEE Int. Conf. ASSP, Albuquerque

[140] HEITZ F. and BOUTHEMY (1990b): Multimodal motion estimation and segmentation using Markov random fields. Int. Conf. Pattern Recognition, Atlanta City, pp. 378–383

[141] HEITZ F. and BOUTHEMY (1992): Multimodal estimation of discontinuous optical flow using Markov random fields. Submitted to: IEEE Trans. PAMI

[142] VAN HEMMEN J.L. and KÜHN R. (1991): Collective phenomena in neural networks. In: Domany E., van Hemmen J.L. and Schulten K. (eds.) Physics of Neural Networks. Springer, Berlin Heidelberg New York, pp. 1–105

[143] HILLIS W.D. (1988): The connection machine. The MIT Press, Cambridge/Massachusetts London/England

[144] HINTON G.E. and SEJNOWSKI T. (1983): Optimal perceptual inference. Proc. IEEE Conference on Computer Vision and Pattern Recognition, pp. 448–453

[145] Hinton G.E., Sejnowski T. and Ackley D.H.F (1984): Boltzmann machines: constraint satisfaction networks that learn. Technical Report, CMU-CS-84-119, Carnegie Mellon University

[146] Hjort N.L. (1985): Neighbourhood based classification of remotely sensed data based on geometric probability models. Tech. Report no. 10/NSF, Dept. of Statistics, Stanford University

[147] Hjort N.L. and Mohn E. (1985): On the contextual classification of data from high resolution satellites. Proceedings of the 18th International Symposium on remote Sensing of the Environment, Paris, pp. 1693–1702

[148] Hjort N.L. and Mohn E. (1987): Topics in the statistical analysis of remotely sensed data. Invited paper 21.2, 46th ISI Meeting, Tokyo, September 1987

[149] Hjort N.L., Mohn E. and Storvik G.O. (1987): A simulation study of some contextual classification methods for remotely sensed data. IEEE Transactions on Geoscience and Remote Sensing, vol. GE 25, no. 6, 796–804

[150] Hjort N.L. and Taxt T. (1987): Automatic training in statistical pattern recognition. Proc. Int. Conf. Pattern Recognition, Palermo, October 1987

[151] Hjort N.L. and Taxt. T (1987): Automatic training in statistical symbol recognition. Research Report no. 809, Norwegian Computing Centre, Oslo

[152] Hoffmann K.H. and Salaman P. (1990): The optimal annealing schedule for a simple model. J. Phys. A: Math. Gen. **23**, 3511–3523

[153] Holley R.A. and Stroock D. (1988): Simulated annealing via Sobolev inequalities. Comm. Math. Phys. **115**, 553–569

[154] Holley R.A., Kasuoka S. and Stroock D. (1989): Asymptotics of the spectral gap with applications to the theory of simulated annealing. J. Funct. Anal. **83**, 333–147

[155] Hopfield J. and Tank D. (1985): Neural computation of decisions in optimization problems. Biological Cybernetics **52**, 141–152

[156] Horn R.A. (1985): Matrix analysis. Cambridge University Press, Cambridge New York New Rochelle Melbourne Sidney

[157] Horn B.K.P. (1987): Robot vision. The MIT Press, Cambridge (Massachsetts), London (England); McGraw-Hill Book Company, New York St. Louis San Francisco Montreal Toronto

[158] Horn B.K.P. and Schunck B.G. (1981): Determining optical flow. Artificial Intelligence **17**, 185–204

[159] Hsiao J.Y. and Sawchuk A.A. (1989): Supervised textured image segmentation using feature smoothing and probabilistic relaxation techniques. IEEE Trans. PAMI, vol. 11, no. 12, 1279–1292

[160] Huber P. (1985): Projection pursuit. Ann. Statist. **13**, 435–475

[161] Hunt B.R (1973): The application of constrained least squares estimation to image restoration by digital computers. IEEE Transactions on Computers, vol. C-22, no. 9, 805–812

[162] Hunt B.R. (1977): Bayesian methods in nonlinear digital image restoration. IEEE Transactions on Computers, vol. C-26, no. 3, 219–229

[163] Hwang C.-R. and Sheu S.-J. (1987): Large time behaviours of perturbed diffusion Markov processes with applications, I, II and III. Technical Report, Inst. of Math., Academia Sinica, Taipei, Taiwan

[164] Hwang C.-R. and Sheu S.-J. (1989): On the weak reversibility condition in simulated annealing. Soochow J. of Math. **15**, 159–170

[165] Hwang Ch.-R. and Sheu Sh.-J. (1990): Large-time behaviour of perturbed diffusion Markov processes with applications to the second eigenvalue problem for Fokker-Planck operators and simulated annealing. Acta Applicandae Mathematicae **19**, 253–295

[166] HWANG C.-R. and SHEU S.-J. (1991): Remarks on Gibbs sampler and Metropolis sampler. Technical Report, Inst. of Math., Academia Sinica, Taipei, Taiwan, R.O.C

[167] HWANG C.-R. and SHEU S.-J. (1992): A remark on the ergodicity of systematic sweep is stochastic relaxation. In: Barone P., Frigessi A., Piccioni M. (eds) Stochastic models, statistical methods, and algorithms in image analysis. Lecture Notes in Statistics, vol. 74. Springer, Berlin Heidelberg New York, pp. 199–202

[168] HWANG C.-R. and SHEU S.-J. (1991c): Singular perturbed Markov chains and the exact behaviors of simulated annealing processes. Technical Report, Inst. of Math., Academia Sinica, Taipai, Taiwan, to appear in: J. Theoretical Probability

[169] HWANG C.-R. and SHEU S.-J. (1991d): On the behaviour of a stochastic algorithm with annealing. Technical report, Institute of Mathematics, Academia Sinica, Nangkang, Taipai, Taiwan 11529, R.O.C.

[170] INGRASSIA S. (1990): Spettri di catene di Markov e algoritmi di ottimizzazione. Thesis, Università degli studi di Napoli

[171] INGRASSIA S. (1991): A geometric bound on the rate of convergence of a Metropolis algorithm. Preprint, Dipartimento di Matematica, Università di Catania, Viale Andrea Doria, 6 - 95125 Catania (Italy)

[172] IOSIFESCU D.L. and THEODORESCU R. (1969): Random processes and learning. Grundlehren der math. Wissenschaften, Bd. 150. Springer, New York

[173] IOSIFESCU M. (1972): On two recent papers on ergodicity in nonhomogeneous Markov chains. Ann. Math. Statist. **43**, 1732–1736

[174] ISAACSON D.L. and MADSON R.W. (1976): Markov chains theory and applications. Wiley & Sons, New York London Sydney Toronto

[175] JÄHNE B. (1991a): Digitale Bildverarbeitung (in German), 2nd edition. Springer, Berlin Heidelberg New York London Paris Tokyo

[176] JÄHNE B. (1991b) Digital image processing. Concepts, algorithms and scientific applications. Springer, Berlin Heidelberg New York

[177] JENG F.-C. and WOODS J.W. (1990): Simulated annealing in compound Gaussian random fields. IEEE Trans. Inform. Theory **36**, 94–107

[178] JENNISON CH. (1990): Aggregation in simulated annealing. Lecture held at "Stochastic Image Models and Algorithms", Mathematisches Forschungsinstitut Oberwolfach, Germany, 15.7–21.7.1990

[179] JENSEN J.L. and MØLLER J. (1989): Pseudolikelihood for exponential family models of spatial processes. Research reports no. 203, Department of Theoretial Statistics, Institute of Mathematics, University of Aarhus

[180] JENSEN J.L. and MØLLER J. (1992): Pseudolikelihood for exponential family models of spatial processes. Ann. Appl. Prob. **1**, 445–461

[181] JOHNSON D.S., ARAGON C.R., MCGEOCH L.A and SCHEVON C. (1989): Optimization by simulated annealing: an experimental evaluation, Part I (graph partition). Operations Research **37**, 865–892

[182] JOHNSON D.S., ARAGON C.R., MCGEOCH L.A and SCHEVON C. (1989): Optimization by simulated annealing: an experimental evaluation, Part II (graph colouring and number partitioning). To appear in: Operations Research

[183] JOHNSON D.S., ARAGON C.R., MCGEOCH L.A and SCHEVON C. (1989): Optimization by simulated annealing: an experimental evaluation, Part III (the travelling salesman problem). In preparation

[184] JULESZ B. (1975): Experiments in the visual perception of texture. Scientific American **232**, no. 4, 34–43

[185] JULESZ B. et al. (1973): Inability of humans to discriminate beetween visual textures that agree in second-order statistics. Perception **2**, 391–405

[186] KAMP Y. and HASLER M. (1990): Recursive neural networks for associative memory. Wiley & Sons, Chichester New York Brisbane Toronto Singapore

[187] KARSSEMEIJER N. (1990): A relaxation method for image segmentation using a spatially dependent stochastic model. Pattern Recognition Letters **11**, 13–23

[188] KASHKO A. (1987): A parallel approach to graduated nonconvexity on a SIMD machine. Dep. Comput. Sci., Queen Mary Colledge, London, England

[189] KASTELEYN P.W. and FORTUIN C.M. (1969): Phase transitions in lattice systems with random local properties. J. Phys. Soc. Jpn. [Suppl. 11]

[190] KEILSON J. (1979): Markov chain models – rarity and exponentiality. Springer, Berlin Heidelberg New York

[191] KEMENEY J.G. and SNELL J.L. (1960): Finite Markov chains. van Nostrand Company, Princeton/New Jersey Toronto London New York

[192] KHOTANZAD A. and CHEN J.-Y. (1989): Unsupervised segmentation of textured images by edge detection in multidimensional features. IEEE Trans. PAMI, vol. 11, no. 4, 414–421

[193] KIFER Y. (1990): A discrete-time version of the Wentzell-Freidlin theory. Ann. Probab. **18**, 1676–1692

[194] KINDERMANN R. and SNELL J.L. (1980): Markov random fields and their applications. Contemporary Mathematics, vol. 1. American Mathematical Society, Providence, Rhode Island

[195] KIRKPATRICK S., GELATT C.D. Jr. and VECCHI M.P. (1982): Optimization by simulated annealing. IBM T.J. Watson Research Center, Yorktown Heights, NY

[196] KIRKPATRICK S., GELATT C.D. Jr. and VECCHI M.P. (1983): Optimization by simulated annealing. Science **220**, 671–680

[197] KITTLER J. and FÖGLEIN J. (1984): Contextual classification of multispectral pixel data. Image and Vision Computing **2**, 13–29

[198] KITTLER J. and ILLINGWORTH J. (1985): Relaxation labelling algorithms – a review. Image and Vision Computing **3**, 206–216

[199] KLEIN R. and PRESS S.J. (1989): Contextual Bayesian classification of remotely sensed data. Comm. Statist. – Theory Methods **18**, 3177–3202

[200] KNUTH D.E. (1969): The art of computer programming. Volume 2/Seminumerical Algorithms. Reading, Massachusetts; Melo Park, California; London; Don Mills, Ontario

[201] KOZLOW O. and VASILYEV N. (1980): Reversible Markov chains with local interaction. In: Dobrushin R.L., Sinai, Ya.G. (eds.) Multicomponent Random Systems. Academy of Sciences Moscow, USSR; Marcel Dekker Inc., New York and Basel

[202] KÜNSCH H. (1981): Thermodynamics and the statistical analysis of Gaussian random fields. Z. Wahrscheinlichkeitstheorie und Verw. Gebiete **58**, 407–421

[203] KÜNSCH H. (1984): Time reversal and stationary Gibbs measures. Stochastic Process. Appl. **17**, 159–166

[204] KUSHNER H.J. (1974): Approximation and weak convergence of interpolated Markov chains to a diffusion. Ann. Probab. **2**, 40–50

[205] VAN LAARHOVEN P.J.M. and AARTS E.H.L. (1987): Simulated annealing: theory and applications. Kluwer Academic Publishers, Dordrecht, Holland

[206] LAKSHMANAN S. and DERIN H. (1989): Simultaneous parameter estimation and segmentation of Gibbs random fields using simulated annealing. IEEE Trans. PAMI, vol. 11, no. 8, 799–813

[207] LALANDE P. and BOUTHEMY P. (1990): A statistical approach to the detection and tracking of moving objects in an image squence. 5th European Signal Processing Conference EUSIPCO 90, Barcelona

[208] LASOTA A. and MACKEY M.C. (1995): Probabilistic properties on dynamic systems. Cambridge Univ. Press, New York

[209] LASSERRE Y.B., VARAIJA P.P. and WALRAND J. (1987): Simulated annealing, random search, multistart or SAD. Systems Controll Letters **8**, 297–301

[210] LI X.-J. and SOKAL A.D. (1989): Rigorous lower bound on the dynamic critical exponent of the Swendson-Wang algorithms. Phys. Rev. Letters 63, 827–830

[211] LIN S. and KERNIGHAN B.W. (1973): An effective algorithm for the travelling salesman problem. Oper. Res. **21**, 498–516

[212] LUENBERGER D.G. (1989): Introduction to linear and nonlinear programming. Addison-Wesley, Reading MA

[213] MADSON R.W. and ISAACSON D.L. (1973): Strongly ergodic behaviour for non-stationary Markov processes. Ann. Probab. **1**, 329–335

[214] MALHORTA V.M., KUMAR PRAMODH M. and MAHESHWARI N. (1978): An $O(|V|^3)$ algorithm for finding the maximum flows in networks. Inform. Process. Lett. **7**, 228–278

[215] MARR D. (1982): Vision. W.H. Freeman and Company, New York

[216] MARROQUIN J., MITTER S. and POGGIO T. (1987): Probabilistic solution of ill-posed problems in computational vision. J. Amer. Statist. Assoc. **82**, 76–89

[217] MARSAGLIA G. (1968): Random numbers fall mainly in the planes. Proc. Nat. Acad. Sci. **60**, 25–28

[218] MARSAGLIA G. (1972): The structure of linear congruential sequences. In: Zaremba S.K. (ed.) Applications of Number Theory to Numerical Analysis. Academic Press, London, pp. 249–285

[219] MARTINELLI F., OLIVIERI E. and SCOPPOLA E. (1990): On the Swendson-Wang dynamics I, II. Preprint

[220] MASE SIGERU (1991): Discussion on the paper by Besag J., York J. and Mollié A. : Bayesian image restauration with two applications in spatial statistics. Ann. Inst. Statist. Math. **43**

[221] MCCORMICK B.H. and JAYARAMAMURTHY S.N. (1974): Time series models for texture synthesis. International J. of Computer and Information Sciences **3**, 329–343

[222] MEES C.E.K. (1954): The theory of the photographic processes. Macmillan, New York

[223] MEHLHORN K. (1984): Data structures and algorithms 2: graph algorithms and NP-completeness. EATC Monographs on Theoretical Computer Science. Springer, Berlin Heidelberg New York

[224] MÉTIVIER M. and PRIOURET P. (1987): Théorèmes de convergence presque sure pour une classe d'algorithmes stochastique à pas décroissant. Probab. Th. Rel. Fields **74**, 403–428

[225] METROPOLIS N., ROSENBLUTH A.W., ROSENBLUTH M.N., TELLER A.H. and TELLER E. (1953): Equations of state calculations by fast computing machines. J. Chem. Phys. **21**, 1087–1092

[226] MITRA D., ROMEO F. and SANGIOVANNI-VINCENTELLI A. (1985): Convergence and finite-time behavior of simulated annealing. Proc of the 24th Conference on Decision and Control, Ft. Lauderdale, FL, Dec. 1985, pp. 761–767

[227] MITRA D., ROMEO F. and SANGIOVANNI-VINCENTELLI A. (1986): Convergence and finite-time behavior of simulated annealing. Adv. Appl. Probab. **18**, 747–771

[228] MITTER S.K. (1986): Estimation Theory and Statistical Physics. In: Hida, Ito (eds.) Stochastic Processes and their Applications, Proceedings of the International Conference held in Nagoya, July 2–6, 1985. Lecture Notes in Mathematics, vol. 1203. Springer, Berlin Heidelberg New York, 157–176

[229] MÜLLER B. and REINHARDT J. (1990): Neural networks. An introduction. Springer, Berlin Heidelberg New York London Paris Tokyo Hong Kong Barcelona

[230] MURRAY D.W., KASHKO A. and BUXTON H. (1986): A parallel approach to the picture restoration algorithm of Geman and Geman on an SIMD machine. Image and Vision Computing **4**, 133–142

[231] MUSMANN H.G., PIRSCH P. and GALLERT H.-J. (1985): Advances in picture coding. Proc. IEEE **73**, 523

[232] NAGEL H.-H. (1981): Representation of moving objects based on visual observations. IEEE Computer, 29–39

[233] NAGEL H.-H. (1985): Analyse und Interpretation von Bildfolgen. Informatik Spektrum **8**, 178, 312

[234] NAGEL H.-H. and ENKELMANN (1986): An investigation of smoothness constraints for the estimation of displacement vector fields from image sequences. IEEE Trans. PAMI-8, 565

[235] NEUMANN K. (1977): Operations Research Verfahren. Band II: Dynamische Programmierung, Lagerhaltung, Simulation, Warteschlangen. Carl Hanser Verlag, München Wien

[236] NIEMANN H. (1983): Klassifikation von Mustern. Informatiklehrbuchreihe. Springer, Berlin Heidelberg New York Tokyo

[237] NIEMANN H. (1990): Pattern analysis and understanding. Springer Series in Information Sciences, vol. 4. Springer, Berlin Heidelberg New York

[238] OGAWA H. and OJA E. (1986): Projection Filter, Wiener Filter, and Karhunen-Loeve Subspaces in Digital Image Restoration. J. Math. Anal. Appl. **114**, 37–51

[239] PARK S.K. and MILLER K.W. (1988): Random number generators: good ones are hard to find. Comm. Assoc. Comput. Mach. **31**, 1192–1201

[240] PERETTO P. (1984): Collective properties of neural networks, a statistical physics approach. Biological Cybernetics **50**, 51–62

[241] PESKUN P.H. (1973): Optimum Monte Carlo sampling using Markov chains. Biometrika **60**, 607–612

[242] PICKARD D. (1976): Asymptotic inference for an Ising lattice. J. Appl. Probab. **13**, 486–497

[243] PICKARD D. (1977): Asymptotic inference for an Ising lattice II. Adv. in Appl. Probab. **9**, 479–501

[244] PICKARD D. (1987): Inference for discrete Markov field: The simplest nontrivial case. J. Amer. Statist. Assoc. **82**, 90–96

[245] PICKARD D. (1979): Asymptotic inference for an Ising lattice III. J. Appl. Probab. **16**, 12–24

[246] POSSOLO A. (1986): Estimation of binary Markov random fields. Department of Statistics, University of Washington, Technical Report

[247] PRATT W.R. (1978): Digital image processing. Wiley & Sons, New York Chichester Brisbane Toronto

[248] PRUM B. (1984): Processus sur un réseau et mesures de Gibbs. Applications. Masson, Paris New York Barcelona Milan Mexico Sao Paulo

[249] PRUM B. and FORTET J.V.C. (1991): Stochastic processes on a lattice and Gibbs measures. Kluwer Academic Publishers, Dordrecht Boston London

[250] REINELT G. (1990): TSPLIB – A Traveling Salesman Problem library, Report No 250, Augsburg. To appear in: ORSA Journal on Computing

[251] REINELT G. (1991): TSPLIB – Version 1.2. Report No 330, Augsburg

[252] RIPLEY B.D. (1976): The second-order analysis of stationary point processes. J. Appl. Probab. **13**, 255–266

[253] RIPLEY B.D. (1977): Modelling spatial patterns. J. R. Statist. Soc., Series B 39, 172–212
[254] RIPLEY B.D. (1981): Spatial statistics. Wiley & Sons, New York Chichester Brisbane Toronto Singapore
[255] RIPLEY B.D. (1986): Statistics, images, and pattern recognition. Canad. J. Statist. **14**, 883–1111
[256] RIPLEY B.D. (1987a): Stochastic Simulation. Wiley, New York
[257] RIPLEY B.D. (1987b): An introduction to statistical pattern recognition. In: Phelps R. (ed.) Interactions in Artificial Intelligence and Statistical Methods. Gower Technical Press, Aldershot, pp. 176–189
[258] RIPLEY B.D. (1988): Statistical inference for spatial processes. Cambridge University Press, Cambridge New York New Rochelle Melbourne Sidney
[259] RIPLEY B.D. (1989a): The use of spatial models as image priors. In: Possolo A. (ed.) Spatial Statistics & Imaging. IMS Lecture Notes, 29 pp
[260] RIPLEY B.D. (1989b): Thoughts on pseudorandom number generators. In: Lehn J. and Neunzert H. (eds.) Random numbers and simulation, 29 pp
[261] RIPLEY B.D. and TAYLOR C.C. (1987): Pattern recognition. Sci. Prog. Oxf. **71**, 413–428
[262] ROCKAFELLAR K.T. (1970): Convex analysis. Princeton University Press, Princeton, New Jersey
[263] ROSSIER Y., TROYON M. and LIEBLING TH.M. (1986): Probabilistic exchange algorithms and Euclidean Traveling Salesman problems. OR-Spektrum **8**, 151–164
[264] ROYER G. (1989): A remark on simulated annealing for diffusion processes: SIAM J. Control. Optim. **27**, 1403–1408
[265] SCHUNCK B.G. (1986): The image flow constraint equation. CVGIP **35**, 20–46
[266] SENETA E. (1973): On the historical development of the theory of finite inhomogeneous Markov chains. Proc. Cambridge Phil. Soc. **74**, 507–513
[267] SENETA E. (1981): Non-negative matrices and Markov chains, 2nd edition. Springer, New York Heidelberg Berlin
[268] SHEPP L.A. and VARDI Y. (1982): Maximum likelihood reconstruction in positron emission tomography. IEEE Trans. on Medical Imaging **18**, 1225–1228
[269] SIARRY J. and DREYFUS G. (1989): La méthode du recuit simulé. Paris: IDSET
[270] SILVERMAN B.W. (1986). Density estimation for statistics and data analysis. Chapman and Hall
[271] SOKAL A.D. (1989): Monte Carlo methods in Statistical Mechanics: Foundations and new algorithms. Lecture Notes, Lausanne
[272] SONTAG E.D. and SUSSMANN H.J. (1985): Image restoration and segmentation using the annealing algorithm. Proceedings of the 24th Conference on Decision and Control, Dec. 1985, Ft. Lauderdale, FL, pp. 768–773
[273] STRANG G. (1976) Linear algebra and its applications. Academic Press, New York
[274] SWENDSEN R.H. and WANG J.-S. (1987): Nonuniversal critical dynamics in Monte Carlo simulations. Physical Review Letters **58**, 86–88
[275] TROUVÉ A. (1988): Problèmes de convergence et d'ergodicité pour les algorithmes de recuit parallélisés. C.R. Acad. Sci. Paris **307**, Série I, 161–164
[276] TSAI R.Y., HUANG T.S. (1984): Uniqueness and estimation of 3-D motion parameters of rigid bodies with curved surface. IEEE Trans. PAMI-6, 13
[277] TSITSIKLIS J.N. (1988): A survey of large time asymptotics of simulated annealing algorithms. In: Fleming W., Lions P.L. (eds.) Stochastic Differential Systems, Stochastic Control Theory and Applications. New York, pp. 583–599

[278] TSITSIKLIS J.N. (1989): Markov chains with rare transitions and simulated annealing. Math. Op. Res. **14**, 70–90

[279] TUCKEY Y.W. (1971): Exploratory data analysis. Addison-Wesley, Reading, Massachusets

[280] TUCKWELL H.C. (1988): Elementary applications of probability theory. Chapman and Hall, London

[281] TYAN S.G. (1981): Median filtering: Deterministic properties. In: Huang (ed.) Two-dimensional Digital Signal Processing II. Springer, Berlin Heidelberg New York

[282] VARDI Y., SHEPP L.A. and KAUFMAN L. (1985): A statistical model for positron emission tomography. JASA **80**, 8–20 and 34–37

[283] VASILYEV N. (1978): Bernoulli and Markov stationary measure in discrete local interactions. In: Dobrushin R.L., Kryukov V.I. and Toom A.L. (eds.) Locally interacting systems and their application in biology. Springer Lecture Notes in Mathematics, vol. 653. Springer, Berlin Heidelberg New York

[284] WEBER M. and LIEBLING TH.M. (1986): Euclidean matching problems and the Metropolis algorithm. ZOR **30**, A 85.A 110

[285] v. WEIZSÄCKER H. and WINKLER G. (1990): Stochastic integrals. An introduction. Vieweg & Sohn, Braunschweig Wiesbaden

[286] WENG J., HUANG T.S. and AHUJA N. (1987): 3-D motion estimation, understanding, and prediction from noisy images. IEEE Trans. PAMI-9, 370

[287] WINKLER G. (1990): An Ergodic L^2-theorem for simulated annealing in Bayesian image reconstruction. J. Appl. Probab. **28**, 779–791

[288] WRIGHT W.A. (1989): A Markov random field approach to data fusion and colour segmentation. Image and Vision Computing **7**, No 2, 144–150

[289] YOUNES L. (1986): Couplage de l'estimation et du recuit pour des champs de Gibbs. C. R. Acad. S. Paris, t. 303, série I, n° 13

[290] YOUNES L. (1988a): Estimation pour champs de Gibbs et application au traitement d'images. Université Paris Sud Thesis

[291] YOUNES L. (1988b): Estimation and annealing for Gibbsian fields. Ann. Inst. Henri Poincare **24**, no. 2, 269–294

[292] YOUNES L. (1989): Parametric inference for imperfectly observed Gibbsian fields. Prob. Th. Rel. Fields **82**, 625–645

[293] ZHOU Y.T., VENKATESWAR V. and CHELLAPPA R. (1989): Edge detection and linear feature extraction using a 2-d random field model. IEEE Trans. PAMI **11**, 84–95

Index

Springer-Verlag and the Environment

We at Springer-Verlag firmly believe that an international science publisher has a special obligation to the environment, and our corporate policies consistently reflect this conviction.

We also expect our business partners – paper mills, printers, packaging manufacturers, etc. – to commit themselves to using environmentally friendly materials and production processes.

The paper in this book is made from low- or no-chlorine pulp and is acid free, in conformance with international standards for paper permanency.

SPRINGER NATURE

GPSR Compliance

The European Union's (EU) General Product Safety Regulation (GPSR) is a set of rules that requires consumer products to be safe and our obligations to ensure this.

If you have any concerns about our products, you can contact us on ProductSafety@springernature.com

In case Publisher is established outside the EU, the EU authorized representative is:

Springer Nature Customer Service Center GmbH
Europaplatz 3
69115 Heidelberg, Germany

FSC
www.fsc.org
MIX
Papier | Fördert
gute Waldnutzung
FSC® C083411

Zeitfracht Medien GmbH
Ferdinand-Jühlke-Straße 7
99095 Erfurt, Deutschland
produktsicherheit@kolibri360.de